THE NEW
MEDICAL
MARKETPLACE

THE NEW MEDICAL MARKETPLACE

A PHYSICIAN'S GUIDE

TO THE HEALTH CARE SYSTEM IN THE 1990s

Revised and Updated Edition

by Anne M. Stoline, M.D.

and Jonathan P. Weiner, Ph.D.

with Gail Geller, Ph.D.
and Eric K. Gorovitz, M.P.H.

The Johns Hopkins University Press
Baltimore and London

The Johns Hopkins University Press
2715 N. Charles Street
Baltimore, Maryland 21218-4319
The Johns Hopkins Press Ltd., London

Originally published, 1988, as *The New Medical Marketplace: A Physician's Guide
to the Health Care Revolution*, The Johns Hopkins University Press.

A catalog record for this book is available from the British Library.

Library of Congress Cataloging-in-Publication Data
Stoline, Anne, 1961–
    The new medical marketplace: a physician's guide to the health care
  system in the 1990's / by Anne M. Stoline and Jonathan P. Weiner,
  with Gail Geller and Eric K. Gorovitz. — Rev. and updated ed.
      p. cm.
  Includes bibliographical references and index.
  ISBN 0-8018-4582-3 (hc : alk. paper). — ISBN 0-8018-4583-1 (pbk.
  alk. paper)
    1. Medical economics—United States.   I. Weiner, Jonathan P.
II. Title
    [DNLM: 1. Delivery of Health Care—economics—United States.
2. Economics, Medical—trends—United States. 3. Health Policy-
-trends—United States.   W 74 S875n 1993]
RA410.53.S76   1993
338.4'73621—dc20
DNLM/DLC   92-48457
for Library of Congress   CIP

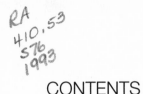

CONTENTS

FOREWORD

The scientific and technical aspects of medical practice have been undergoing a continuous revolution for more than half a century, but until recently, the system for delivering medical care in the United States as well as the position of physicians within that system had not changed very much. Students and new physicians could concentrate on acquiring the medical information and skills they needed, secure in the knowledge that they would enter a stable medical care system where they would be free to practice their profession as they saw fit under whatever arrangements they chose. The role of the physician as the center of power in the system was accepted without question.

All that has changed now. An economic crisis has developed that is reshaping the structure of American health care and profoundly affects the way doctors work. With the problem of cost also have come related problems of access to care and the maintenance of quality. Social, political, and legal forces impinge on the practice of medicine as never before, and physicians confront ethical and economic problems that were undreamed of even a decade ago. In turn, these have necessitated changes in their style of practice. Until recently, solo, fee-for-service practice dominated the scene, but new arrangements now are coming to the fore. Very soon, most young physicians will practice in some kind of group setting, often on a salaried basis. In many cases, physicians are being asked to share financial risks with insurers or are being hired directly by the insurers to provide care to beneficiaries, thus creating new and disturbing conflicts of interest between doctors and patients. Even in fee-for-service practice, competitive economic pressures have encouraged entrepreneurial behavior among many physicians, creating a commercial climate in medicine unlike anything seen before. Third-party payers now attempt to control costs by "managing" the medical care they pay for; increasingly, intrusive utilization review and new requirements for prior approval of costly medical decisions are beginning to restrict physicians' freedom to practice and are adding to their administrative burdens.

This revolution seems to have taken most of the medical profession by surprise. Immersed in their own practices and relatively uninformed about the gathering social and economic forces, physicians did not see the handwriting on the wall, were unprepared for what happened, and could do little more than watch in frustration as their influence waned and control of their future gradually was taken over by others. Not surprisingly, their level of unhappiness is high, and their expressions of dissatisfaction with the present state of medical practice abound.

Physicians need not be pawns or simply react to changes initiated by others, however. I believe there is still time for them to take constructive actions that will defend traditional professional values and promote the interests of their patients, but to do this, they will need to learn the objective facts about, and understand the social and economic forces behind, the current health care revolution. That is why this book is so important. In clear and succinct style, Stoline and Weiner (along with their colleagues) take the reader on a rapid tour of the changing medical scene. They show why change is inevitable, and they explain both the inadequacies and the contradictions of our present nonsystem. Reading this book, one cannot fail to see the problems and gain insight into their possible solutions. No detailed answers are provided, but most of the ingredients for intelligent policy-making are here.

This book should be part of a required course for medical students, who are given lamentably little education about the new social climate in which they will practice. It also could be read with much benefit by physicians both in training or in established practices who want to understand what has been happening to them and why.

Of course, this understanding should be followed by thoughtful and constructive action. That will require more collective initiative and moral conviction than we have seen so far, but no useful action is possible without the kind of insights provided here. As I write this Foreword, the United States, at last, seems ready to undertake major health care reforms. Although the exact shape of these reforms is yet undecided, it seems clear that effective plans for reform must deal with the issues that this book so clearly defines.

I am enthusiastic about *The New Medical Marketplace* because it provides information that is needed by physicians now more than ever but is almost impossible to find so neatly and attractively packaged in one place. If enough doctors and medical students read this book and then ponder its lessons, we might even see the medical profession become a major participant in the efforts to improve the present state of affairs. Such efforts, if based on the clear vision afforded by books like this, might even have a chance of succeeding.

Arnold S. Relman, M.D.
Editor-in-Chief Emeritus,
The New England Journal of Medicine
Professor of Medicine and of Social Medicine,
Harvard Medical School

PREFACE TO THE REVISED EDITION

Since the first edition of this book was published in 1988, the problems facing the U.S. health care system have multiplied. Costs continue to spiral, barriers to access remain for many Americans, and technical knowledge is burgeoning faster than either the public or medical professionals can manage to absorb it.

Several of these problems have created a need for this new edition. During the last 4 years, some new policies have been implemented, among them Medicare's resource-based fee schedule for physician reimbursement and several state plans augmenting health care coverage for the uninsured. Many powerful trends mentioned in the last edition have now become entrenched; these include the push toward cost-effectiveness and quality improvement, practice guidelines, and managed care. Moreover, there has been a resurgence of the debate regarding the future organization of the U.S. health care delivery system. Today, health care reform tops the political agenda.

Although this revised edition has been significantly updated, it retains the background information necessary for those just learning about the U.S. health care system. The order of information is identical to the first edition, but the organization has been changed. This edition is divided into four parts. Part I, "Socioeconomic Revolution in the Health Care System," provides an historical background on the health care system, tracing the roots of current problems in financing and delivery of care; it also contains a chapter on basic health care economic principles. Part II, "The Organization and Financing of Today's Health Care System," describes major cost control initiatives aimed at patients and health care providers, followed by a description of resulting changes in the health care system. Part III, "Care, Cost, and Conscience," looks at current clinical issues from the medical professional's perspective; it divides health care into its technical, resource allocation, and ethical components and examines each of these aspects in turn. This section includes a greatly expanded chapter on ethical issues and covers the new movements to improve the quality and outcome of treatment in some detail. Part IV, "Societal Issues and the New Medical Marketplace," highlights health care issues facing our society, including malpractice, access to care, and society-wide choices concerning resource allocation; it contains an expanded discussion of national health insurance that is commensurate with the increased political attention currently on this issue.

Physicians' reactions to the policy issues that face the U.S. health care system were a major theme of the first edition of this book. Although the health care system has continued to evolve since then, many physicians are no more ready to accept these changes. Health care providers react with bewilderment, resentment, and—above all—anxiety to the numerous cost-control measures implemented by payers and policymakers in an attempt to bring health care costs under control. Medical students and residents worry about where the profession is heading. More than ever, college students are reluctant to enter medical training.

Some perceive imposition of this new medical marketplace on the medical profession mostly by external forces, but physicians are not exactly "innocent bystanders." The cost-containment problem was caused to a significant degree by their actions and inactions as well as by their practices and conventions. As a result, adaptation and involvement by individual clinicians and the professional organizations representing them is needed.

It is not too late for physicians and other health care providers to make a positive influence on the ongoing health care revolution. Medical professionals have the clinical knowledge that is necessary to make these modifications, and it is appropriate that clinicians actively contribute to that change. Indeed, it is essential that professional voices be heard on a wide range of critical issues.

The perspectives of a practicing physician, a health policy analyst, an ethicist, and a law student are incorporated in the authorship of this book. In addition to the input of our two clinical coauthors on the previous edition, the authors had the considerable benefit of advice from a range of consultants within the Johns Hopkins Medical Institutions, people expert in the areas of decision analysis, medical ethics, health economics, nursing, and medical history. Although the text that follows is written for physicians, medical students, and other clinicians and trainees, it also will be helpful to anyone who is interested in America's evolving medical care delivery system. Policymakers, health care administrators, corporate benefit managers, and insurance executives can find clarification of the many complex issues treated in this book. Consumers of medical care will also benefit from this information, whether they be individual patients or persons with community-level responsibilities.

This book explains what has happened to the U.S. health care system and why. It creates a basis for discussion of current health policy issues, but without attempting to provide all the answers. Our hope is that an increased understanding of these changes will help clinicians to cope with the many challenges the new system offers to medical practice, financing, and ethics. This text provides a beginning to the education of the current generation of physicians as well as those for whom they care. We have attempted to present the material as simply as possible, without misrepresenting the complex issues at stake. May it ease the new way for all.

ACKNOWLEDGMENTS

The development of the first edition of this book was supported, in part, through grants from the National Fund for Medical Education and the W.K. Kellogg Foundation to the Office of Medical Practice Evaluation of the Johns Hopkins Medical Institutions. We also are grateful for the continued support of Peter Dans, M.D., and Mary Mussman, M.D., M.P.H., who coauthored the first edition of the book.

In addition, we thank the numerous people who assisted in the preparation of this book. Many people at the Johns Hopkins Hospital, the Johns Hopkins Schools of Medicine and Public Health, and other institutions helped to identify and prioritize the masses of material that were synthesized to form this work. Among these people are Gerard Anderson, Ph.D., Uwe Reinhardt, Ph.D., James Studnicki, Sc.D., and Andrew Sumner, M.D.

The computer-generated graphics in this text were created by Ethan Weiner.

The grant from the National Fund for Medical Education that in part supported the development of the earlier version of this book was sponsored by the AT&T and BankAmerica Corporations.

For critiquing earlier drafts, we thank Elizabeth Fee, Ph.D., Richard Frank, Ph.D., Daniel Hardesty, M.D., the late Harry Klinefelter, M.D., Laura Morlock, Ph.D., Marie Stoline, R.N., Mary Torchia, M.D., M.P.H., and Richard Torchia, M.D. We also are grateful to the numerous readers and reviewers of the first edition who provided feedback on its strengths and weaknesses.

For supporting this project in diverse ways, we extend our thanks to our editors, Anders Richter and Wendy Harris of the Johns Hopkins University Press, to Bev Siegel of the Johns Hopkins Health Services Research and Development Center, and, in particular, to our families and friends.

THE NEW
MEDICAL
MARKETPLACE

PART I

SOCIOECONOMIC REVOLUTION IN THE HEALTH CARE SYSTEM

The medical objectives of an era emanate from two formative influences. The first relates to the state of the art in the medical science of the period, which provides an understanding of disease processes and therapeutic modalities for successful intervention. The second is society's expectation of health care. These two influences coalesce to make explicit the social purpose of the system. Each era of medical objectives builds on the last. The eras overlap considerably.

Alvin Tarlov

A revolution in the organization and provision of medical care is under way in the United States. Major modifications have recently been made in reimbursement to both hospitals and physicians, and additional modifications are planned. Government and businesses now have an unprecedented influence on the health care system. In short, the atmosphere in which medicine currently is practiced is profoundly different from that of even 10 years ago.

The changes now under way in the U.S. health care system were necessitated by a unique combination of social, political, and technologic forces that have deep historical roots in both American society and the health care sector. Part I explores the roots and results of these changes as well as the context in which they occurred to educate medical practitioners about the new medical marketplace.

Chapter 1 examines major landmarks in the evolution of medical care—from science to service delivery—during the last hundred years. The revolution in medical care was set in motion over two decades ago by a rapid inflation of health care costs, and by the year 2000, U.S. medical care expenditures are expected to exceed $5,500 per capita—a total of over $1500 billion, accounting for 15 percent of the nation's annual gross domestic product (GDP). No other nation has ever spent anywhere close to this much on health care, and many contend that no nation can without critically shortchanging other sectors of society.

This escalation of costs has prompted an evaluation of the benefits obtained from our massive commitment of resources to health care. Comparisons with other countries have not been favorable. For example, in 1990, U.S. per-capita health care costs were almost three times higher than those of Great Britain, yet average life expectancy and most other health indicators were comparable in the two countries. Such comparisons further fueled the cry for cost control. By the late 1970s, changes in political priority and social attitudes combined to create conditions for what has been termed *the health care cost crisis,* and Chapter 2 explores the causes of this crisis as well as the responses to it by government, corporate employers, and insurers—the bankrollers of the enterprise.

Chapter 3 provides a brief overview of major economic principles; these form the basis for the cost-controlling interventions of the last 20 years. An understanding of both the differences and similarities between health care and other products aids in our understanding of the difficulty in controlling expenditures in the medical marketplace.

Most societal change is evolutionary and incremental. An overall view of society's functions and purposes—in Kuhn's term, a *paradigm*—is widely accepted at any given time. As its implications are increasingly explored, progress of sorts occurs, but with it a kind of dissonance or instability owing to shifts in societal beliefs and patterns of living. This instability leads to more or less modest changes in the paradigm: as new ways are gradually accepted, former beliefs are modified or replaced. In contrast, the development of an entirely new paradigm, either for society as a whole or some facet of it, may lead to revolutionary change. Thus, a "watershed" period exists, during which a new paradigm gains acceptance, and this is followed by an era of relative stability until another paradigm appears.

The U.S. health care system is currently undergoing such a revolutionary change. This transition has been under way for some time, and it is unclear how long the transition will take. However, if we are uncertain of the future, we *can* perceive relevant historical factors that influence it. Because the causes of this transition originated in past events, the present revolution can be understood better when the circumstances leading to it are considered.

CHAPTER 1

HISTORICAL BACKGROUND

What's past is prologue.
William Shakespeare, *A Midsummer Night's Dream*

Entering the Twentieth Century

The Industrial Revolution of the 1830s brought much of the U.S. population into the cities in search of steady employment and a better life, but their dreams often were shattered by the harsh reality of poor housing, inadequate food, unclean water, and unsafe working conditions. Life on the farm, though somewhat better, was far from idyllic as well; not only farmers but also their wives and children did backbreaking work for long hours with very little return. For most Americans, poor sewage disposal and crowded living conditions facilitated the spread of infectious diseases, which were the major cause of both sickness and death in the nineteenth century. The average life expectancy in 1900 was only 47 years, in large part because of high infant and child mortality.

Before the turn of the century, the predominant involvement of government in health care was in the military. In 1775, funds were authorized to build a hospital for the Revolutionary Army. In 1798, the Marine Hospital Service (forerunner of the U.S. Public Health Service) was created to care for merchant seamen who contracted communicable—mainly sexually transmitted—diseases during their travels. Although the federal government's involvement in health care for civilians began to expand at this time as well, most medical care spending went toward city, county, and state public health programs. Health policy focused on environmental and community health.

The American Public Health Association, founded in 1872, worked to establish community health standards, and civic reformers clamored for such changes. Some, like improvements in housing and food, were related only indirectly to disease but very directly related to citizens' health. A number of legislative reforms were passed, including the first Food and Drug Act. Municipal health departments were created, and visiting nurse services were provided. Most important were programs to provide clean water supplies and proper waste disposal. These actions were instrumental in improving social conditions and the average life expectancy. In the words of Oliver Wendell Holmes, a prominent late-nineteenth century physician, "The bills of mortality are more affected by drainage than this or that medical practice" (Ackerknecht 1982, p. 210).

There were only a few effective compounds in the pharmacopoeia of the 1890s, notably digitalis, morphine, and the smallpox vaccine. In an address to the Massachusetts Medical Society, Holmes exempted opium, wine, and anesthetics, then stated: "I firmly believe that if the whole materia medica, *as now used,* could be sunk to the bottom of the sea, it would be all the better for mankind–and all the worse for the fishes" (Evans 1978, p. 439).

Medical practice remained unsophisticated at the turn of the century, primarily because few disease models as we know them had been developed. Much important scientific research had been done, however, and hints of a revolution to come were evident. Improvements in medical practice had little currency, in part because the concept of professionalism had not yet been applied to medicine; there was no medical profession as such to respond to the new research. For example, although microbiology was gaining acceptance as a discipline thanks to pioneer researchers like Pasteur and Semmelweiss, the notion of antisepsis was slow to take hold, and even at the turn of the century, most surgeons still operated with bare hands.

Diffusion of knowledge was incomplete, in part because of a lack of consensus on medical theory and disease processes that led to a wide variety of educational approaches. Schools with differing views of medical care—among them allopathy, osteopathy, homeopathy, botany, and eclecticism—coexisted in a state of fierce rivalry. Prospective students faced a bewildering choice among some 160 medical schools. Few of these required a high school diploma for admission or provided students with any grounding in science, and many were in business chiefly for profit. The typical medical school program lasted 2 years and consisted mainly of lectures; patient contact was a neglected aspect of most programs. (The

American Medical Association (AMA), established in 1847, was composed primarily of allopathic practitioners.*)

In this era, most physicians used what medical knowledge they had to benefit the sick, but some merchandisers were less scrupulous. No laws prohibited false claims in drug labels, so bottled preparations labeled as cures for cancer legally could be sold and were. Also, because narcotics had not yet been brought under government control, "soothing syrups" for babies contained morphine, many preparations contained cocaine, and the active ingredient in a popular concoction known as "Lydia Pinkham's Tonic" was ethanol.

As might be expected, some self-styled healers, less politely known as *quacks,* used consumer ignorance to profit financially. As to the origin of this term, "*Quacks* is short for *quacksalvers,* or people who applied salves of quicksilver (mercury). 'Quacking out' [or advertising] in the marketplace, they stood in contrast to regular physicians who weren't supposed to advertise themselves. The essence of quackery was retailing 'secret remedies,' often called 'patent medicines,' which meant not that the formula itself was patented but that the name was trademarked" (Shorter 1985, pp. 69–70).

Traditional physicians also often misrepresented their wares, but from less self-serving motives. Having little to offer a sick patient but compassion, and aware that charisma could sometimes transform a worthless nostrum into an effective treatment, physicians regularly wrote detailed prescriptions for inactive compounds and urged them on their patients. "The contents were a deep mystery, and intended to be a mystery. . . . The purpose of this kind of therapy was essentially reassurance. . . . They were placebos, and they had been the principal mainstay of medicine, the sole technology, for so long a time—millennia—that they had the incantatory power of religious ritual" (Thomas 1983, p. 15).

---

*The term *allopathy,* or "other" therapy, drew its label mainly in contrast to *homeopathy,* or "like" therapy. In homeopathy the belief was that "like cured like;" small amounts of drugs that in larger amounts actually caused a disease were used to fight it. This approach relied on eliciting the body's own defensive responses. The allopathic philosophy (the predominant form of medicine to this day) was based on creating a second condition that was incompatible with the patient's presenting disease.

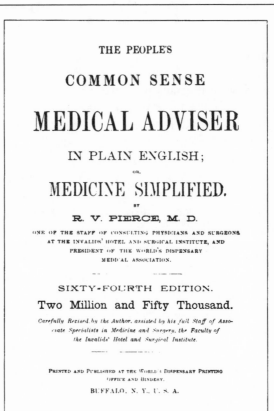

THE PEOPLE'S

COMMON SENSE

MEDICAL ADVISER

IN PLAIN ENGLISH;

OR,

MEDICINE SIMPLIFIED.

BY

R. V. PIERCE, M. D.

ONE OF THE STAFF OF CONSULTING PHYSICIANS AND SURGEONS
AT THE INVALIDS' HOTEL AND SURGICAL INSTITUTE, AND
PRESIDENT OF THE WORLD'S DISPENSARY
MEDICAL ASSOCIATION.

SIXTY-FOURTH EDITION.

Two Million and Fifty Thousand.

Carefully Revised by the Author, assisted by his full Staff of Asso-
ciate Specialists in Medicine and Surgery, the Faculty of
the Invalids' Hotel and Surgical Institute.

PRINTED AND PUBLISHED AT THE WORLD'S DISPENSARY PRINTING
OFFICE AND BINDERY.

BUFFALO, N. Y., U. S. A.

INTRODUCTORY WORDS.

The profession of medicine is no *sinecure;* its labors are constant, its toils unremitting, its cares unceasing. The physician is expected to meet the grim monster, "break the jaws of death, and pluck the spoil out of his teeth." *His* ear is ever attentive to entreaty, and within his faithful breast are concealed the disclosures of the suffering. Success may elate him, as conquest flushes the victor. Honors are lavished upon the brave soldiers who, in the struggle with the foe, have covered themselves with glory, and returned victorious from the field of battle; but how much more brilliant is the achievement of those who overwhelm disease, that common enemy of mankind, whose victims are numbered by millions! Is it meritorious in the physician to modestly veil his discoveries, regardless of their importance? If he have light, why hide it from the world? Truth should be made as universal and health-giving as sunlight. We say, give light to all who are in darkness, and a remedy to the afflicted everywhere.

REMEDIES FOR DISEASE.

Dr. Pierce's Golden Medical Discovery. In addition to the alterative properties combined in this compound, it possesses important tonic qualities. While the Favorite Prescription exerts a tonic influence upon the digestive and nutritive functions, the Golden Medical Discovery acts upon the excretory glands. Besides, it tends to retard unusual waste and expenditure. This latter remedy tones, sustains, and, at the same time regulates the functions. While increasing the discharge of noxious elements accumulated in the system, it promptly arrests the wastes arising from debility, and the unusual breaking down of the cells incident to quick decline. It stimulates the liver to secrete, changes the sallow complexion, and transforms the listless invalid into a vigorous and healthy being. At the same time, it checks the rapid disorganization of the tissues and their putrescent change, while it sustains the vital processes. It is, therefore, an indispensable remedy in the treatment of many diseases.

Dr. Pierce's Pleasant Pellets, being entirely vegetable in their composition, operate without disturbance to the system, diet, or occupation. Put up in glass vials. Always fresh and reliable. As *a laxative, alterative,* or gently acting but searching *cathartic,* these little Pellets give the most perfect satisfaction. Sick Headache, Bilious Headache, Dizziness, Constipation, Indigestion, Bilious Attacks, and all derangements of the stomach and bowels, are promptly relieved and permanently cured by the use of Dr. Pierce's Pleasant Pellets. In explanation of the remedial power of these Pellets over so great a variety of diseases, it may truthfully be said that their action upon the system is universal, not a gland or tissue escaping their sanative influence.

Dr. Pierce's Favorite Prescription. The Favorite Prescription, in addition to those properties already described, likewise combines tonic properties. In consequence of the never ceasing activities of the bodily organs, the system requires support, something to permanently exalt its actions. In all cases of debility, the Favorite Prescription tranquilizes the nerves, tones up the organs and increases their vigor, and strengthens the system. Directions for use accompany every bottle.

Figure 1. Excerpts from Dr. Pierce's widely read consumer guide, first printed in 1895. His institute specialized in mail-order dispensing. (Source: R.V. Pierce, *The People's Common Sense Medical Advisor,* World Dispensary Printing Office, Buffalo, NY 1898.)

The type of health care that patients received was determined by their ability to pay and their geographic location. In cities, wealthy patients were treated in their homes by private physicians; poor people, if able and willing to leave their sickbeds, commonly obtained free services from outdoor dispensaries that were funded by the city and private charities. Those who stayed at home either received visits from a dispensary physician or relied on folk-healing methods. Beginning at the turn of the century, however, publicly funded visiting nurses became an important source of professional home care for the poor, especially for children and pregnant women.

In 1873, fewer than 200 hospitals existed in the United States. Most were in large cities, and approximately one third provided care for mentally ill patients. The word *hospital* derives from the Latin words *hospes,* for "host," and *hospitalis,* meaning "of a guest," and the typical hospital of that era *was* little more than a guest house for people who lacked family or the financial resources to sustain them through an illness. They were also commonly used for the isolation of patients with communicable diseases. A patient with enough money could be admitted to a pay ward or private room, but most were cared for in large charity wards. All in all, the hospital at the turn of the century held little advantage over home care. With its limited techniques, surgery could be performed as easily at home as in the hospital, and the risk of infection from another patient was avoided at home. Also, of course, patients preferred to be at home during convalescence. For all of these reasons, therefore, hospitals were not the main source of care for the affluent *or* the poor at the turn of the century.

Many hospitals were run by religious orders, which held expenses to a minimum. Operating a hospital was viewed as charity work, and affluent citizens often subsidized expenses. Physicians and nurses donated their skills to such hospitals, arranging to visit the wards several times a week; because of their mission to the poor and the poverty of their patient population, few charged for their services.

Physicians at the turn of the century usually had offices in their own homes, and many traveled on horseback or by buggy to make house calls, carrying all the equipment available to them in a single bag. Despite the abundance of medical schools, however, physicians were in short supply in many regions. Workloads were particularly heavy in rural areas.

In 1870, a house call cost between 50 and 75 cents. An office call cost 25 cents. An average hospital stay cost only about $1 per day. Insurance to pay for medical expenses had been instituted in Europe during the Industrial Revolution, but this was not yet common in the United States, except for some unionized immigrant workers in large cities. Financial transactions between patients and their physicians or hospitals typically were direct, with some bills paid in produce, livestock, or services, particularly in rural areas. Most turn-of-the-century physicians were not affluent.

Many physicians settled permanently in one location and cared for their patients—often more than one generation of a family— from birth to death. The personal relationships that developed gave such physicians a respected place in the community, and they were consulted on a wide variety of issues. Indeed, a romanticized image of the seemingly selfless and inexhaustible practitioner, dating from this era, remains our standard for professional dedication. To this day, physicians benefit from this image in the respect they are accorded, yet the very attachment to such an idealized image makes it difficult for physicians and others to be objective about changes in the delivery of medical care. Changes occur anyway, of course, but not all are quickly accepted.

From 1900 to World War II

Paralleling the rising importance of the machine model within the industrial world, medicine moved out of the prescientific era during the early 1900s. Physicians began viewing the body as a composite of individual systems that "could be examined and treated without the rest of the body being affected" (Berliner 1975, p. 576). This shift in thinking paved the way for the advent of medical specialization as well as for research that focused on pathophysiologic processes; there was decreased emphasis on the social causes of disease.

Beginning at the turn of the century, rapid advances were made in diagnosis and therapy. Knowledge increased tremendously, which allowed "diseases to be treated as universal entities rather than as individual afflictions different for everyone" (ibid., p.

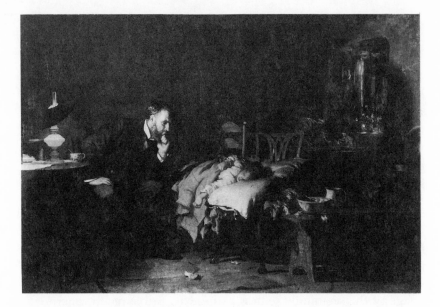

Figure 2. Sir Luke Fildes (1844–1927), *The Doctor*. Oil on canvas, 1891. (Source: The Tate Gallery, London.)

576). X-rays had been recently discovered, and they were soon used in diagnosis. The electrocardiogram was developed in the early 1900s, and new pharmaceuticals were discovered and entered general use. In 1910, arsphenamine was introduced for the treatment of syphilis, and in the 1920s, the discovery of insulin made possible the treatment of diabetes. The development of the sulfa drugs (in 1935) and penicillin (in 1941) provided the first effective treatments against many infectious diseases. Effective therapy for asthma as well as the initial breakthroughs toward an understanding of the allergic process also date from this era.

For patients undergoing surgery, effective anesthetics became readily available, and the widespread acceptance of antiseptic techniques minimized bacterial growth. The discovery of the four major blood groups in 1901 permitted safer blood transfusions as well. These improvements in turn led to great advances in surgical technique, and in the early 1900s, several operations that had been experimental and highly dangerous only a few years earlier now became commonplace. Surgical mortality rates rose initially, but as pioneering surgeons became more proficient at these new techniques, the mortality rates soon declined. For example, before 1890, appendicitis was treated by allowing the inflamed appendix to rupture, form an abscess, and wall itself off before the abdomen was opened. The first successful appendectomy was performed in 1890, and over time, as knowledge of the technique spread and surgeons became skilled in performing it, appendectomy became the new standard of practice. Over a 17-year period, from 1893 to 1910, mortality from appendectomies dropped from 26 percent to 2 percent.

Allopathic physicians thoroughly incorporated scientific attitudes into medical care, and they began to declare themselves as the only legitimate medical practitioners. The explosion of therapeutic advances increased the volume of medical care and heightened its complexity; as a result, the personalized, holistic approach to patient care began to decline during this era. Patients were removed from the social context of their afflictions and were "thought of almost as an abstraction" (ibid.). Whereas patients and physicians had formerly viewed disease similarly, the physician's scientific knowledge now created a disparity between their views. Thus, for example, patients might continue to believe that they could "catch a cold" when their feet got wet, but more and more physicians knew that colds were caused by viruses and bacteria.

All this took time, however, and even decades later, practitioners were still without cures for many common conditions, as Lewis Thomas, who accompanied his physician father on house calls in the 1920s, described. "The general drift of his conversation was intended to make clear to me, early on, the aspect of medicine that troubled him most all through his professional life; there were so many people needing help, and so little that he could do for any of them. It was necessary for him to be available, and to make all these calls at their homes, but I was not to have the idea that he could do anything much to change the course of their illnesses" (1983, p. 13).

While established practitioners were only beginning to feel its effects, scientific progress was having a significant impact on medical education. The modern physician needed a greater range of skills than the old-fashioned medical education supplied. The Association of American Medical Colleges, founded in 1876, had begun to develop stricter standards for medical school members,

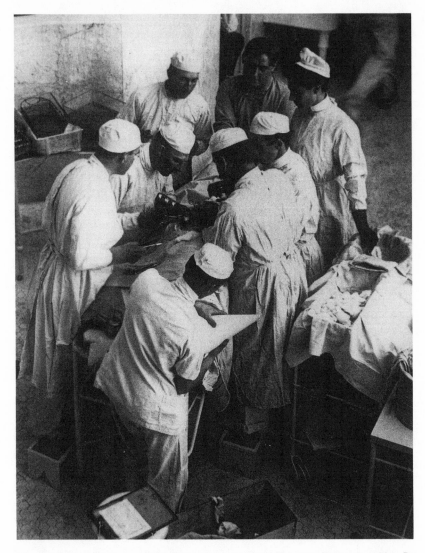

Figure 3. A surgical operation at the Johns Hopkins Hospital, Baltimore, 1904. Dr. William S. Halsted is the lead surgeon in the center. (Source: The Chesney Medical Archives of the Johns Hopkins Medical Institutions.)

but far more sweeping changes were needed. These changes came with the 1910 publication of the Flexner Report (so called after its main author, Abraham Flexner) that codified a general shift in society's approach to educating physicians. Based on a study sponsored by the Rockefeller and Carnegie Foundations, the Flexner

Report has been called the single most important document in the history of American health care.

Two years (preferably 4) of undergraduate college education, including courses in the basic sciences, now became the requirement for admission to a medical school. This requirement made it much more difficult for a relatively poor person to obtain a medical education, however, and it thus altered the social structure of the profession. In addition, all medical schools from that point on took a common approach to the study of both patient and disease: the AMA and allopathic medicine had emerged as the victors of the competition among the medical "sects."

The association of medical schools with universities also dates from this time. Medical schools developed into research centers that specialized in the application of sophisticated technology, and the role of patient care was reduced in importance. The duration of the medical school program also increased to 4 years. The number of medical schools had already been decreasing, and as schools that could not meet the new standards closed, this decline in the numbers both of schools and their graduates continued (Fig. 4).

For many years, no serious shortage of physicians existed, and the old system remained essentially in effect. Shorter described the typical physician of the preantibiotic era as possessing "almost courtly good manners" and added that "around 1930, 56 percent of all GPs [general practitioners] made [house calls]. They were frequent during an episode of illness and accumulated to an impression of caring" (1985, p. 209). Eventually, however, the transformation of medical education caused a reduction in the supply of practitioners. The number of medical schools and the physician-to-population ratio both reached a plateau during the 1920s and 1930s.

The concept of physicians practicing jointly in a group was introduced by the Mayo family in Minnesota during the late nineteenth century, but most physicians in the 1920s and 1930s practiced alone. Less than one in a hundred practiced in a group of three or more. At this time, the frequency of house calls began to decline as well. Not only did the lower physician-to-population ratio make home visits impractical for overworked practitioners, but the apparatus of adequate medical care was increasingly too complex to be transported in a bag.

Scientific advances had only begun to affect the patient–practitioner encounter outside the hospital. Within the hospital, how-

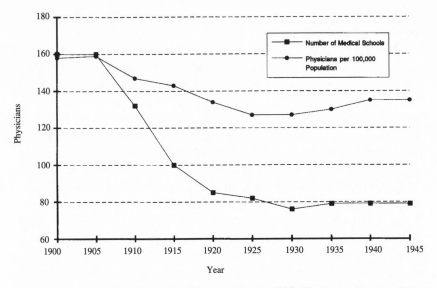

Figure 4. Medical schools and physician manpower, 1900–45. (Source: Data from Fein 1962.)

ever, much changed during this period. Doctors began to require new equipment, services, and support personnel. Introducing the latest technology benefited both the hospital and the physician: the former because it attracted physicians and patients, and the latter because it enabled the provider to practice up-to-date medicine. Hospitals added diagnostic laboratories and radiologic services in the early decades of the twentieth century, and aseptic surgical suites also became common during this time.

As it became apparent that good outcomes could result from hospital treatment, people became more willing to stay in the hospital. A government commission reported, "The removal of the death-house stigma from the hospital was probably the most important factor in influencing the change in the public attitude toward the institution" (Commission on Hospital Care 1947, p. 49). The hospital soon eclipsed the home, for both wealthy and poor patients, as the preferred site for the treatment of serious illness. The presence of illness replaced poverty as the basis for hospital admission, and the daily inpatient census came to represent a greater cross-section of the community. When this happened, the hospital became a community asset and, as such, a focus of local support and pride. By the 1920s, more than two thirds of patients paid at least some portion of the bill for care they received. As more affluent people used the hospital and were able to pay for their medical care, hospitals began operating from a patient-revenue base instead of relying chiefly on philanthropy. Still, most physicians charged only those patients who could pay and donated their services to those who could not.

Partly as a result of the hospital's increasing complexity, hospital charges rose; the costs of new advances were included in medical care bills. The average length of stay decreased dramatically, in part because hospitals were no longer used exclusively for long-term housing of indigent patients, but more importantly because scientific advances led to early cures of some diseases that previously had been left to run their natural course. Because the length of stay decreased and the costs increased, the average cost per day increased over 200 percent from 1900 to 1920 and another 38 percent between 1920 and 1940 (Table 1).

When it became possible for hospitals to be run profitably, entrepreneurs were encouraged to build them. The number of hospital beds increased substantially during this time, but population growth as well as the increased role of the hospital in medical care also contributed to this trend. The Great Depression led to a decrease in the 1930s; however, there were over four times as many hospital beds in 1941 as in 1909.

Socioeconomic conditions also influenced the development of the health care industry during this era. In the Great Depression, both hospitals and physicians were unable to collect fees from unemployed patients. Many people forewent elective procedures, and many chose to stay at home during an illness instead of seeking hospital care. Large numbers requested charity care, thus driving

Table 1. Hospital Costs and Length of Stay, 1900–44

Year	Average cost per admission	Average length of stay (days)	Average cost per day
1900	$38	32	$1.19
1920	48	13	3.70
1940	56	11	5.09
1944	65	10	6.50

Source: Adapted from Commission on Hospital Care 1947, p. 545.

up hospital debts. After decades of unprecedented growth, the limited flow of dollars put a considerable strain on health care providers and the delivery system itself.

Public hospitals obtained enough government funding to remain open despite their bad debts, but proprietary hospitals (many of them founded during the booming economy of the 1920s) were hit hard. In an effort to remain financially viable in the face of decreased occupancy rates, such hospitals decreased their charges, reduced the wages of their employees, appealed to philanthropic sources of funding, and closed beds; some limited admissions to emergency cases only. Even so, many proprietary hospitals did not survive, and the relative glut of hospital beds diminished.

With the rising cost of medical care as well as an unstable economy, people turned to health insurance as a way to minimize their risk of financial hardship in case of a serious illness. The health insurance industry, a multibillion-dollar giant today, grew from humble beginnings in 1929. In that year, the first group health insurance plan was started in Baylor, Texas, where some 1500 schoolteachers were enrolled in a plan that formed the basis for the Blue Cross Insurance Company; for $6 per year, enrollees received the benefit of 21 days of hospitalization coverage.

By assuring payment for a hospital stay, health insurance benefited both the hospitals and patients. Thus, although ostensibly created primarily to assist the patient, health insurance also was a direct outcome of the financial crisis that the hospital sector experienced during the Great Depression. Some years later, similar insurance programs were developed (eventually called Blue Shield) to cover physicians' professional services.

Another important development was the establishment of the Veterans Administration (VA) that offered veterans of World War I treatment for service-related injuries or diseases at government expense. This was an important turning point in the history of health policy: for the first time (outside of a war situation), total medical care for a designated group of entitled persons became a public sector responsibility. This set a precedent for broader measures in the future.

The composition of society also changed during this era. The early 1900s brought a wave of immigrants, most of whom found employment in unskilled, poorly paid jobs, to the United States.

Many Americans of all origins lost their employment during the Great Depression as well. More affluent citizens could purchase health insurance (and often did so), but poor citizens could not. And with both the shortage of physicians and the expensive hospital bills, their needs for health care were inadequately met. Figure 5 plots family income against physician contacts in the early years of the Depression; the wealthiest Americans received more than twice as much care as the poorest.

As charity care moved from the realm of moral responsibility to a social concern, the federal government sought to bring poor citizens under a new umbrella of limited protection. The first major effort in the health field was the Sheppard-Towner Act of 1921, which provided grants to the states for maternal and child health programs. Its objectives were not significantly different from those of the popular child labor legislation of that time, but the bill was still controversial, particularly in the medical community: "Many physicians opposed it. They claimed that there would be undue interference in state affairs and regimentation of medical practice" (Anderson 1985, p. 93).

During the 1930s, access to health care again became an issue. In 1927, the Committee on the Costs of Medical Care was formed to look into what many felt were excessive health care costs and to explore ways of subsidizing medical care for the poor. The comprehensiveness and foresight of this committee's recommendations had considerable impact on national health policy. The Social Security Act of 1935 incorporated some of them; others, however, were not adopted until several decades later. Another government group, the Committee on Economic Security, also was appointed in 1934 to "recommend legislation for a program 'against misfortunes which cannot be wholly eliminated in this man-made world of ours.' One of the issues to be considered by the committee was the problem of personal health services" (ibid., pp. 109–10).

In addition, a third government group, the Technical Committee on Medical Care, further broadened the scope of health policy by recommending grants to states for mandatory health insurance, expanded public health programs, medical care for welfare recipients, health care for children, federal permanent disability insurance, and grants for hospital construction. These recommenda-

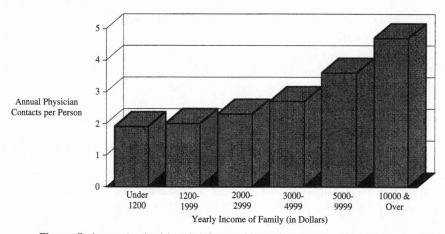

Figure 5. Access to physicians is influenced by patient income, 1928–31. (Source: Data from Committee on the Costs of Medical Care 1932.)

tions were made in a proposal sent to Congress in 1939, but no action was taken during World War II. Within the next 20 years, however, all the committee's recommendations except for mandatory health insurance were enacted into law.

Expenditures on health care were systematically tallied beginning in 1946, and these expenditures were estimated retrospectively as far back as 1929. In 1929, the country spent an estimated $3.5 billion on health care, or 3.5 percent of the gross national product. During the Great Depression, spending for health care decreased, reaching a low point of less than $2 billion in 1933. It increased from that year on, however, and by 1935 totaled some $2.9 billion, or 4.0 percent of the somewhat shrunken gross national product.

During the New Deal years of the 1930s and 1940s, many politicians and social reformers felt that if the private sector could not provide health insurance to the masses, then the government should. Extensive debates were held on the merits of national health insurance. Because any such legislation would have cut the insurance companies out of the health insurance business, however, the growing insurance industry exerted itself to increase enrollment in private sector health plans. Such was the first of many cycles of debate on the implementation of a national health insurance plan in the United States. This debate has again achieved national prominence in recent years. (Current proposals are discussed in Chapter 12.)

The medical profession also resisted increased government involvement in health care. What was to grow into a long history of AMA–government conflict began with the AMA's official opposition to the Sheppard-Towner Act. While acknowledging the financial advantages of private insurance and public subsidies to both patients and providers, physicians desired to maintain control over the process of medical care. In particular, they did not want third-party payers to set the reimbursement rates; physicians wanted to set these rates themselves. To some extent, this was sheer self-interest, and to some extent also an unwillingness to give up the myth of the benevolent and wise solo practitioner:

Most doctors who opposed the cooperative reforms genuinely believed in the traditional ideals of individualism and freedom for the doctor and patient. Despite the scientific, professional, and economic changes which had swept over the medical profession since 1900, these men were committed to the idealized and emotionalized image of the rural general practitioner as the true representative of medical practice. Just as many industrialists of these years tended to deny real conditions and look upon themselves as benevolent partners with their employees in society's productive processes, many doctors identified themselves with the self-sacrificing and largely mythical GP of earlier decades. Somehow he, despite the fact that he carried almost all his tools in his little black bag and kept his accounts in his head, supplied the best type of medical care to his patients. And it was he who, by fulfilling his role of family doctor, by preserving the doctor–patient relationship, and by caring for the poor and unfortunate without payment or complaint, upheld the finest traditions of professional service. (Hirshfield 1970, pp. 34–5)

In this era, the house call remained the emblem of professional dedication even as new technologies were demonstrating their superior effectiveness. The practitioner's influence on the larger aspects of health care was on the wane, however. The new era could no longer be denied: despite physicians' efforts to maintain control of the health care industry, the influence of private insurers and politicians had begun to increase.

From World War II to 1978

Social, economic, and scientific changes continued to influence the development of medical care in this era. For example, concerns about patient autonomy have their roots early in this period, resulting from Nazi atrocities that included human torture in the name of "medical research." Post-war examination of these activities led to the development of the Nuremburg Code, an international policy statement that prohibited human research without the consent of the subjects. In the United States, medical research got a boost after World War II, when funding dedicated to the Office of Scientific Research and Development (which coordinated the atomic bomb project) was transferred to research through the National Institutes of Health (NIH).

The NIH has existed, albeit in several different forms, since 1887. In 1944, Congress gave the NIH "general legislative authority to conduct research" (Spingarn 1976, p. 22). Strong financial backing of the NIH began after World War II and continued through the 1960s: "The medical research renaissance ... flowered in Bethesda [Maryland] during the 1950s and 1960s. Fact and legend mingle here, but it is true that a combination of cirumstances then made NIH the great and productive leader among the world's health research institutions. An expanding economy, a favorable political ambience, a consensus stemming largely from World War II technological success that scientific research can pay off big, and a set of remarkably effective health leaders in both public and private sectors, all worked smoothly in the Institutes' behalf" (ibid., p. 5).

In part as a result of such public and private support, medical science continued to advance in this era. Relman (1988) termed the period from the late 1940s through the 1960s the *Era of Expansion*. Research efforts in oncology focused on surgery, radiation, and chemotherapy. Vaccines were developed to counter polio and tuberculosis. Pharmacologic treatment of mental illness also began in the 1950s with the development of the major tranquilizers (now termed *neuroleptics*). Surgical developments included the heart–lung machine and cardiac catheterization, and mechanical ventilation, introduced in the 1950s, improved resuscitation techniques. Organ transplantation became possible in the 1960s as well. The government funded important work in genetics, neurosciences, and a myriad of other areas. Biomedical research continued to be an unquestioned federal budget priority through the early 1970s.

Not only did such investigations revolutionize our scientific understanding of human physical function, but they also had social and medical consequences. For example, with the development of in vitro fertilization, embryos and fetuses came to be thought of in an entirely new light, thus stimulating great debate about the societal implications of this new technology. The role of patient autonomy grew further during this time as well, and such developments successfully challenged the authority of physicians to make unilateral medical decisions. They also set the stage for later challenges to the patient–physician relationship, most of them based on economic considerations.

The general population continued to benefit during these years from the ongoing improvements in environmental and social factors as well as from advances in medical science. Figure 6 summarizes the dramatic increase in life expectancy that has occurred during the twentieth century. In 1989, the average life expectancy for a U.S. citizen stood at 75.2 years, up from approximately 50 years at the turn of the century. Figure 7 compares the top ten causes of death in 1900 and 1983, and it reveals a dramatic shift in etiology from infectious diseases in the historical era to the indirect effects of social problems (e.g., accidents, some cases of suicide) and lifestyle choices (e.g., smoking, lack of exercise, high-fat diet, alcohol abuse) today.

Technologic expansion during this era also affected medical care in many ways. As scientific sophistication increased the complexity of care, clinicians needed more finely honed technical skills. Moreover, the volume of medical knowledge increased exponentially, thus motivating medical students to specialize as a means of gaining a sense of mastery over the material. Soon, specialty care became more lucrative than primary care, with a physician's prestige increasingly associated with his or her degree of specialization as a result. In 1945, approximately half of all U.S. physicians were general practitioners; by 1978, this figure had fallen to approximately 12 percent, a trend essentially that was unchanged during the 1980s.

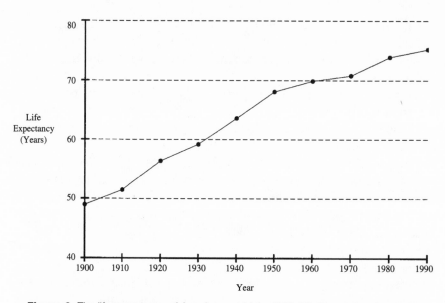

Figure 6. The life expectancy of Americans at birth, 1900–90. (Source: Data from National Center for Health Statistics 1991.)

One effect of this trend toward specialization was to reinforce the drift away from personalized medical care. As a battery of sophisticated tests became available, many physicians began substituting them for the close, hands-on examination the GP used in earlier years. The field of medical ethics took clearer shape during this era as well, being seen by some as a moral counterbalance to the increasing use of technologic interventions in medical treatment, and indeed, scientific advances have increased the number of difficult moral decisions that confront both medical practitioners and patients. In 1958, Pope Pius XII discussed the ethical justifications for removing patients from ventilators, and in the mid-1960s, it became necessary to formally redefine death in terms of brain function rather than heart and lung function.

The mode of health care delivery also changed during these years. Group practice became much more common; solo practitioners were fewer, and house calls were rare. A new type of practice arrangement became common in some areas of the country: the prepaid plan. The first large *prepaid group practice* (PPGP) was started in 1933 by a California physician named Sidney Garfield,

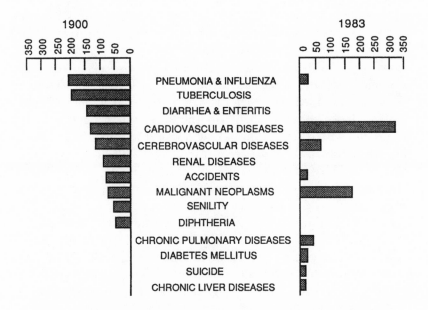

Figure 7. A comparison of the top 10 causes of death among Americans, 1900 and 1983. Rates represent deaths per 100,000 people. (Source: Data from National Center for Health Statistics 1987.)

who contracted to provide comprehensive medical care to 5000 workers who were building an aqueduct in return for $1.50 per worker per month from the employer and 5 cents per day from each worker. In 1938, Dr. Garfield contracted with the Kaiser Corporation for prepaid care of the workers building the Grand Coulee Dam as well as their families (10,000 people in all), and during World War II, Kaiser shipyard workers also were cared for by this plan. Kaiser's experience with this arrangement was so successful that the corporation entered the health care business after the war and eventually enrolled millions, mainly on the West Coast, in its PPGPs.

Health care delivery was also affected by a physician shortage, which surfaced in the 1940s as a health policy issue. One problem was that rural areas and inner cities were inadequately served. Another was that primary care physicians were becoming a rare commodity. Still, owing in part to AMA opposition, legislation to increase the number of U.S. physicians was not passed until the early 1960s. The Health Professions Education Assistance Act of 1963 authorized funds to support the construction of new teaching facilities, and existing medical schools were also given funds for student loans and operating expenses. Additional legislation in 1971 rewarded schools that increased their enrollment. Billions of federal dollars were spent on these growth programs in the 1960s and 1970s. In addition, new laws made it easier for foreign medical graduates to practice; in the early 1970s, almost as many foreign as U.S. graduates entered practice in the United States. The training of alternative primary care providers, such as physician assistants and nurse practitioners, was encouraged as well, and as a result of these manpower policies, the number of physicians in active practice increased by one third between 1960 and 1975.

A hospital shortage existed in this period as well. During the Great Depression, many hospitals went bankrupt, and World War II halted the construction of new facilities. The shortage was particularly acute in rural areas, where many people had no access to hospital care. The Hill-Burton Act of 1947, which authorized federal subsidies to states to modernize existing hospitals and construct new ones, first addressed this problem. Hospitals receiving grants had to provide annual charity care amounting to between 2 percent and 5 percent of their operating budgets. During the next three decades, grants under this law paid for the construction or modernization of 6500 health care facilities, and the nation's hospital-bed capacity approximately doubled.

Modern hospitals bore little resemblance to their predecessors. Research advances and federal money increased their technologic sophistication, and as religious orders became less a part of the employee force, the missionary aspect of the hospital diminished in importance. Also, for the first time, labor problems surfaced: hospital workers demanded higher wages, and employee strikes led to the unionization of support workers and nurses. Inevitably, costs rose. Average daily hospital rates rose from $5 per day in 1940 to $15 per day in 1950 and more than $200 per day in 1978.

Payment for medical care underwent several changes during this era. First, health insurance premiums came to be paid mainly by employers. This development was catalyzed by organized labor,

which became a powerful force during World War II; wartime collective bargaining led to the concept of fringe benefits, of which
health insurance coverage was (and is) a major component. Many
employers agreed to pay the costs of employees' health insurance
as part of their wage package at this time, and organized labor
maintained its strength after the war. In part reflecting the growth
of insurance as an employment benefit, only 9 percent of the population in 1940 was covered by some form of hospital insurance;
eight years later, this figure was 50 percent (Fig. 3).

When federal legislation in 1954 exempted employers' payments
for health insurance from corporate taxes, employers were effectively encouraged to steer dollars to fringe benefits rather than to
salaries. By 1958, nearly 30 percent of all health insurance enrollees were in collectively negotiated plans.

Things did not go as well for the poor, however. While certain
of payment from the middle- and upper-class patients who were
largely covered by insurance, many hospitals would not admit the

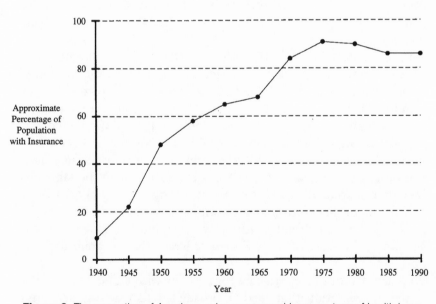

Figure 8. The proportion of Americans who are covered by some type of health insurance, 1940–90. (Source: Data from Health Care Financing Administration 1991; Health Insurance
Association of America 1991.)

poor, or hospitals transferred them to municipal facilities that were often second rate when they were seriously ill. Many impoverished families, particularly in rural areas, had no access to adequate health care. Fifty percent of aged people had no health insurance, and another 25 percent had inadequate coverage.

This situation was intolerable to the members of the liberal Great Society movement in the 1960s. A "War on Poverty" was declared, and health care was proclaimed to be a citizen's right. Access to care became a prominent social issue, and many believed that public funds should be used to provide medical care of the highest possible quality to the underprivileged population.

The Office of Economic Opportunity (OEO) was a government unit that was developed to lead the so-called War on Poverty. When indigent participants in OEO programs were screened, a significant number were found to have untreated diseases. As a result, the OEO allocated funds to projects that would effect "basic changes in the way that health services were delivered to the poor" (Sardell 1983, p. 485). One such project was the Neighborhood Health Center Program, which was designed to provide comprehensive health care services to people living in target neighborhoods.

In the politically tense atmosphere of that time, the momentum for social reform increased. The Medicaid and Medicare programs were created in 1965 and took effect in 1966, subsidizing health care for the U.S. poor and elderly (with other groups added later, such as the permanently disabled). Medicare Part A offered federal hospital insurance for persons over 65 years of age, and benefits included acute care hospitalization, limited nursing home care, and other institutional services. Medicare Part B, with the same eligibility requirements as Part A but requiring a financial contribution from enrollees, covered professional fees for medical and surgical services. Medicaid, with a wider range of benefits than Medicare, was developed as a joint federal–state program for the poor.

Concern about access to care for patients with kidney disease resulted in legislation that further broadened federal responsibility for medical care. In 1973, an End-Stage Renal Disease Program, which pays for kidney transplants or dialysis treatment for beneficiaries, was incorporated into Medicare. End-stage renal patients are the only group of Medicare beneficiaries who are not required to be either elderly or fully disabled to qualify for coverage; their care is subsidized because of their particular disease. Victor Fuchs's 1974 book, *Who Shall Live?*, revealed how hospital committees were choosing patients to receive the limited number of available kidney transplants, reflected societal concerns at that time, and described the political climate that led to this important Medicare policy change.

These large-scale government programs, following some 30 years of debate about public sector financing of health care, effectively transferred primary responsibility for health care within the public sector from the local to the federal level. With their passage, the AMA lost a major battle in its war to maintain full professional independence in the health care field. However, despite the initial misgivings of many physicians about Medicare and Medicaid, their benefit to both patients and providers soon became apparent, and organized medicine came to support them.

In seven decades, the U.S. health care industry had been transformed from a prescientific, individualistic cottage industry into a monolithic, publicly subsidized system. The concern over access to health care and support for its expansion, which had contributed to the creation of this industry, continued for several years, but serious questions then arose about the value of the system and, in particular, its costs.

The price of medical care was already climbing twice as fast as the cost-of-living index when the Medicare and Medicaid programs went into operation in mid-1966. The introduction of those programs was like firing a booster rocket. Physicians' fees, which had been going up by less than 3 percent annually, began rising more than twice as fast. The steep climb in hospital charges became even steeper. (Editors of *Fortune* 1970, p. 19)

This quote, which uses jargon from the space program, captures the tenor of the times. Having successfully placed a man on the moon, the United States was in an optimistic mood. Other ambitious domestic programs had been implemented, including the War on Poverty and two major health programs, and society supported these projects. The price for significant reform and expensive technologic innovation, however, was a dramatic escalation in federal expenditures.

Medical care remained a top social priority throughout the 1960s and early 1970s, but by the mid-1970s, priorities shifted from the creation of new programs to the maintenance of existing ones. Some were actually dismantled; for example, Hill-Burton grants were changed to loans in 1970, and the program terminated entirely in 1974. However, despite these measures, it was still estimated that by 1980 the nation had over 100,000 excess beds in acute care hospitals. In addition, increases in biomedical research spending were also tempered in the late 1960s. Until 1968, for example, Congress had always granted the NIH more dollars than were requested, but in that year, only the requested amount was granted. In later years, requested amounts were slashed.

The spiraling costs of health care set the stage for a new movement in the late 1970s: the era of cost control, and the following chapters further discuss the motivation for both the public and private sectors to rein in expenditures.

CHAPTER 2

FROM 1979 TO THE PRESENT: THE ERA OF THE HEALTH CARE COST CRISIS

> The current battle follows a decade or two of dreams and delusions during which both parties to the fray seem to have believed sincerely that a nation that defied the law of gravity to go to the moon could also defy the most fundamental laws of economics.
>
> *Uwe Reinhardt*

Open-ended, largely unbridled budgets for medical care characterized U.S. health policy in the 1960s, but by the end of that decade, there were already hints of a change in political attitude toward the U.S. health care delivery system. First, the positions of government and other payers underwent a subtle change, and then society at large became not-so-subtly concerned about the costs of health care.

Causes of Increasing Health Care Costs

The rapid escalation of health care prices during the 1960s and beyond had many causes. General inflation was a major factor; the cost of most goods and services in the economy increased. The health care sector, however, consistently experienced a more severe rate of inflation than did the rest of the economy. Inflation in medical services outpaced that in all other sectors of the economy (including food, housing, apparel, transportation, entertainment, and other goods and services) every year during the 1980s. Furthermore, the gap in the annual percentage change in the inflation rate between health care and other services increased in the 1980s, as medical care prices continued to rise 6.5 percent to 7.5 percent annually while the overall consumer price index slowed to an annual increase of between 1.9 percent and 4.8 percent.

Greater scientific and technologic sophistication, resulting in more complex services, also contributed to these price increases. This same factor increased hospital prices significantly as well because of the costs associated with purchasing equipment, training specialized employees, and maintaining complex machines. The overall effect of technology on the health care sector is probably mixed, however, because as in other industries, providing a product more quickly (or of better quality) will often decrease its costs. The potential benefit in terms of improved quality of life should also be factored into the economic assessment.

Demographic factors contributed to the increased costs of health care as well. Not only has the U.S. population continued to grow, the average age of this population has been rising. Today, over 12.5 percent of the U.S. population is over 65 years of age, and this proportion will increase substantially in the coming decades. Elderly people have a higher incidence of chronic diseases, thus necessitating more tests, treatments, and hospital admissions. On average, the annual medical care for a person over 65 years of age costs more than 2.5 times that of a 35-year-old.

Private insurance was already covering a significant percentage of the U.S. population, and both Medicare and Medicaid subsidies enlarged the patient population by many thousands who previously could not afford such care. For both public and private sector programs, policy decisions about services to be covered profoundly affect the costs of health care. The end-stage renal disease (ESRD) component of the Medicare program provides a dismaying example of the financial effect that expanding coverage creates. Before this benefit was added, most people with ESRD died because of a lack of funds for treatment. When coverage for ESRD was added to the program in 1974 it was estimated that expenditures for this benefit would level off at approximately $200 *million* annually; the actual figure for 1986, however, was $2.5 *billion.**

---

*In less than 10 years, the number of people obtaining services increased 12-fold. After this very high initial growth in enrollment, the net rate of growth slowed, because the annual mortality of ESRD is approximately 20 percent, even with dialysis and transplantation. Expenditures continue to increase, however, because of the growing number of enrollees rather than increasing charges. The annual growth of charges slowed significantly after a cap on reimbursement for dialysis was instituted and also reflects greater success over time with kidney transplantation.

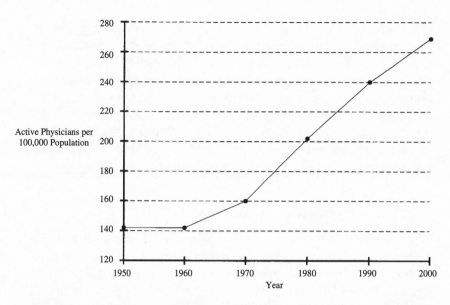

Figure 9. Physician manpower (including both M.D.s and Doctors of Osteopathy), 1950–2000. A projection is used for the year 2000. (Source: Data from American Medical Association 1991a, 1991b; U.S. Department of Health and Human Services 1990.)

Some analysts felt that a surplus of providers contributed to the cost problem. Figure 9 shows the increase in the number of physicians from 1950 through 1990 as well as an estimate for the year 2000. The manpower policies of the 1960s and 1970s were so successful that by 1980 the problem had shifted from a shortage to surfeit. In that year, a blue-ribbon panel—the Graduate Medical Education National Advisory Committee (GMENAC)—forecasted not only a significant oversupply of physicians in most surgical and medical subspecialties, but an overall "surplus" of 12 percent by 1990 and 21 percent by 2000.

The trend predicted by GMENAC proved to be true. The number of physicians in active practice increased by another one third between 1975 and 1990, and although projections vary, many experts believe that the United States already has more practicing physicians than it needs or can afford.

These concerns are mitigated, however, by the changing demographics of this physician population. First, the number of women in the medical field is increasing rapidly, and women tend to work fewer hours and fewer years than men, effectively reducing the average total physician work-hours. Second, there is an overall trend among younger physicians to work fewer hours per week, which is thought to reflect changing personal priorities among these professionals. Another important consequence of the physician oversupply was a contribution to the decreased political power of the AMA (in that health care became more of a "buyer's market"). The AMA and the American Hospital Association (AHA) traditionally have been two strong opponents of cost-control initiatives.

The Increasing Costs of Health Care

Perhaps more than any other illustration in this book, Figure 10 demonstrates why concerns about the costs of health care have profoundly influenced recent health care policy. Both as a percentage of GDP and in actual dollars, health care expenditures began climbing significantly after the Great Society legislation of the 1960s. This trend continued through the 1970s, 1980s, and into

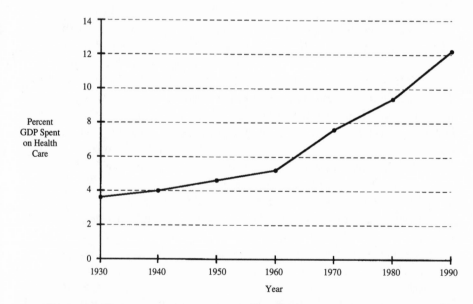

Figure 10. The percentage of the U.S. gross domestic product that is spent on health care, 1930–90. (Source: Data from Health Care Financing Administration 1987; Levit et al. 1991.)

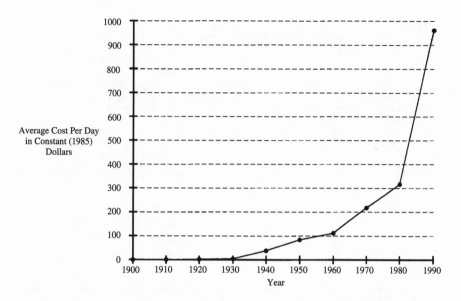

Figure 11. The average cost of a day in a hospital, 1900–90. (Source: Data from Health Insurance Association of America 1987, 1991.)

the 1990s. The absolute amounts involved are huge; since at least 1984, health care has been the third-largest U.S. industry (after food and housing). In 1991, U.S. health care expenditures totaled over $738 billion, or 13 percent of the GDP for that year.

From 1965 to 1975, increased intensity of care *and* price inflation were comparable contributors to the growth in health care spending. From the mid-1970s through the late 1980s, higher prices have been the major cause of increased expenditures. Figure 11 illustrates the cumulative effect over time of all factors on hospital costs per day.

Table 2 presents a series of additional indicators of health care expenditures. Every measure in this table shows a tremendous increase in cost over the last two decades.

Who's Paying?

Figure 12 summarizes the current sources of funds spent on U.S. health care. In 1965, only 20 percent of health care spending came from public funds (including local, state, and federal govern-

Table 2.   Health Care Expenditures, 1930–90

Year	Total U.S. expenditures (billions)	Per-capita expenditure	Per-capita expenditure in 1985 dollars	Percentage change in real per-capita expenditure over a 5-year period
1930	$ 3.5	$ 29	$ 240	—
1935	2.9	23	176	–27%
1940	4.0	30	225	+28
1945	6.0	55	310	+38
1950	12.7	82	359	+16
1955	17.7	105	413	+15
1960	26.9	146	516	+25
1965	41.9	207	687	+33
1970	75.0	350	952	+39
1975	132.7	591	1,158	+22
1980	248.1	1,054	1,353	+17
1985	422.6	1,710	1,710	+26
1990	666.2	2,566	2,112	+24

Source: Data from Sorkin 1986; Levit and Cowan 1991.

ment subsidies and reimbursements). After implementation of the Medicare and Medicaid Programs, public spending jumped 70 percent over the next 5 years, to 34 percent of total spending. Since then, the contribution from public funds gradually but

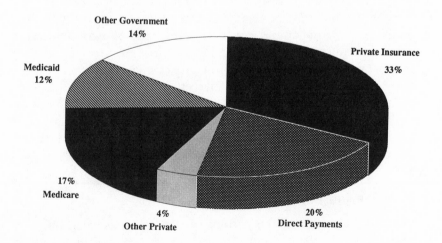

Figure 12. Sources of health care expenditures in the United States, 1990. (Source: Data from Levit et al. 1991.)

steadily increased, finally reaching a plateau above 40 percent in the late 1970s. (Of course, because government revenue derives from taxes, public sector expenditures ultimately are borne by taxpayers in the private sector.) Private sector sources, payments from patients, and third-party reimbursements account for the other 60 percent, but out-of-pocket payments currently account for only 20 percent of the total.

Despite the growth in public sector programs, the percentage of disposable income that Americans spend on medical care has continued to rise over time. The Health Insurance Association of America (HIAA) estimates that in 1960, 5.7 percent of disposable personal income went to medical expenses, rising to 7.7 percent in 1970, 9.7 percent in 1980, and 11.7 percent in 1989. The peak occurred in 1988, at 12.7 percent, approximately half of which paid for health insurance premiums. This inexorable rise reflects the steep inflation in health care prices as well as the greater average intensity of services per person.

Figure 13 presents a breakdown of how today's typical health care dollar is spent. Approximately 40 percent goes to hospitals, and the proportion of hospital services paid for by government sources (mainly Medicare and Medicaid) is approximately 55 per-

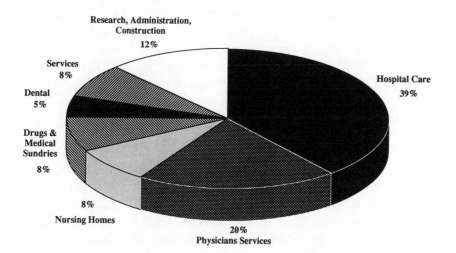

Figure 13. The distribution of health care expenditures in the United States, 1990. (Source: Data from Levit et al. 1991.)

cent. For this reason, hospitals were the first area targeted for cost-control measures.

Public Sector Programs

Medicare is the largest health care program in the United States in terms of both expenditures and beneficiaries. Data from slightly more than 25 years of operation reveal that the number of enrollees in the program increased approximately 60 percent, from 20 million to more than 33 million. During that time, expenditures increased more than 21-fold, from $4.7 billion to over $100 billion. Over half of all Medicare outlays are spent on hospital care.

Close to 100 percent of America's elderly people are enrolled in the Medicare program. Because of rising health care costs, however, these people have not been helped as completely as the Great Society legislators envisioned. The government annually spends many billions of dollars to cover their medical expenses, but elderly Americans continue to pay a significant percentage of their income (approximately 10 percent) for health care. Public funds now pay approximately two thirds of the health care costs for those aged 65 and older, and to aid this elderly population further with their medical costs, Congress *increased* Medicare subsidies with passage of a catastrophic health care package in 1989. Expansion of a federal health program was a rare event in the 1980s; however, this legislation was repealed in 1990 because of strong lobbying by groups like the American Association of Retired Persons (AARP), whose members strongly objected to the increased premiums that were to have been charged those elderly people at higher income levels.

Enrollment in the joint federal–state Medicaid program has doubled, from 12 million people in 1969 to 25.2 million in 1990. Outlays for Medicaid increased more than 15-fold during this period, to $75.2 billion in 1990, and of the total program budget allocated by each state, 50 percent to 73 percent is paid from state coffers (the percentage based on the individual state's wealth) and the remainder from federal funds. On average, Medicaid now consumes 14 percent of state governments' budget outlays. While the program has grown, however, so has the number of poor people in the United States. (Chapter 12 discusses the effectiveness of Medicaid in covering the health care costs of the poor.)

The other major federal health care program, the Department of Veterans Affairs (VA) (formerly the Veterans Administration), has grown substantially over the years as well, becoming very costly in the process. In 1985, the VA was the third-largest federal agency, with 220,000 full-time employees and an annual budget of $27 billion. Since then, both the budget and number of employees have increased, particularly since the VA achieved Cabinet-level status in 1989.

Medicare Part A is in financial trouble. Financed by a trust fund, this program's payouts have so greatly outpaced revenue that (according to one projection) no funds will be left by the early years of the twenty-first century. Current federal law prohibits using general revenue sources to subsidize the program, so other solutions to the problem must be found. Backed by general revenues, the VA, Medicare Part B, and Medicaid are in better financial shape, but policymakers understandably are concerned about outlays for these programs as well.

The Crisis in Corporate Health Care Costs

Employers are another significant category of payer in the U.S. health care system, because they subsidize employee health insurance premiums. During the last two decades, employers became concerned with escalating health care costs. After steep rises in the amount paid for employee health care during the 1970s, employers' outlays doubled again from 1980 to 1986, to $90 billion, and reached $145 billion for employee group health insurance premiums in 1989. In 1990, employers paid over $186 billion for health care, or almost 30 percent of overall expenditures. These outlays include employee health insurance premiums, mandatory contributions to the Medicare hospital insurance trust fund, workers' compensation medical premiums, temporary disability medical insurance, and industrial in-plant services.

Examining their operating expenses, many corporate executives realized the extent to which health care costs were reducing their profit. Consider the following corporate discoveries of the early 1980s:

- Ford paid the equivalent of $300 per vehicle for worker health care in 1983.
- AT&T paid $1.6 billion in medical and dental premiums for workers in 1983.
- The cost of employee health benefits for the Armstrong Tile Company increased 40 percent *each year* from 1978 to 1983.
- Chrysler paid $480 of the price of every new car in 1982 for workers' health care costs, and despite adding many cost-control innovations to their benefits program, these costs increased to $500 per car in 1984.

Inflation in health care prices occurred at a time when U.S. productivity lagged behind other countries' and when many corporations found themselves in fierce competition with foreign manufacturers. Health care costs were higher than many companies could easily manage. Since World War II, employers simply had paid the bill for employee health insurance premiums, but in the 1980s, corporate executives began to look for alternative health insurance arrangements for their employees. Widespread private sector concern with the issue of health care costs began at this time.

Corporate financing problems worsened in 1990 when the Financial Accounting Standards Board (FASB) determined that employers' balance sheets should reflect the liabilities represented by the health care that these employers promised to retirees. The General Accounting Office estimated this liability to equal $227 billion. This change in accounting procedure was intended to ensure that corporate financial statements more accurately reflected companies' actual financial situations; in the process, billions of dollars must be encumbered to cover the health care costs of retired workers.

Driven by economic necessity to derive innovative solutions in order to continue providing health care fringe benefits, employers soon made new proposals. Today, "business people are becoming the most important influence in the re-design of the health care system. They have become the new and potent fourth party. This new party on the scene is pressing for a thorough re-design of the delivery system" (Freedman 1985, p. 579).*

To cease providing employee health insurance altogether might have been a simpler solution, but the tax exemption for such insurance was a significant advantage for both the employer and employee. Union opposition to such a move of course was significant as well.

Perhaps the most common strategy that large corporations adopted was *self-insurance*. Not only can employers lower insurance expenses by assuming the risk themselves, but as such programs are exempt from most government regulations mandating the extent of coverage, additional savings are achieved. Under this arrangement, usually administered by a private insurance company or a third-party administrator (TPA), all or most employee claims for medical care are paid out of funds that the corporations set aside from their general operating budgets. This approach has grown in popularity over the years; it was estimated that in 1992 over 50 percent of U.S. employees with company-sponsored benefits were covered by some form of self-insurance plan. An analogous situation had occurred earlier in the automobile industry; when manufacturers realized that the steel they needed was too expensive as well as inefficiently produced, they took control of the steel production.

Despite action taken in the early 1980s when initial cost concerns developed, employer outlays for employee medical care have continued to escalate: it is estimated that employers' spending has increased 15 percent to 20 percent annually since 1987. By 1990, it was estimated that the overall health care costs of U.S. corporations exceeded their post-tax profits by 8 percent. This reflects the idiosyncracies that are inherent in the health care market, which lacks the influence of traditional market forces that are present in other industries such as steel manufacturing.

*The health care insurance transaction involves several *parties*. The *first* and *second* parties are the patient and the clinician. The *third* party is the payer, which traditionally was an insurance company or government program.

The Commercial Insurance Industry and Cost Control

Because commercial insurance companies pass along any increased health care costs to their consumers in the form of higher premiums, one might expect such increases not to trouble these companies, but when premiums rose too high, many people elected to risk the occurrence of a serious illness and pay their medical expenses out of pocket. Moreover, an increasing number of corporate clients were switching to self-insurance. Another threat to the insurance industry was posed by the competition from alternative care delivery systems such as health maintenance organizations (HMOs), which typically offer expanded health care coverage at prices equal to or lower than conventional insurance plans. These conditions catalyzed the interest of Blue Cross/Blue Shield in fighting the inflation of health care prices. The "Blues," which control approximately half of the private insurance market, led the way for other commercial insurers.

As a result of these developments, insurance companies joined with corporations and public policymakers to limit increases in the cost of health care. These three parties have been called "the new triumvirate" of U.S. health care, and this union has created a relatively cohesive vehicle for health care cost containment.

International Comparisons

When discussing a society's expenditures on health care, how are we to know how much is enough and how much is too much? One way to assess this is by comparing one country's outlays to those of other countries having similar economic systems and similar health indices. Table 3 shows spending levels, the availability of health care resources, and statistics on several health markers for the United States and eight other developed countries having free-enterprise industrial economies. All of these countries enjoy health indicators that at least equal, and in most cases exceed, those of the United States, and U.S. expenditures exceed those of all other countries listed. It is at least arguable, therefore, that "adequate" health care could be provided in this nation at lower cost. (This issue is discussed further in Part III).

The ratio of health care spending to GDP stabilized in the early 1980s in Canada, France, the United Kingdom, Japan, Italy, and Germany, but it has continued to rise in the United States. Thus, the gap in spending between the United States and these countries continues to widen. Whether or not these other health care systems will begin to face economic problems of a degree comparable to those in the United States is unclear. Other countries have greater social homogeneity than the United States, however, and France, which may have the widest range of socioeconomic diversity in Europe, is beginning to experience health care budgetary problems that may be attributable to this factor.

Social Attitudes Play a Role

The interests of society in containing the costs of health care vary according to how one defines "society." Taxpayers want to pay lower taxes; purchasers seek lower premiums; and patients want the best health care, which may not be the least expensive or most efficient. These are all the same people, however, and their priorities change as their roles change. As recently as 1982, the patient's view was the dominant one; in an opinion poll conducted that year, more than half of the people surveyed favored increased gov-

Table 3.   Health and Health Care Characteristics of Nine Industrialized Countries

Country	Infant mortality,* 1987	Expected male longevity at birth, 1987 (years)	Health care costs per capita, 1988 U.S. dollars	Health care costs as a percentage of GDP, 1988	Active physicians per 100,000 population, 1987	Acute care hospital beds per 1,000 population, 1987
United States	10.1	71.5	$2,354	12%	220	5.1
Australia	8.7	73.0	1,093	8	228	5.4
Canada	7.3	72.9	1,683	9	214	6.8
Denmark	8.3	71.8	912	6	256	6.3
Finland	5.8	70.7	1,067	7	221	12.3
Japan	5.0	75.9	1,035	7	150	13.0
Sweden	6.8	73.8	1,361	9	161	10.2
United Kingdom	8.8	71.7	836	6	164	7.2
Germany	8.3	71.8	1,232	8	280	11.0

Source: Data from Schieber 1990; National Center for Health Statistics 1991
*Deaths per 1000 live births

ernment spending on health. As Anderson pointed out in the mid-1980s, "the American people want choices, easy access, and the latest technology rather than low cost. To the public, the relationship of health care services to the GNP is an abstraction that has no bearing on their daily lives" (1985, p. 23).

As insurance premiums and medical expenses continued to rise, however, public opinion began to change. People began to perceive rising health care costs as a problem. They continued to value good health care, but more and more of them could not afford it. Some 68 percent of those polled in a 1985 survey named cost as the greatest single problem that faced the health care industry, and the media drove this message home with references to the health care cost "crisis." Soon, the average American was very aware of this problem.

This attitude arose in part from misgivings about whether money for medical care was being well spent. U.S. life expectancy, which had been increasing since record-keeping began, reached a plateau from the mid-1950s to the late 1960s, "leading some to wonder whether more medical care made any real difference in human well-being or survival" (Blendon and Rogers 1983, p. 1880).

The Development of Political Consensus

During the early 1960s, Congress passed legislation supporting generous allocations to the health care sector, but while the federal financial commitment to health care was increasing, the economy was changing for the worse. The Johnson Administration's effort to finance both the Vietnam War and the new domestic programs proved too ambitious, and it led to severe inflation. The idealism of the Great Society began to fade as budget realities became clearer. Energy and national defense issues became prominent. Health care was no longer a top priority.

Economic troubles continued into the 1970s. The national debt grew alarmingly, and productivity slowed, exacerbating the effects of inflation on the economy. It became popular to cite the failures of the Great Society (such as increased costs) rather than its successes (such as assistance for the indigent). Health care stood out as an area where savings could be made—the more so, critics argued, because sharp increases in health care costs had not brought the expected reductions in morbidity and mortality rates. Legislators grew less interested in health as a social issue and more interested in keeping the costs of health care down. For the first time, politicians supported slowing the growth of the health care sector instead of offering *carte blanche* for its expansion.

By the time of the Reagan Administration, the role of health care in the economic picture was even clearer. Federal expenditures had continued to rise: 10 percent of the federal budget was spent on health care by 1984, up from 5 percent in 1961. President Reagan brought a free-enterprise philosophy to the White House, and his priorities were lowering taxes, increasing defense spending, and otherwise minimizing the government's role in all industries, including health care. Reagan thought federal spending on health care was far too high, and his main health policy goal during the eight years of his presidency was cost containment. His successor, George Bush, took a similar approach to these issues.

Control of Health Care Costs

The tides of support for health care had begun to shift in the 1970s. In the 1980s, the atmosphere of financial crisis made the arguments for cost control more persuasive. The era of cost control dates from that time, and the following quotation captures the spirit of this new time.

Although there is no magic formula for determining a precise limit on what a country can afford to spend for health care, there is a limit. Every dollar spent on health care is a dollar that cannot be spent on something else. No set of expenditures can rise faster than the gross national product forever. At some point, health-care expenditures must slow down to the rate of growth of the gross national product. (Thurow 1984, p. 1569)

Through subsidies for research, medical schools, hospitals, and patient bills, the federal government long since had become the largest single payer of health care costs. It was accordingly the logical candidate to take the lead in reducing costs. Federal policymakers initiated efforts to gain control of the health care sector, and state and private payers soon joined their efforts.

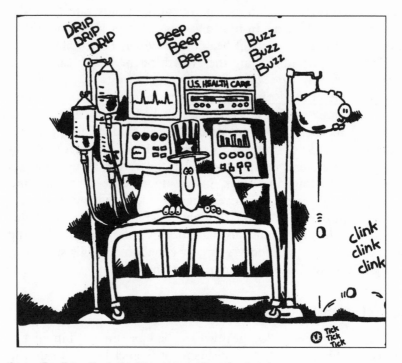

(Source: Tom Toles, *The Buffalo News*, Universal Press Syndicate.)

It has not been easy to bring such a large and politically power-ful industry under legislative control. The health care sector is composed of numerous constituents with diverse goals and agen-das. Strong political pressure from within the health care industry has affected the reform process through the protection of some programs from budget cuts; for example, funding for the Hill-Burton program, which subsidized hospital expansion, continued until 1974 despite a growing federal concern over an impending surplus of hospital beds.

Health care reform is a highly charged social and personal issue as well, so consensus on problems and the appropriate solutions is difficult to achieve. The great size and decentralization of the U.S. government also hampered a streamlined approach to reform: new policies and regulations sometimes worked in opposition to the existing ones. For example, the federal government encouraged the expansion of class sizes in medical schools to address the problem of underserved populations, while at the same time, it was reducing investment in the infrastructure necessary to deliver care to these populations.

Furthermore, health care economics is enormously complicated. Some economic problems, such as the cost consequences of the ESRD program (discussed in Chapter 1), were not recognized in a timely manner. Other trends, such as the effects of the number of physicians on the market economy, are subject to multiple interpretations. All of these complicating factors present formidable barriers to health care reform.

Nevertheless, health care financing and organization are evolving within the constraints set by policymakers and the major third-party payers. Cost control measures by government (both as payer and regulator), the business sector, and the health insurance industry, respectively, are examined in the following chapters.

CHAPTER 3

HEALTH CARE AS A MARKET COMMODITY

> Economics is the science of proving that
> what works in the real world can actually work in theory.
> And . . . health economics is the science of proving
> that what works in the real world can't work in health care.
>
> *David Himmelstein*

Because cost-containment interventions are based on various theories concerning the behavior of the health care market, a brief digression to examine basic health care economics is necessary. However, as the nature of the medical care product is in many ways capricious, it will become apparent that health care economic theory is inconsistent with other consumer markets. These differences between the markets for health care and those for other products help to clarify why some cost-containment measures are effective while others fail.

Balance of Supply and Demand

Economists use the theory of supply and demand to describe the relationship among three variables: the price, availability, and demand for a product. *Demand* for a given product is the volume or amount that is purchased, and demand (D) is influenced by several factors, including the price of the product, the prices of goods or services that could be substituted for it, consumer income, and consumer tastes or preferences. The quantity (Q) of a product that producers offer is its supply (S), and supply, like demand, usually is responsive to price (P). In general, the price of a product rises as the demand for it increases; the inverse also occurs: if demand decreases, the price will fall in response, which in turn leads to a reduced supply.

Numerous medical services constitute the products of the health care market. Those offering these products, such as hospitals and physicians, are termed *providers* in the health care industry. Those who purchase their services, including patients, government, and insurance companies, are the *consumers.*

A demand curve illustrates the theoretic relationship between price and demand, as shown in Figure 14. The intersection of the lines reflects the *theoretic* equilibrium point that determines the most efficient levels of product supply and demand.

These classic supply-and-demand relationships do apply for some products in the health care market. For example, many ophthalmologists, opticians, and optometrists offer competitive rates for eye examinations and glasses; prospective customers might compare prices before choosing a provider.

Most medical services, however, are not governed by simple laws of supply and demand. The unpredictable nature of medical services confounds the application of traditional economic theory to the problems of health policy. Some of the practical issues in

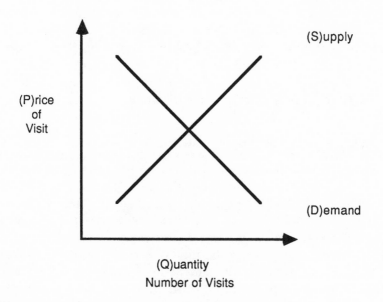

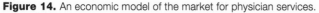

Figure 14. An economic model of the market for physician services.

employing the theory of supply and demand within the health care market are outlined below.

The Uniqueness of the Product

First, medical care is a uniquely valuable product. It directly affects the quality of a person's life and, at the extreme, can mean the difference between life and death. As a result, we must expand the strict sense of demand to include the *need* for the product when examining health care. Many ethicists who are concerned with theories of distributive justice (discussed in Chapter 10) argue that health care should be delivered on the basis of need, not the ability to pay, in cases where care is *required*, and not simply *desired* (as in many plastic surgery procedures). In contrast, classical economic theory deals with products that consumers have the *option* to purchase.

Health care is unique in another sense as well. Classic economic theories base their assumptions on the consistent nature of the product that is supplied, but medical services are heterogeneous (in essence, tailor-made for each patient depending on the illness and the decisions made during the patient–provider encounter). A medical service may be circumscribed fairly well, such as suturing a laceration, but just as often the product is nebulous, such as spending an hour reassuring a healthy but anxious patient that the brain tumor he or she imagines in fact does not exist. The differing nature of these services must be quantified if they are to conform to the theory of supply and demand.

The Inefficient Allocation of Health Care

Classic theories suggest that the demand for a product is based on the consumer's willingness and ability to pay for it; however, a number of circumstances complicate this assumption. In some cases, the overall effect is to increase the demand. For example, third-party insurance coverage decreases the price that is paid directly by the consumer at the time of service. Referring to Figure 14, insurance decreases the patient's out-of-pocket price, thereby shifting the equilibrium point of the supply-and-demand curve to the right; in the case of fully insured services or charity care, the effect of cost on patient demand is eliminated entirely. Other factors also serve to artificially decrease demand. For example, patients who need medical care but are unable to afford it, and who do not receive charity care, shift the equilibrium point to the left.

Supply-side factors inhibit the efficient allocation of health care resources as well. Classic theory suggests that the supply of a product is based on the producers' willingness to offer it at a given price. Noneconomic factors, like geographic location, influence the availability of medical care services and providers: more physicians choose to live in urban areas; as a result, health care (particularly specialty care and new technology) is unavailable in some rural areas at *any* price. Consumers also depend on other types of access to care, such as the availability of 24-hour emergency departments.

Another consideration making a supply-and-demand analysis difficult is the value that society, in the aggregate, derives from the health of its individual members. Termed an *external effect,* this affects neither the consumer who purchases the service nor the provider who supplies it. The classic example of a medical service with an external effect is vaccination: although the patient benefits from the service, that benefit is less than the advantage that is enjoyed by society as a whole when all of its members are vaccinated. Thus, if some people are unable or unwilling to pay for vaccinations, then the product is supplied anyway and the public sector pays the bill.

Consumer Dependency

The supply-and-demand model also assumes a buyer who is knowledgeable, which is a dubious assumption when it comes to health care. Health care consumers, therefore, depend on providers to tell them what services they should purchase. While patients usually recognize their need for care in cases of pain, bleeding, impaired function, or other abnormalities, they often do not know what specific care they need. Alternatively, the need for medical care may be subtle or hidden, as in essential hypertension (known as "the silent killer"), asymptomatic tumors, and numerous other painless conditions that nevertheless may harm the patient seriously. Furthermore, emotional needs and other personal characteristics can affect the need for care, thus leading patients to seek more or less care than their physical condition necessitates.

Elasticity of demand is a term for the relationship that exists between the cost of and the consumer's demand for a service. If there is elasticity, demand is sensitive to price, that is, as the price of a service rises or falls, the demand will change concomitantly. Demand is *inelastic* when service utilization is not directly affected by a change in the price of that service.

Some medical services are price elastic, but many of them are not. The classic case of price inelasticity in health care is a life-or-death situation, such as the arrival in an ambulance of an unconscious trauma victim. Medical care is provided on the assumption that the patient, if awake, would request it, regardless of its price. (This example admittedly is oversimplified: other factors, such as the value inherent to human life, also contribute to the decision of providing care in this situation.)

Another cause of price inelasticity in the health care market is the low degree of product interchangeability. If steak costs too much, then we can buy hamburger instead. If a patient needs an appendectomy, however, then what can be substituted to achieve a benefit that is comparable to the surgical procedure?

Thus, in the case of medical care, consumer demand is different from consumer need. An example of a cost-control method that ignores this difference is the insurance policy that denies reimbursement for emergency room visits if the presenting problem is not clinically deemed an "emergency" (i.e., urgent and life-threatening). Patients cannot always differentiate between their subjective demands and their demands that are based on medically verifiable need.

Creation of Demand by Providers

A corollary to consumer dependency is the ability of providers to *create* demand, for example, by scheduling return appointments or recommending surgery. This ability on the supplier's part complicates the relationships between supply, demand, and price. It also raises an important ethical question: to what extent are patients helped by physician-initiated medical care, and to what extent is the initiation in the practitioner's self-interest? According to

Wilensky and Rossiter, "Physician initiation is inducement only when services are recommended above and beyond what the patient would be willing to pay for if the patient knew as much as the physician" (1983, p. 259). The difference between initiation and inducement is subtle but critical: initiation is appropriate, and inducement is a violation of professional ethics.

Ethical considerations aside, however, the health care consumer is largely dependent on the producer for information concerning that consumer's condition and possible treatment and is influenced heavily by the producer's recommendations. In effect, the producer acts as the consumer's agent in purchasing medical services, which makes the relationship between doctor and patient very unlike the usual producer–consumer relationship.

This control of demand by providers is one reason why the dramatic increase in the number of hospitals and physicians has not led to price wars among them. During the 1970s, an increase in the national supply of physicians occurred simultaneously with increasing prices *and* higher demand for medical services, a trend that continued into the 1980s and early 1990s. Several studies found that the number of practitioners in a given area correlated directly with both health care prices *and* the quantity of services provided. For example, the number of certain surgical procedures performed in one Vermont community correlated with the number of surgeons there and not necessarily with the incidence of surgically correctable disease.

On a related theme, Roemer, a physician and health policy researcher, carried out a study on demand in the health care industry. He found a direct correlation between the number of hospital beds in a given area and the use of those beds when all other variables that were likely to affect their usage were held constant. "Roemer's Law" accordingly states that hospital beds will fill up to the extent that they are available; in effect, "the supply of beds creates a demand for those beds" (Feldstein 1983, p. 89). (Roemer's Law, however, has not held true in recent years. Cost containment *has* resulted in the closure of low-occupancy hospitals.)

Classic supply-and-demand theory would have predicted that as the supply of physicians and the quantity of services they provided increased, competition among the providers would reduce their prices. Instead, the health care market has accommodated without much difficulty additional providers, who have been financially successful, but not all researchers agree on the implications of these studies. Some believe that physician inducement is a relatively minor factor in consumers' decisions to use medical services; other factors, such as the increasing complexity of services, may have contributed to increasing prices (or costs) as well. This effect in part may be caused by the large percentage of specialists in our system. In Canada, more than half of all physicians are GPs or family physicians, whereas the comparable figure in the United States is less than 15 percent.

Barriers to Competition

A prerequisite to the application of market theory is that competition exist among suppliers of the same product. According to this theory, production improves and the per-unit cost decreases as more products are provided. In general, however, this is not true of appendectomies, or even of annual check-ups. The one-on-one nature of most health care products is a key reason why health care providers have had a difficult time competing primarily on the basis of price. Also, of course, "the unpredictable and acute nature of many health problems often precludes 'shopping' for health services. A person afflicted by life-threatening symptoms is hardly in a position to search the market for the 'best deal'" (Hsiao and Stason 1979, p. 23).

Another factor affecting competition in this field is the relative lack of competitive pricing for its professional fees. Historically, health care practitioners set their own fees without regard to those of other practitioners; they charged what they thought fair or what the market would bear. Until recently, as is discussed in Chapter 6, complex third-party price-setting mechanisms allowed for such practices and thus, in effect, supported them.

Norms of behavior have also contributed to independent fee-setting: it was long considered unprofessional not only to disparage another practitioner's services or fees but to advertise one's own. For many years, the code of professional ethics of the AMA and other professional associations prohibited advertising. Consequently, it was difficult for a consumer to base a decision on price.

When medical care prices did not decrease in the 1970s, despite an increasing supply of active physicians and hospital beds, it became clear that a simple competitive model was inadequate to describe the health care market. Enthoven, a health economist, noted that physicians have acted in various ways to suppress competition; among other things, they obstructed the use of PPGPs and other lower-cost providers, refused to grant hospital privileges to practitioners who discounted their fees, and boycotted insurance companies that put ceilings on reimbursement rates. Also in part because of an active and well-funded lobby in Washington, they generally were successful in keeping their reimbursement rates high.

It is the goal of antitrust legislation to prevent such behavior and to promote competition. The medical profession, however, was exempt from antitrust regulation until 1975, when the Supreme Court upheld a lower court's ruling that the Virginia state bar association could not establish or enforce a minimum fee schedule for lawyers. By treating the legal profession like other trades, this court decision paved the way for the medical profession to be considered a "trade" as well.

The Federal Trade Commission then successfully sued the AMA to remove its prohibition on advertising. Physicians and hospitals now may advertise their services, and many of them now do. Indeed, marketing efforts have become an important aspect of profitable private practice management in the 1980s and 1990s, but while the prohibition against advertising is now illegal, the reluctance to advertise is still discernable, reflecting the tradition within the medical profession. Unfortunately, however, antitrust legislation has affected adversely the medical profession's ability to regulate itself, because any attempt to impose internal standards—whether planning the class sizes of medical schools, regulating the behavior of peers, or policing state licensing criteria—may lead to an allegation of antitrust activity.

Competition is not applicable to every facet of the health care industry, but economists consider it relevant for some aspects, such as shopping for health insurance. For example, the goal of Enthoven's "Consumer-Choice Health Plan" was to create competition between alternative insurance packages by giving tax credits or vouchers to taxpayers and direct subsidies to low-income citizens for the purchase of health insurance. His plan was submitted to the Carter Administration in 1978 as part of their consideration of national health insurance proposals. The Enthoven plan was not adopted, but it did prompt discussion concerning the role of competition within the health care sector. A revised version of Enthoven's plan, labeled "managed competition," is under consideration by the Clinton Administration.

Thus, in several fundamental ways, medical services deviate from the assumptions that underlie market economic theories. The uniqueness of the product, its value to the consumer and society, inefficient allocation of resources, consumer dependency on the provider, price inelasticity, product heterogeneity, low substitutability, demand creation by providers, barriers to competition—is it any wonder that the task of predicting the behavior of the health care market is so formidable?

Despite these complications, however, both payers and policymakers in the era of cost containment have initiated a wide variety of cost-controlling approaches. Some attempted to regulate the market and others to increase competition. Most reforms intended to correct one or more of the market imperfections that this chapter discussed; specific measures are explored in the following chapters.

PART II

THE ORGANIZATION AND FINANCING OF TODAY'S HEALTH CARE SYSTEM

You can only hope to find a lasting solution to a conflict
if you have learned to see the other objectively, but,
at the same time, to experience his difficulties subjectively.

Dag Hammarskjöld

S ince the 1940s, medical care has usually involved a one-to-one interaction between a patient and a private practitioner. Uninsured patients paid the provider directly, and fees for insured patients were paid directly by a remote insurance company. Several factors under this insurance arrangement contributed to inflation and the rapid growth of expenditures. Under fee-for-service (FFS) reimbursement, both doctors and hospitals were paid (for the most part) whatever they requested. The growth of medical technology offered new tests and treatments that physicians too commonly incorporated into their practice in an additive rather than a selective manner; rote test ordering contributed to the escalation of health care expenditures. Broader changes, such as the implementation of Medicare and Medicaid legislation as well as the growth and aging of the U.S. population, also contributed to the health care cost crisis that blossomed in the 1970s.

As health care costs rose because of both inflation and technologic improvements, consumers sought greater insurance coverage, shielding both patients and physicians from rising expenditures. Not shielded, however, were the government, employers, and insurance companies; in fact, these parties together pay approximately 80 percent of the nation's current medical bill. Bolstered by their market strength (and backed by concerned health care consumers), this new triumvirate of U.S. health care financing is using its buying power increasingly to restrain the upward spiral of costs. Several cost-control methods were implemented in the 1980s and 1990s that fundamentally modified the delivery of health care, and the exchanges that now occur within the health care system comprise a complex lattice of financial and administrative interactions in which unregulated, unnegotiated FFS payment is the exception and not the rule.

This trend puts new pressure on medical practitioners. As recently as 15 years ago, an understanding of both the financing and organization of health care was considered unnecessary for most patients and physicians. In today's new medical marketplace, however, this is no longer true. Cost has become a major variable in the patient–provider equation; in addition to clinical knowledge and ethical factors, an awareness of health care financing and organization has become indispensable to health care providers. Insurance beneficiaries also often must negotiate complex systems and regulations to qualify for their health care benefits.

After describing the financial structure of the system, Part II delineates the major regulatory and reimbursement changes that have been implemented by payers and policymakers. Chapter 4 focuses on those changes affecting the incentives of insurance beneficiaries, and Chapters 5 and 6 examine the major types of provider reimbursement and describe several major new payment methods. Chapter 7 examines the health care system in overview and assesses the major changes that were catalyzed by the era of cost containment.

This part opens with Dag Hammarskjöld's quote, because our intent is to increase our readers' understanding of the perspectives and concerns of both payers and policymakers; later sections focus on the response of patients and providers. Given the complexity of the situation, wisdom, diplomacy, and knowledge—in the spirit proposed by the former United Nations' Secretary General—will be required on everyone's part if the system is to reach a new equilibrium.

CHAPTER 4

COSTS: THE CONSUMER'S PERSPECTIVE

Medical bills are expensive; a hospital stay of moderate length can easily cost more than a new automobile. Moreover, people become ill unpredictablely, which makes it desirable for them to pool their risks with others. A large majority of Americans now have health insurance for these and other reasons. The availability of this third-party coverage, as well as its structure, have had a profound impact on the U.S. health care system.

To most people, the workings of third-party payers take place in the proverbial "black box." Consumers pay insurance premiums or taxes into the box, and their coverage emerges from it. Health care practitioners submit claim forms for the services they provide, and the box (usually) provides their reimbursements. The dynamic environment in which this black box operates has been largely ignored by the patients as well as the medical care providers who benefit from it. Their ignorance is understandable, because until recently, the expansion of benefits to both providers and patients has characterized U.S. health care policy, but like most kinds of ignorance, this has had its costs.

Structure of Health Insurance Benefits

Approximately 87 percent of all Americans have some type of insurance coverage for medical care. Approximately two thirds of all families are insured by private insurers, HMOs, or other prepaid plans and 20 percent by government-sponsored programs. The rest, approximately 13 percent, lack insurance coverage of any kind.

Conventional insurance programs are considered *indemnity* programs. Indemnity refers to compensation for loss or damage, because the insurer agrees to protect the beneficiary against what he or she otherwise would have to pay for their medical care. Most private indemnity insurance policies cover hospitalization and its associated professional fees; additional benefits typically include diagnostic services such as laboratory and radiologic tests. Many consumers also purchase a *major medical* policy, which covers services such as office visits to physicians and the portion of hospital bills exceeding a predetermined limit (frequently set at $50,000), that the core policy excludes. Indemnity policies rarely cover any care that is not directly related to an illness; preventive services are usually excluded for this reason. Neither do most policies cover long-term care, such as that provided by nursing homes, for any extended period of time.

Insurance premiums are priced according to *actuarial risk,* which is calculated statistically on the basis of the expected occurrence of illness. The actuarial risk of having a given condition varies according to the characteristics of the population subgroup being considered. For example, the risk of having a stroke increases with a person's age, and the incidence of stroke also varies by race.

The insurer's risk is more predictable, and premiums accordingly lower, when expenses are dispersed among a large number of insured people. Similarly, an insurance company's administrative overhead is lower when dealing with a single corporation that employs 1000 people compared with having to deal with 1000 individuals. Companies therefore prefer to cover large groups, such as all the employees of a given firm, and any individual consumer purchasing a policy outside of such a group usually faces either prohibitive premiums or limited coverage.

Fixed premiums assure a consumer a degree of predictability regarding their health care costs, but most insurers require their policyholders to pay a portion of the costs incurred when health care services are received. Insurance companies favor such cost-sharing arrangements not only because they reduce the company's payout, but also because the additional cost may influence policyholders and their dependents (together usually known as *beneficiaries* or *enrollees*) to consider whether the medical care they seek is actually necessary.

Cost-sharing provisions take a variety of forms. One is *co-insurance,* in which the patient pays a predetermined percentage of the medical bill. For example, with a 20 percent co-insurance rate, the beneficiary pays 20 percent of the *approved* cost of the service. (The amount on the bill, however, is often greater than the amount the insurance company allows. Given that co-insurance usually is calculated based on an approved charge, the patient may be responsible for all charges above this amount.)

Another type of cost-sharing is *co-payment,* in which the patient pays a fixed dollar amount per unit of service, such as $5 per visit, regardless of what the physician charges. Still another is a *deductible,* in which the enrollee first pays the deductible amount (often in the range of $200 to $500) out-of-pocket before any insurance benefits are paid. Most policies have an upper limit on such cost-sharing, known as a *stop-loss;* beyond this point (for example, $2000), the insurance will cover all expenses. Insurers often set a limit on their financial risk by setting a maximum amount of coverage (for example, $1 million). This maximum is sometimes also known as a *stop-loss* (because the cap stops the insurer's loss), thus the term is context dependent.

These arrangements frequently occur in combination. For example, a patient receives his or her first medical bill of the year, totaling $1000; the services received are covered by an insurance policy that stipulates an annual deductible of $200 with a 20 percent co-insurance rate thereafter. Therefore, the patient is responsible for paying $200 (the deductible) plus 20 percent of the remaining $800 (the co-insurance) for a total of $360. The insurance company pays $640. If the next bill that same year is $200, then the patient only pays the co-insurance of $40 and the insurance company pays the rest because the annual deductible has been met.

The nonprofit Blue Cross/Blue Shield companies differ in several ways from for-profit, private (or commercial) insurance companies. One difference can be linked to the early role that hospitals played in developing such insurance plans. The "Blues" traditionally have not required co-insurance or deductible payments for inpatient care; accordingly, their policyholders often pay higher premiums. Also, although the Blues (and other nonprofit companies), like any business, do their best to make sure that their revenues exceed their expenses, they differ in that all excess revenue is reinvested in the company and is *not* paid out to shareholders.

This, as well as certain tax advantages, help to keep their premiums competitive with plans that make greater use of cost-sharing and to maintain their market share of approximately 50 percent of the private insurance business.

The Method of Capitation Payment

Some indemnity insurance plans reimburse the beneficiary for covered services that the beneficiary pays for out-of-pocket; others reimburse the provider on the consumer's behalf. Almost all indemnity plans determine reimbursement on a FFS basis *after* the care has been delivered, but a very different payment arrangement is growing in importance within the United States. Under this scheme, known as *capitation,* an organization of health care providers is paid in advance on a per-capita basis for health plan enrollees, who must then obtain all nonemergency care from that organization (i.e., patients must pay out-of-pocket for any unauthorized care they seek from outside providers).

In a capitation plan, enrollees or their employers pay a predetermined fee for 1 year of coverage. Benefits typically are comprehensive, including preventive care (such as well-child check-ups), office visits, prescription drugs, and hospital care as necessary. Capitation plans rarely, if ever, require deductibles or co-insurance, but small copayments (on the order of $5) may be required for some services.

Such an arrangement usually occurs only within nontraditional delivery settings, the predominant form of which is the HMO. Therefore, from a provider's perspective, capitation is often viewed more as an organizational arrangement than as an insurance program; from the patient's perspective, however, capitation is both an organizational arrangement *and* an insurance mechanism. Like conventional insurance, capitation protects patients against financial loss from an illness, and of course, the prepayment is analogous to purchasing an insurance premium. Capitation also has important effects on the health care delivery process, because patients under capitation schemes are generally restricted to those providers who participate in the program (and clinicians are generally restricted in the way that they may provide care).

Studies have shown capitation plans to be less expensive than other types of insurance. In part, this reflects financial incentives to the practitioner who usually is rewarded for efficient use of resources. Total costs, including premium payments plus out-of-pocket expenses, average 10 percent to 40 percent lower for HMO enrollees than for beneficiary groups with comparable health status who are covered under conventional indemnity insurance plans. Thus, it is not surprising that increasing enrollment in capitated plans has been considered as a possible solution to the health care cost crisis, and enrollment has been increasing rapidly, more than doubling since 1984 (approximately 15 million) to 34 million in 1990.

Barriers to Obtaining Private Insurance Coverage

Blue Cross/Blue Shield plans historically have been based on a community rating, which means that the actuarial rate of the entire insured population is used. A different way to calculate actuarial rates, and one that generally is used by the commercial insurers (and increasingly by the Blues as well), is *experience* rating, in which premiums are determined by the past use of the particular employer group.

For small employers using insurance based on an experience rating, trouble may begin when a number of employees grow ill, especially with conditions that are expensive to treat, like acquired immune deficiency syndrome (AIDS), cancer, or severe heart disease. Because the company's "experience" then increases, the premium increases, and the company may no longer be able to afford coverage. The insurer may offer to reduce the premium if the sick employee is exempted from the policy; such exclusions, however, often place the excluded employee in a "Catch-22," because many plans bar coverage for individuals with pre-existing conditions. The excluded employee therefore cannot get coverage elsewhere. "Experience rating segments the population into low-risk groups with low premium costs, to whom the industry heavily markets its insurance products through employers, and a smaller number of high-risk individuals who become virtually uninsurable because of the high premiums charged for them" (Brown 1988, p. 579).

Legislation to reform the insurance industry has been proposed to eliminate this type of problem by barring exclusion for pre-existing conditions. (Reform proposals are discussed more fully in Chapter 12.)

The Effects of Insurance Coverage

Most insurance—including fire, theft, and life—covers against the risk of unexpected occurrences, but health insurance differs in that most people expect they will need medical services. Fire and life insurance policies generally prohibit policyholders from acting to get a return on their investments (for example, by denying coverage in cases of beneficiary foul play). With health insurance, however, it is to the consumers' economic advantage to seek a return on their premiums by obtaining health care: by getting, as it were, what was paid for (which is not to say that people *want* to get sick). This has been termed the *more-is-better* incentive of health insurance. The tendency to use, and perhaps overuse, a health insurance policy because of the strong financial incentive to do so has been labeled by economists the *moral hazard phenomenon* (which is somewhat of a misnomer, as it describes what is an economic and not a moral issue).

More-is-better incentives are particularly compelling for an enrollee with what is termed *first-dollar coverage,* that is, a policy with minimal or no co-insurance or copayments and without a de-

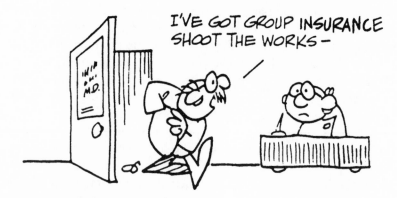

I'VE GOT GROUP INSURANCE SHOOT THE WORKS—

(Source: King Features Syndicate, Inc.)

ductible. Most capitation plans are essentially of this sort; the enrollee has no financial disincentive to use the HMO as there is no significant additional cost once the capitation payment is made. The financial survival of the organization therefore requires that the effects of the more-is-better tendency be limited. Among the nonfinancial barriers that HMOs sometimes use to limit services are time delays between making the appointment and the actual visit (for nonurgent conditions), telephone triage, physician gatekeepers (who must authorize services), and limits on the number of visits for certain conditions (e.g., psychiatric).

The Effects of Cost-Sharing on Demand

The extent and type of cost-sharing that is incorporated into an insurance policy influence the consumer's demand for health care services. For example, purchase of a policy with the typical 20 percent co-insurance provision results in an 80 percent decrease in the patient's out-of-pocket costs when medical services are obtained, and providers must substantially increase their charges before patients with such coverage feel the financial effects of the costs they incur. A patient with a steep deductible faces two very

Table 4. Statistics on the Use and Costs of Medical Services by Type of Service, 1991

Type of medical service	Estimated use per year per person	Approximate percentage of population receiving services per year	Typical cost per unit of service	Approximate percentage of all costs borne directly by individuals	Approximate percentage of U.S. health care costs
Hospital admission	0.10	8%	$5,500	10%	39%
Physician services					
Ambulatory visit	5.30	78	50	50	12
Surgery	0.20	15	800	20	5
In-hospital visit	0.60	8	45	20	3
Medication/drugs*	4.50	60	19	70	6
Dental visit	2.00	56	35	70	5
Nursing home admission	0.05	0.5	30,000†	50	8

Source: Data from American Medical Association 1991; Health Care Financing Administration 1991; Health Insurance Association of America 1992; National Center for Health Statistics 1992
  *Prescribed out of hospital.
  †Cost per year.

different economic incentives—not to use care before the deductible is met, then to use care freely thereafter. These phenomena have had significant effects on health care expenditures, facilitating both inflation in the price of medical services and the increased use of such services by policyholders. Table 4 presents some detailed information on typical uses and costs of different types of service in 1991.

The Rand Health Insurance Experiment was an extensive, federally financed study conducted by the Rand Corporation between 1974 and 1982. Some 2000 families living in six cities were randomly assigned to one of 14 insurance plans with four degrees of cost-sharing, ranging from 0 percent to 95 percent. For the plans with some degree of cost-sharing, differing upper limits were set on annual out-of-pocket expenditures ranging from 5 percent to 15 percent of family income to a maximum of $1000. The study found that members of families with lower cost-sharing percentages visited physicians more frequently and entered the hospital more often than did members of families with higher percentages; in other words, the less the family had to pay for care, the more care they sought. Table 5 summarizes these findings. On the basis of both this study and others, one expert concluded that a typical insurance policy approximately *doubles* the demand for services over what would occur without a policy.

The ESRD Program demonstrated that coverage decisions have important budgetary consequences, and the Rand Experiment showed that cost-sharing provisions do as well. These are important factors for health insurance executives, whose major objective

Table 5. The Effect of Cost-Sharing on the Demand for Medical Care

Co-insurance paid by consumer	Total expenditure*	Ambulatory expenditure*
0% (free care)	$401	$186
25†	346	149
50†	328	120
95‡	254	114

Source: Data from the Rand Experiment. Newhouse et al. 1981
*Current (1974–1978) dollar averages per person, per year across four sites.
†With a family stop-loss of $1000.
‡Family pays 95 percent up to a $450 deductible.

is to set competitively priced premiums that will cover all services that are supplied to beneficiaries while still leaving some surplus as a return to investors. Thus, their objective is to forecast, and if possible decrease, beneficiaries' use of medical services.

Consumer Contributions to Public Sector Programs

Medicare and Medicaid are the public sector's insurance programs. Nearly every U.S. citizen over the age of 65 is enrolled in Medicare Part A, and more than 97 percent also are enrolled in Part B. Those who set policy for the public sector programs, analogous to the goals of private sector insurers, attempt to budget funds that are adequate to cover expenses.

Medicare Part A is supported by a trust fund that is replenished annually by Social Security payroll taxes paid by both employers and employees. Eligible enrollees pay no premiums for Part A, but they are required to pay a significant deductible as well as co-insurance. A single deductible is paid for all hospital services that are used during a defined benefit period, and a new benefit period begins when the patient has been out of the hospital for 60 days.

Medicare Part B is considered a supplemental insurance program. The Part B monthly premium originally was designed to pay for half of the program's costs; federal funds were to pay for the other half. This has not been the case, however, and today, revenues from beneficiaries (including premiums, co-insurance, and deductibles) constitute only 25 percent despite repeated increases in both premiums and deductibles. Federal funds from a separate trust fund that is financed by general tax revenues pay 75 percent of the program's costs, and less than 2 percent derives from interest earned in that trust fund.

Medicaid technically is considered an *entitlement* or *assurance* (not an *insurance*) program because those eligible receive coverage without paying into the plan. Enrollees pay no premiums or co-insurance, but some states do require a small copayment for prescription drugs and other services. Medicaid is funded entirely by public sources, and the percentage of funding contributed by federal, state, and local sources varies by state. The proportion paid by a given state is calculated according to that state's per-capita income relative to national per-capita income. As a result, the federal share is higher in poor states. Overall, approximately half of the financing comes from federal sources and half from state sources. Medicaid programs in most states are suffering severe budget shortfalls and, in more than one instance, bankruptcy; therefore, many programs currently are relying on sources such as provider taxes, private donations, and regulatory loopholes that generate more federal funds. For example, some states receive "donations" from Medicaid-recipient hospitals, then use those donations in calculating the state-raised proportion of funding, which increases the federal matching contribution. The state then provides funds back to the hospital, in effect getting more federal money without any real increase in state funding. Some Medicaid administrators claim that these "creative financing" methods have become crucial to the survival of the program, but the Health Care Financing Administration (HCFA) is attempting to regulate such practices.

Cutting Costs through Cost-Sharing

When consumers bear some responsibility for the costs of health care, the inflationary effects of the moral hazard phenomenon are diminished. A variety of efforts have been made by government, private insurers, and employers to control costs by decreasing the incentives to use medical services. Two methods in particular have been used to pare down the insulation between patients and their bills: providing fewer benefits for the same premium price; and increasing the required payments for co-insurance, deductibles, and the like. The first approach places consumers at direct financial risk when they receive care that is not covered. The second raises the threshold above which they will seek care for covered services and also decreases the insurer's outlays.

The public sector has made extensive use of cost-sharing to keep its expenditures down. HCFA has regularly increased the deductible that must be paid by Medicare Part A beneficiaries before their coverage is activated. In fact, the deductible has gone up every year since the inception of the Medicare program, and in 1992, it was $652. The Part B monthly premium for Medicare in

1992 was $31.80, with an annual deductible of $100 and a co-insurance rate set at 20 percent of "allowed" charges (except for psychotherapy, which requires a 50 percent copayment).

The intended disincentive effect of Medicare cost-sharing is undercut, to some degree, by the additional insurance coverage that is available to most beneficiaries. The vast majority of Medicare enrollees (approximately two thirds) purchase supplemental private insurance, often termed *medi-gap* insurance, to pay for their Medicare deductibles and co-insurance charges. The medi-gap industry has been the target of complaints for almost 20 years, and accusations that salespeople pressure senior citizens into buying policies that are often expensive, worded in confusing terms, or do not provide coverage as promised culminated in recent federal insurance reform legislation. Now, 10 standard policies will replace the approximately 250 variations that are currently on the market. This should make comparison shopping easier for the consumer.

Medicare enrollees who are indigent qualify for a limited type of Medicaid enrollment that pays for their Medicare co-insurance, premiums, and deductibles. As a consequence of medi-gap insurance and Medicaid supplementation, cost-sharing is not a significant disincentive against using services for most beneficiaries of Medicare.

One way the public sector could increase its revenues would be to eliminate tax exemptions on health insurance premiums, thereby increasing both employer and employee cost-sharing. Billions of dollars in potential federal and state revenues are lost each year by these exemptions: it was estimated that nearly $50 billion was lost in 1990. Congress has threatened several times to impose a tax on employers' contributions to benefit packages, but intense lobbying has successfully blocked such action. In 1982, the amount of tax-deductible personal medical care expenses (which include contributions toward health insurance premiums) was reduced, but employers' deductions were preserved.

More employers have chosen plans that incorporate employee co-payments. Some plans offer employees more- and less-expensive options; those who choose the more costly policy must pay the difference in premium costs out-of-pocket. Corporations also have increased their use of deductibles, and others limit their employees' choice of physicians to so-called "preferred providers" who charge less. Such Preferred Provider Organization (PPO) enrollment increased from 1.3 million in 1984 to over 38 million in 1992. (Chapter 7 discusses PPOs further.)

A few employers have implemented innovative plans that indirectly incorporate cost-sharing. One such plan offers each employee minimal coverage (for example, hospitalization coverage alone) but also sets up a special account containing additional funds that are intended to pay for medical services the employee's policy does not cover. If the employee uses medical care, then the bills are paid from that account. At the end of the year, a portion of any unused money in this account is returned to the employee as a bonus. This gives employees a direct incentive to minimize their use of medical care.

Many businesses also have started occupational health clinics and health promotion programs. Many of these programs are expansions of *employee assistance programs,* which are services provided within a corporation that focus primarily on employees' mental health problems and substance abuse. Employers expect all of these programs to result in healthier, happier employees who require less medical care and, therefore, incur lower health care costs.

Other Consumer-Oriented Controls

In addition to cost-sharing provisions, most insurers have incorporated programs, termed *utilization review,* that are designed to decrease the use of specific kinds of service. These programs are part of a trend known as the "managed care movement," which encompasses several methods of overseeing resource utilization. During the 5-year period between 1984 and 1989, the percentage of FFS insurance companies that used managed care strategies grew from less than 5 percent to half of the market. The methods described below are directed primarily at the consumer's decisions about medical resource use; additional methods that focus on the provider's decisions are discussed in later chapters.

One example of utilization review is the second surgical opinion program, where if a surgical procedure is advised, the program pays for consultation with a second surgeon. If the two surgeons disagree, then the program will pay for a third consultation. Some insurers (or employers) require a beneficiary to obtain a second opinion before undergoing any major elective procedure; others simply offer the second opinion as an option. An estimated 20 percent of all patients in such programs do not undergo the surgery that was initially recommended: the process identifies some patients for whom surgery is avoidable, and others likely are dissuaded from surgery in response to a disagreement among consultants. The cost-saving intent of this program is apparent in that the insurers seek to protect themselves from paying for unnecessary procedures; however, it is not known whether such programs pay for themselves.

Another cost-containment method uses the fact that outpatient procedures are less expensive than the same services are when provided in a hospital (as there is no daily bed-charge). Some payers have introduced programs to encourage the use of outpatient facilities; for example, since 1982, Medicare has paid for 100 percent of the physician's fee for ambulatory surgery but only 80 percent for inpatient surgery (in a designated group of procedures), thus creating a strong incentive for patients to use outpatient facilities when possible. Also in 1982, Medicare issued a list of procedures that would be reimbursed *only* on an outpatient basis barring special contraindications.

Many large, self-insured corporations now hire nonphysician reviewers (sometimes known as *case managers**) to monitor the use of expensive major services such as extended hospitalizations or rehabilitation therapy. The purpose of these reviewers is to see that the corporation, in essence, gets its money's worth. "Corporations and insurers are quick to point out that they never tell an employee not to have a hysterectomy or forbid anyone from entering the hospital to see if that lesion is cancerous. All they do is, at times, decline to pick up the full bill for a procedure they deem unnecessary. The patient, they insist, can do as he pleases" (Kleinfield 1986, p. F3). Of course, financial considerations will frequently prohibit a patient from obtaining medical care if insurance will not cover that care; therefore, such corporate policies *do* have consequences for employees' health.

---

*Note that this term is used in different contexts, with slightly different meanings.

Another arrangement, usually known as *the gatekeeper system* (and also termed *case management*), is used by many HMOs and some state Medicaid plans to cut down on duplication of services and unnecessary referrals. In this system, a primary-care physician (or organization) is selected (or appointed) to act as care coordinator for the beneficiary. The patient must call the gatekeeper before any nonemergency care is received from other providers, or those services might not be reimbursed. Outside of HMOs, the gatekeeper usually receives a monthly payment in addition to any FFS reimbursement. Rather than "managed care," however, the federal government and some companies now use the more positive-sounding term *coordinated care* for these methods.

Also of note, little information is available on the effectiveness of these strategies in containing the costs of or effects on the quality of medical care. Managed care programs, which are resisted by providers and advocated by payers, are controversial, and the results of studies are mixed. Some research shows that these programs do not save any money (in that increased third-party administrative costs negate any savings), but it is impossible to know how health care costs would have grown without them.

Additional Corporate Retrenchments

The public sector has the legislative power to regulate its expenditures successfully, and it has reduced its share of some health care costs. Many of these costs have been shifted to the private sector; as a result, corporations have experienced even steeper rises in their costs of health care. In fact, from 1980 to 1987, corporate health care expenses as well as individual insurance premiums were the two fastest growing sources of health care financing. Corporate management thus has been forced into further action to reduce the costs of employee medical care.

Employees of large corporations traditionally have been assured of health coverage even after retirement; when added to Medicare coverage (for retirees over the age of 65), this valuable asset provides essentially free health care. "Like active employee health programs, retiree medical benefit programs were often introduced years ago, and the corporate costs (essentially booked on a pay-as-you-go basis) were relatively inexpensive when compared with the total compensation package" (LeBlanc 1991, p. 31).

With increasing health care costs and an ever-growing number of retirees, however, corporate liability for this particular benefit has grown enormously. As noted in Chapter 2, the FASB requirement that corporations include these future costs in their current balance sheets has transformed many corporations' bottom lines from black to red ink. As a result of both increased health care costs and modified accounting procedures, reducing retiree medical coverage has become another method of cost containment, and many corporations are cutting back on these benefits for future employees. In addition, corporations now are less likely to provide coverage for the spouses and dependents of full-time workers and are less likely to cover part-time or temporary workers as well.

Employees have reacted to these changes with contract disputes between labor and management. In fact, the majority of major labor strikes in 1989 were caused by disputes over health insurance benefits. Nevertheless, because these changes will provide corporations with both current and future savings, these trends in corporate coverage of health care costs are likely to continue.

In addition, thousands of people employed by companies that went bankrupt have been left without current or future health insurance coverage. Other ways to pay for the coverage of individuals who are affected by these policy changes and corporate closures will be necessary, and it is likely that both out-of-pocket costs and public sector expenditures will increase.

Additional Public Sector Retrenchments

The Reagan Administration, as part of its effort to decrease government spending, took several steps to reduce federal expenditures and involvement in health care. President Bush continued this approach during his term in office. The Neighborhood Health Center Program was phased out, but since then, direct funding to approximately 600 free-standing Community Health Centers has been reinstated. The National Health Service Corps, which subsidized the medical education of providers who were willing to practice in underserved areas, also was cut back significantly.

Regarding the Medicare program, the Reagan Administration sought to decrease both the number of beneficiaries and of reimbursable services. One proposal was to raise the age of eligibility for the Medicare program, and this idea found some support in 1985, when Congress increased the age of eligibility for full Social Security retirement benefits from 65 to 67 (commencing in the year 2000). The age of eligibility for Medicare benefits, however, has not yet been raised.

The Reagan Administration's attitude toward cost containment within the Medicaid program was similar. This administration sought to reduce the number of enrollees and of services covered. At the state level, Medicaid expenditures were reduced by decreasing the income level above which families did not qualify for Medicaid. The income level below which a family was considered "medically indigent," which applies to families with incomes above the cutoff level for Medicaid coverage but with sufficiently large medical expenses to qualify them for Medicaid, also was decreased. The number of services covered (within the limits set by federal guidelines) was reduced as well.

Given the demonstrated savings in capitated plans, the Reagan Administration encouraged Medicare beneficiaries to enroll in Medicare HMOs and *competitive medical plans* (CMPs), which are primarily HMOs that do not meet HCFA's federal qualifications (as described in Chapter 6). The HMO experiment with Medicare beneficiaries began in the early 1980s, but the number of elderly people who have enrolled in HMOs has been modest. As of 1990, over 1.25 million beneficiaries (or 3 percent of the Medicare population) were enrolled in approximately 90 such "risk-contract" plans. Surveys of Medicare HMO enrollees have shown them to be satisfied with their HMOs, but in mid-1987, after a handful of plans were found to be offering poor-quality care, federally funded PROs that were established previously to monitor Medicare-supported hospital care began to monitor risk-contract HMOs. There have been other problems with the program as well, deriving from its policy of continuous open enrollment (i.e., people can sign up or leave the plan at any time during the year) in contrast to closed enrollment, whereby enrollment is permitted only during designated times. Nor has the program encouraged efficiency as its payments are based on FFS-sector funding levels in the geographic area surrounding the HMO.

Recent efforts include tax changes requiring wealthy elderly people to pay more for their health care coverage. State Medicaid programs are also relying more heavily on HMOs and utilization review arrangements.

The Effectiveness of Public Programs

How well are government programs meeting the intents of their original enabling legislation? The goal of Medicare was to protect elderly persons against health care expenses, but out-of-pocket costs for Part B recipients are increasing very quickly, nearly doubling in the last 10 years. These costs are rising faster than annual Social Security benefits, so health care is taking a larger and larger portion of elderly people's income. To its credit, however, Medicare enrolls nearly all those who are eligible.

In contrast, less than half of the nation's poor, who constitute some 14 percent of the population, are covered by the Medicaid program. The goal of Medicaid, which is to provide medical care to the poor on welfare, has not been reached; in fact, it is estimated that only 20 percent of the program's funding is used for this group. Nursing home coverage, mandated since 1972, now applies to approximately one third of Medicaid beneficiaries and consumes approximately two thirds of the program's funds. Elderly people account for the largest share of Medicaid payments (37 percent), but they represent approximately 14 percent of all Medicaid recipients. Blind and disabled persons also account for a disproportionate share of total payments (36 percent of payments for 14 percent of all recipients). In contrast, recipients in families with dependent children account for only 24 percent of total Medicaid payments but represent 70 percent of all recipients (HCFA 1991).

Federal legislation implemented in 1990 mandated that Medicaid, as a step toward fulfilling its original intent, cover women who were pregnant and either at or below 133 percent of the federal poverty level with an option to cover such women up to 185 percent of the federal poverty level. An assets test for Medicaid eligibility has been waived by 48 states and the District of Columbia, and Medicaid coverage has also been expanded to children in families earning up to 100 percent of the poverty level. All children born after September 30, 1983, are covered by this policy change, which provides coverage until the child's 18th birthday. (The issue of access is explored further in Chapter 12.)

The Medicare program has been affected significantly by cost-containment measures as well. Congress and the Bush Administration agreed to $43 billion in Medicare savings between 1991 and 1995, and 16 percent of federal reductions in spending during the last decade have come from Medicare even though it represents only 7 percent of the total federal budget. As a result, "Medicare is suffering from the paradox of being clinically able, but financially unable, to fulfill its mission of caring for those in need" (Ginsburg and Prout 1990, p. 644).

Summary

Theoretically, patients who are required to pay more for their health care will seek less of it, and in turn, practitioners will provide fewer services; in reality, increased cost-sharing by patients has had only a moderate effect on medical costs, particularly hospital costs. Results from the Rand Corporation Study confirm that consumers are less responsive to cost-sharing for acute-care hospital services than for ambulatory services, probably because it is the physician and not the consumer who usually makes the decision concerning hospitalization. "While individuals may choose their physicians, doctors usually determine the kind and quantity of health services individuals consume. While doctors may have some knowledge of the individual's financial resources, there is little evidence that these considerations have much influence on the type of care prescribed" (Sorkin 1975, p. 23). Furthermore, the need for hospitalization implies a more serious physical condition, thus resulting in less discretion for the patient about whether or not to receive care.

Despite its potential for savings to third-party payers, the same mechanism by which increased cost-sharing can decrease a patient's use of medical care can also decrease his or her access to that needed care. This could potentially delay the identification and treatment of diseases, which may be more expensive in the long term (thus defeating the purpose of cost containment as well as reducing the quality of care). Analyses of Rand Experiment data showed that cost-sharing reduced patient demand for both necessary and unnecessary care, and Mechanic has termed cost-sharing "a crude and irrational way to make allocation decisions" (1991, pp. 249–50).

Rice (1991) pointed out that cost-sharing is also undesirable from a public policy perspective because it is *regressive*, meaning that the burden is greatest on those who are least able to pay, in contrast to *progressive* cost-control mechanisms that impose greater burden on those having more resources. By affecting the poor more than the wealthy, cost-sharing potentially erects barriers to necessary care.

Consumer-focused cost controls can and do help to reduce costs, but for all of these reasons, clear limits on how much they can accomplish exist. As the following chapters demonstrate, third-party payers accordingly have chosen to focus most of their cost-control efforts on the *providers* of care.

CHAPTER 5

COSTS: THE PROVIDER'S PERSPECTIVE

Insurers reimburse providers* for medical services in various
ways. The most common arrangement in the United States has
traditionally been fee-for-service (FFS), whereby a fee is charged
for each separate service provided, such as a day in a hospital
bed, a visit to a physician's office, or a specific laboratory test. Payment is made after the services are received.

Overall, physicians receive approximately 80 percent of their
revenue from third-party payers and 20 percent directly from their
patients. The percentages vary according to the physician's specialty, location, and other factors. Because third-party reimbursement is usually higher than the sum an individual patient could afford to pay out-of-pocket, both patients and providers benefit
from health insurance coverage.

Paying the Hospital

Once charity facilities, nearly all U.S. hospitals now receive payment for their services. These payment arrangements are often
complex, but they can be understood better by recognizing that

---

A distinction must be made between the *real-resource costs* of treating
patients and the *monetary* transfers occasioned by the treatment. The
real-resource costs of a treatment consist of time physicians and other
health workers devote to it, and of supplies, equipment, brick and mortar used up in the process. The monetary costs are measured by the
amount of money patients directly or indirectly funnel to the owners of
these real resources. Clearly, these monetary costs can rise without a
commensurate increase in real-resource costs. For example, if a cardiac

*Hospitals and related institutions, free-standing clinics, physicians, and nonphysician
providers with the legal authority to bill independently are, for the purposes of this discussion, included in the definition of *provider*.

surgeon decides to raise his or her fee for a coronary bypass from $5,000 to $8,000, only the monetary cost of the treatment rises; its real-resource cost does not. (Reinhardt 1985, p. 56C)

The difference between costs and charges is relevant, because hospitals are reimbursed by some payers on a "cost-plus" basis. In this case, *cost* refers to the direct cost of the specific service provided, as well as a percentage of the hospital's fixed or indirect costs, such as labor, capital investment, and maintenance. Other indirect expenses, such as medical education and technology acquisition, have also been factored into some payers' cost formulas. The *plus* refers to a percentage of profits above and beyond expenses that the payer adds to the hospital's reimbursement.

From 1965 through 1983, the Medicare program paid hospitals on a cost-plus basis, and Medicaid programs in several states continue to do so. The original Medicare Part A legislation stipulated that reimbursement was to cover service fees plus 2 percent: hospitals were to receive a 2 percent mark-up on the costs that they incurred. This original arrangement resulted from a political compromise negotiated in 1965 between Congress and the hospital lobby. It reflects not only the political strength of the AHA and the AMA at the time, but also the laissez-faire attitude of government and other third-party payers toward the health care industry. (A subsequent amendment to this legislation removed the additional 2 percent.)

In previous eras, many insurers paid exactly what providers billed. Today, however, this arrangement is much less common. Patients without insurance may be expected to pay their bills in full even though many are unable to do so, but third-party payers use a variety of seemingly arcane procedures to determine how much of the bill they will pay. Techniques differ, but all payers use the spread between costs and charges (between real-resource costs and monetary costs) as their basis for determining payments.

As in most markets, powerful buyers can negotiate lower payments per unit of product than their less-powerful competitors can. As an insurer's market share (the percentage of the potential pool of patients that it covers) increases, this ability to negotiate discounted reimbursement levels also increases. In contrast, small insurers and self-paying patients have no such bargaining leverage. Not always as well understood as it is today, this approach was not applied by payers and policymakers before the cost crisis. Thus, although Medicare controlled a huge share of the market from its inception, policymakers did not wield this potential power effectively during the 1960s, and they exerted their influence only tentatively during the 1970s. (This changed in the era of cost containment, as the following chapter describes.)

The same thing occurs in the private sector. Whereas most commercial insurers must base their reimbursements largely on charges, the Blues, because of their market power in each state (usually about half of all privately insured persons), can base their reimbursements on costs. Also, because of the Blues' long-standing and close relationship with hospitals, many plans have special reimbursement agreements with individual institutions. The resulting leverage minimizes payouts. This strengthens the Blues' ability to offer competitive premiums, which has traditionally been more of a challenge for them because of the comprehensive benefits and first-dollar coverage they offer.

Paying the Physician

Payers using the FFS reimbursement system calculate payment amounts in various ways. Three of the most common are the usual-customary-reasonable (UCR) method, the customary-prevailing-reasonable (CPR) method, and fee schedules. Despite their titles, most health financing experts, however, consider these existing methods to be anything but "reasonable."

The private sector uses UCR, with CPR as the analogous method for public sector programs. UCR was developed in the early 1960s by private insurance companies and later served as a model for developing the CPR formula, which until recently was the exclusive method used by Medicare Part B and by many state Medicaid programs for reimbursement of professional fees. (From 1991 through 1995, however, Medicare will base payments only partially on CPR, at which point it is expected to be phased out completely.) These methods use differing terminology, but in other respects, they are substantially the same. Payers using either UCR or

CPR establish a multifactorial database that includes the provider's payment history (known as the provider's *profile*) for all practitioners whom they reimburse. Table 6 outlines the major features of UCR and CPR payment.

In the private sector, most Blue Shield plans select a cutoff (such as the 90th percentile) of charges for a given service within a geographic area to be the *customary* charge. Enormous variability exists among plans, however, and some Blue Shield plans have differing arrangements for different accounts. Some insurance companies using UCR–CPR methodology use the 92nd percentile. Medicare Part B bases its prevailing fee on the 75th percentile, and legislatively determined limits are placed on yearly increases.

Under Medicare's CPR method, the *reasonable* fee, in general, is the least of the customary fee, the prevailing fee, or the actual charge. After the patient's deductible has been met, Medicare pays 80 percent of this approved amount, and the patient pays 20 percent. In an analogous fashion, the reimbursed amount for private insurance companies using UCR is the least of the usual fee, customary fee, and actual charge.

One serious drawback of the UCR–CPR payment method is that it encourages fee inflation. Not only do a practitioner's fees determine reimbursement in the present (as the *actual* component of the fee), but one year's fees determine the following year's *custom-*

Table 6. A Comparison of the Components of the UCR and CPR Physician Reimbursement Systems

Component of methodology	CPR*	UCR†
Average past fee, based on individual physician's "historic" fee profile	Customary fee	Usual fee
Percentile (e.g., 75% or 90%) of the charges submitted by all physicians in a designated area for "similar" services	Prevailing fee	Customary fee
Charge submitted to insurer for service provided	Actual or submitted charge	Actual or submitted charge
Maximum allowable fee reimbursed to provider	Reasonable fee or approved charge	Reasonable fee or reimbursed charge

*Used by Medicare.
†Used by private insurers.

ary fees. Today's charge also influences a geographic area's average *prevailing* fee level. When these fee-padding incentives are aggregated across all practitioners in an area, fees can become badly inflated. If patients complain, then some providers explain that the fee on the bill is for the insurance company only; a second, lower fee is what will actually be accepted for the patient's portion of the bill. (This arrangement is separate from the *sliding-fee schedule* that providers sometimes offer to patients with low incomes.)

Another drawback of UCR–CPR reimbursement is that it offers no incentive to translate gains in efficiency into lower charges. For example, when a new lens extraction technique reduced the operating time for cataract surgery to an average of 20 minutes, ophthalmologists' fees generally remained at the levels set when the procedure took much longer and placed the patient at much higher risk. This issue was ultimately addressed by legislation in the late 1980s, when Medicare targeted the levels of reimbursement for this as well as 10 other procedures for downward adjustment.

Still another problem is that UCR–CPR reimbursement is a complex paradigm that requires, among other things, annual updating of the customary and prevailing charges. Because fee levels are in continuous flux, it is rarely possible to determine in advance how much an insurer will pay for a given service. This is a disadvantage for both patients and physicians.

Indeed, under the UCR–CPR method, very different amounts might be paid at any one time for the same service or a similar one, depending on the provider's specialty, the geographic area, and the delivery setting. As might be expected, urban rates are generally higher than those in rural areas, specialists receive higher payments than do primary-care practitioners, and visits or procedures performed in-hospital may generate greater reimbursements than those same services when provided in outpatient settings.

One of the chief reasons for income differences among physicians is that insurers have traditionally reimbursed *procedures* at higher rates than *cognitive services* such as physical or psychiatric examinations. Primary-care practitioners provide the majority of cognitive services, whereas specialists (depending on their area of expertise) perform most of the expensive procedures; thus, for example, surgeons receive a much greater percentage of their income from third-party insurance companies than do primary-care physicians.

Therefore, it should come as no surprise that in 1989 U.S. surgeons earned an average net income (after expenses and before taxes) of $220,000, which is more than twice that of pediatricians.

It would be reasonable to ask that if two or more practitioners provide the same services or services of similar complexity, should their reimbursement be the same? A study in the early 1980s found that even after adjustments were made for the complexity of the service, overhead, and other factors that could affect the service's price, GPs were reimbursed an average of $40 per hour, compared with $200 per hour for surgical specialists. Most observers would probably agree that surgeons deserve a higher hourly wage—but higher by a factor of five? Questions such as these became crucial to policymakers in the late 1980s as they grappled with the health care cost crisis.

Patients' Financial Responsibility under UCR–CPR

Because most people have health insurance, direct payment to physicians from patients makes only a minor contribution to total health care expenditures; with cost-sharing, however, even insured patients face out-of-pocket costs for medical services. In addition, a patient with coverage for a service is not assured that the total charge for that service will be paid by the insurer, nor is the patient assured that the provider will accept a lower reimbursement as payment in full. Thus, patients with coverage under a UCR–CPR system usually have a significant financial responsibility.

Many practitioners do accept the insurer's *approved* or *reasonable* amount as their payment in full. This feature of UCR–CPR insurance reimbursement is known as *accepting assignment*. The provider accepts the insurance company's payment as full coverage for the insurer's portion of the fee (usually 80 percent after co-insurance). For example, if the provider charges $100 for a service and the insurance company's approved fee for the service is $90, then the company pays 80 percent of that amount (or $72). The patient is responsible for 20 percent of the approved fee (or $18). The provider who does not accept assignment would bill the difference between the charged fee and the combined reimbursement to the patient ($10 in this case, for a total cost to the patient of $28). This practice is known as *balance billing*.

Arrangements for accepting assignment are found in both the public and the private sectors. Three states now require that physicians accept assignment for all Medicare patients. Since 1986, physicians and other medical professionals have become Medicare *participating physicians* by agreeing to accept assignment for all services and beneficiaries for 1 year. The *nonparticipating physician* does not accept assignment, or does so only on a claim-by-claim basis; patients of nonparticipating physicians are billed not only the 20 percent co-insurance but also any amount that exceeds Medicare's approved fee.

Medicare has offered several incentives designed to encourage physician enrollment in this program. In 1986, participating physicians were granted prevailing charge increases 4 percent greater than the increases for nonparticipants. Since 1987, a complex formula known as the *Maximum Allowable Actual Charge* (MAAC) has been used to cap the actual charges of nonparticipating providers; in 1991, their balance billing was limited to 125 percent of Medicare-approved charges (with the exception of evaluation and management services, which can be balance billed to the lower of 140 percent of the Medicare-approved charge or the provider's 1990 MAAC percentage). Medicare plans to reduce these limits to 115 percent of allowed charges by 1993. Whereas unassigned claims were historically billed by the provider to the patient, a 1990 law requires physicians to submit *all* Medicare claims directly to HCFA whether or not assignment is accepted.

Patients would obviously prefer to receive care from physicians who accept assignment, because their out-of-pocket costs are lower. For the provider's part, Medicare facilitates referral by providing a directory to its beneficiaries that lists its participating physicians. Thus, there are a number of advantages to the physician who participates; in fact, the number of participating physicians has increased each year of the program. In 1986, 28 percent of physicians accepted assignment, whereas 1991 HCFA data indicate that 48 percent were participating physicians.

Fee Schedules

Problems with the UCR–CPR method galvanized both payers and policymakers to search for alternative methods of reimbursement.

This in turn led to renewed interest in weighted fee schedules, whereby reimbursement is related to the complexity of the service provided and then set at a fixed amount for everyone providing that service. Fee schedules thus eliminate some of the most flagrant pricing distortions found in the UCR–CPR system.

Fee schedules have always been a minor reimbursement method in the U.S. health care system, even though they are used for physician reimbursement in most Medicaid programs (31 states in 1987) and by several commercial insurance companies. Some older fee schedules are not based on a specific valuation system; these are simply lists of amounts that will be paid as compensation under a health insurance policy—usually a policy providing minimal coverage. Many of these lists were developed simply on the basis of insurers' UCR experience.

Another, more recent type of schedule is based on a more sophisticated approach to the *relative weighting* of different services. Usually termed RVU (Relative Value Unit) or RVS (Relative Value Scale) systems, these weighting methods represent efforts to identify homogeneous "products" within the heterogeneous-care delivery process and to determine fair values for those products. A fundamental task in creating an RVS is identifying an appropriate dimension of worth and value. Variables used as bases for relative scales are physicians' charges; the length of time spent in providing care or performing a procedure; estimates of overhead and other costs of providing a service; and estimates of the degree of skill, level of training, and intensity of effort necessary to perform a service adequately. Developing an RVS is a complicated and value-laden process. Even something as seemingly straightforward as casting a leg is complex. Should a surgeon be paid on the basis of time spent? Skill? The degree of risk taken? Many nonsurgical encounters are to exchange information or reassure a patient. How should the results of these encounters be measured? How reimbursed?

The process involves several steps. First, a *weighting coefficient* for each procedure or service is established. Next, a *dollar conversion factor* is used to create a fee schedule. Multiplying each weighting coefficient by the conversion factor yields a fee for each procedure. Because more complex or time-consuming procedures will have larger coefficients, the resulting fees will be proportionally larger. If necessary, additional coefficients and conversion factors can be applied to account for other elements such as geographic region, physician's specialty, or care setting.

Relative Value Scales provide several advantages over the UCR–CPR method. Unlike UCR–CPR, the RVS approach has no built-in impetus for an automatic annual increase in fees. If properly designed, an RVS will also minimize the price distortions intrinsic to the UCR–CPR method by permitting payers to retain some control over geographic variations in fee levels, the comparability of fees paid to generalists and specialists, and the relative value of both technical and cognitive services. Current antitrust law states that physician organizations cannot sponsor or derive fee schedules, because of the potential for the creation of a price monopoly. (The incorporation of this reimbursement method into Medicare's new fee schedule, termed the *Resource-Based Relative Value System* (RBRVS), is described in the following chapter.)

Capitation and Salary

Paying a physician by either capitation or salary offers a major alternative to FFS payment. In a capitation scheme, a practitioner or a provider organization agrees to care for enrollees in return for an arranged per-capita fee. Historically, these arrangements were first used by large group practices, which became known as PPGPs. In areas where PPGPs gained a foothold, some solo physicians formed their own prepayment arrangements as a way to maintain an independent practice. These physicians often formed associations that were coordinated by local medical societies and termed *Independent* (or *Individual*) *Practice Associations* (IPAs).

In 1972, the term *health maintenance organization* was applied by the Nixon Administration to both PPGPs and IPAs in the hope that this affirmative name would make capitation plans more palatable to skeptical patients and providers. Today, many types of HMO provide hospitalization, professional fees, and other covered services out of their revenue from prepaid premiums. Some health care practitioners in HMOs are paid by salary or receive a per-capita payment, many others are paid on a FFS basis, and still others are paid by a combination of FFS and capitation.

Salaried physicians often receive a productivity-based incentive payment as well.

To encourage noncapitated practitioners to minimize their use of medical services, these practitioners almost always share some financial risk with the HMO. For example, some portion (20 percent) of their FFS reimbursement may be withheld until the end of the year, at which time it is determined whether their use of services during that year has been efficient. Alternatively, the clinician may receive a fixed dollar amount, a fixed percentage of surplus funds in the risk pool, a bonus based on productivity, a percentage of the organization's profits, or payment based on some combination of these options at year's end. Some organizations reward efficient providers through increases in their fee schedules or by allowing these physicians to become investors in the organization. If inefficiencies are found (for example, "excessive" hospitalization or referral to specialists), then part or all of the withheld amount may be kept by the HMO or the provider may forfeit the bonus.

A 1986 survey of HMOs found that two thirds withhold funds from their primary-care physicians, most often 11 percent to 20 percent of the payment (Hillman et al. 1989). This money is then returned on the basis of provider efficiency. Other financial risks such as future payment reductions, were imposed by one third of HMOs, and forty percent required their primary-care physicians to pay for outpatient laboratory tests directly from their capitation payments or a fund that included capitation payments. Only 20 percent of HMOs, however, held physicians at *individual* financial risk; the majority used a system of *pooled* risk.

Contractual arrangements within HMOs are often very complex and lead to correspondingly complex arrangements for reimbursement. For example, a physician may be a member of a small private group practice that subcontracts to a larger group that in turn contracts to several distinct HMOs, each HMO using a somewhat different scheme of payment. In fact, there are probably as many ways to arrange reimbursement within an HMO as there are HMOs themselves.

Salary is the final traditional method of physician reimbursement. As the era of the solo practitioner passes, a growing number of physicians receive at least some portion of their income through salary. This trend reflects the growth of HMOs, but many salaried physicians are employed by institutions other than HMOs, among them group practices, hospitals, and clinics. A growing number of group practice arrangements place young partners on full or partial salary as well.

Providers' Incentives and Reimbursement Methods

Although some assert that providers are uninfluenced by their methods of reimbursement, data from numerous sources indicate that this is simply not true. Different payment mechanisms offer practitioners different incentives, and these incentives may significantly influence both the amount and the type of care that a patient receives. Aside from the clinical implications, provider reimbursement incentives have major economic consequences; it has been estimated that physicians make direct decisions affecting 70 percent to 90 percent of all outlays for health care. Thus, even though they receive only approximately one fifth of all dollars spent on medical care themselves, their practices have an immense influence over the rest of these outlays.

Fee-for-service reimbursement invites the provider to offer as many services as the patient's condition may warrant (hypothetically, as many as his or her condition could *possibly* warrant). FFS rewards providers for keeping patients in the hospital and ensuring they receive every test and treatment that technology offers (theoretically, every *conceivable* test, at least up to the levels of the patient's insurance coverage). The simplicity of the FFS concept belies its power to inflate costs. Some economists argue that this method of reimbursement is *the* major cause of our increasing expenditures for health care.

Similarly, cost-plus reimbursement contains no financial incentive to manage hospitals efficiently, because any increase in a hospital's operating costs is passed along to payers in the form of higher charges. Even when effective management, increased patient volume, technological improvements, or increased provider skills reduce *costs,* hospital *charges* rarely are lowered.

The capitation arrangement offers a different constellation of economic incentives. First, the provider organization and/or its individual practitioners bear the financial risk instead of the third-party payer or the consumer. Second, because the capitation payment depends only on the number of people cared for and not the quantity of services, no incentive exists to maximize the volume of services provided. Indeed, this creates the incentive to enroll more members and do less for each, as efficiency results in profits.

Salaried practitioners, like those in capitation plans, receive no financial reward for increasing the number of services provided, but unlike those in capitation plans, these practitioners also are not usually rewarded financially if they care for an increased number of patients. For these reasons, some economists regard the salary method as the most neutral type of reimbursement. As Relman stated, "Salaried practice is certainly compatible with a standard of care at least the equal of that usually found in the traditional fee-for-service arrangement . . . But whether these potential advantages of salaried practice are realized depends heavily on the character and objectives of the organization hiring the physicians" (1988, p. 784).

Cost savings in both capitation and salary systems appear to come largely from lower physician-induced demand. In fact, because capitation offers physicians an incentive to provide less care, there has been considerable concern that HMO patients would not be well served; extensive research in the 1960s and 1970s, however, showed that these patients by and large receive care that equals that received by FFS patients. Recent studies also support these results (e.g., Udvarhelyi et al. 1991). Anecdotal evidence aside, the general differences between care in HMO and in FFS settings appear to be not so much qualitative as quantitative: enrollees in prepaid HMOs receive more ambulatory care and less surgery than FFS patients and are hospitalized less often.

As part of the Rand Health Insurance Experiment, groups of people were randomly assigned to an HMO and several FFS plans; the random assignment eliminated any possibility that HMO cost advantages, if found, might be attributable to a self-selection of healthier people into HMOs. The FFS groups' health care expenditures were found to be higher, largely because the hospitalization rate of the HMO group was 40 percent lower. Because other potentially confounding variables were strictly controlled, the difference in costs between the two systems appeared to be attributable largely to differences in the physicians' incentives to hospitalize their patients.

Another study in New England compared 10 FFS physicians with 17 HMO physicians with respect to ordering electrocardiograms (EKGs) and chest x-rays. In the FFS system, these are both high-cost and high-profit tests; in the HMO system, the providers who order these tests often pay for them out of their own income. On average, it was found that the FFS practitioners ordered 50 percent more EKGs and 40 percent more chest x-rays than the HMO practitioners, which clearly demonstrates the influence that the reimbursement method has over clinical decisions.

Alternative methods of reimbursement have also been shown to affect the inclination of surgeons to operate in equivocal clinical situations, with higher rates of surgery under FFS reimbursement. One study found surgery rates in capitation plans to be 3.5 to 5 per thousand, compared with 6.5 to 7 per thousand in FFS arrangements. A study of federal employees found that surgical procedures in capitation plans were performed at one fourth to one half the rate of the same procedures in FFS plans.

Physicians in the United Kingdom are part of a national health service, under which GPs are paid primarily by capitation and specialists by salary. Among other things, comparative studies have found that U.K. physicians perform surgery at approximately one half the rate of U.S. physicians, and they perform fewer radiologic studies. Such comparisons must be correlated with comparative data on the health status of the two populations as well as the quality and outcome of care to be meaningful, otherwise it cannot be stated whether or not Americans pay too much for health care or what may be a reasonable price for higher-quality care. Nonetheless, arguments both ways have been made for decades.

Today, however, as numerous studies show unnecessary inefficiencies throughout the health care delivery system, both payers and policymakers have reached a consensus that changes are necessary in the way that physicians are reimbursed. Expenditure data from Medicare Part B also support their consensus. Part B accounts for one third of all Medicare expenditures, approximately three quarters of which pay for physician services. For the first half of the 1980s, Part B expenditures increased an average of almost 15 percent annually, only 1 year increasing less than 10 percent. Thus, it should not be surprising that the Medicare program has led the way in developing innovative reimbursement methods. The following chapter describes what has been and is being done to encourage more cost-effective behavior by providers.

CHAPTER 6

COSTS: THE PAYER'S PERSPECTIVE

The role of third-party payers has increased so greatly during recent years that some believe payers exert more influence on medical practice than either patients or providers. Understanding the objectives of payers, which include maximizing their revenue and minimizing their expenditures, is critical to understanding today's process of health care delivery.

Actions taken by payers to influence the behavior of hospital administrators and physicians fall into two overlapping categories: regulatory and competitive. Regulatory interventions seek either to prescribe or prohibit certain kinds of behavior by providers. Competitive interventions neither prescribe nor prohibit; instead, these offer incentives designed to encourage cost-sensitive, competitive behavior.

Planning: A Regulatory Approach

Most developed countries have central agencies, either at the national or the regional level, that control medical care resources and coordinate their allocation. In contrast, the pluralistic United States has decentralized planning agencies (where these agencies exist at all), and these agencies have been at best only modestly successful in influencing investment in health care. Considerations of profit have generally been paramount in determining such investment. As a result, some areas today are burdened with surplus facilities, while others, usually rural or inner-city areas, remain underequipped.

In the 1960s, after the introduction of Medicare and Medicaid, the federal government sought ways to contain costs by preventing unnecessary capital investment. Despite the opposition of powerful political groups such as the AMA and the AHA, sporadic efforts at regional planning were made. In the mid-1970s, the Federal Planning Act authorized the creation of a large-scale network of both local and regional agencies to plan for health care needs on community and state levels. These consumer-dominated, quasi-governmental units, which came to be known as Health Systems Agencies (HSAs) and State Health Planning and Development Agencies, had considerable influence in the certification process for major capital expansion within existing health care facilities, but they had no authority to halt noncapital-intensive projects that they deemed unnecessary. Moreover, providers could ignore these agencies' suggestions regarding what new programs were needed by the community. As a result, the now-defunct HSA program had only modest impact on the growth of the health care sector in most areas before it fell victim to the Reagan Administration's budget cuts in 1986.

The *Certificate-of-Need* (CON) program, federally mandated by Congress as part of the Federal Planning Act, was controlled by state planning units with assistance from local HSAs where present. The program required hospitals and other medical institutions to obtain a *certificate of need* from the state before purchasing major equipment, adding beds, developing new services, or making other capital investments above an established dollar amount. Over time, this amount increased from approximately $100,000 to $1 million or more in many states. Planning boards determined whether proposed investments were necessary and had the authority to turn down projects deemed unnecessary.

Several difficulties arose with the CON process. Many hospitals found innovative ways to skirt its regulations; these included making purchases before the CON regulations were implemented or purchasing more equipment when the number of hospital beds was constrained. Planning boards also invariably included physicians and hospital administrators as well as local citizens (who comprised the majority), all of whom benefited from an investment in state-of-the-art medicine, and the boards were not at any financial risk for their decisions. Given these circumstances, it is unsurprising that these committees only rarely opposed new construction projects. For all these reasons, the Federal Planning Act as well as subsequent programs did little to control investment in, and expansion of, health care facilities. The Reagan Administration dropped CON requirements in 1986, but some states still have either a CON process, a program that is equivalent, or a moratorium on new hospital construction and expansion projects.

Utilization Control: A Regulatory Approach

Chapter 4 discussed the concept known as *utilization review* (UR) (also known as *utilization management*) from the perspective of the patients' use of services. UR can target patients, but it is usually oriented toward the provider, where the main focus is on the provider's clinical decisions. In these circumstances, the patient is usually not penalized financially for services that are unapproved or disallowed; the provider, however, may be.

In contrast to planning, which is used to control capital investments, utilization control seeks to achieve efficiency in the basic units of service that derive from patient–practitioner encounters. Physicians' actual use of health care resources is examined on a case-by-case or a practice-profile basis and then compared to predetermined criteria. When these criteria are set by the same physicians who are being monitored, the review is usually termed *peer review*, even if the first-level reviewer is actually a nurse or medical records technician. The general premise is that if providers are more cognizant of the costs they generate and the resources they control, then these providers will assume a heightened responsibility for efficient use of those resources.

Decisions that provider-oriented UR programs most commonly scrutinize are whether a patient is hospitalized, how long a patient remains in the hospital and, if so, whether major therapeutic procedures (such as surgery) or major diagnostic procedures (such as angiography) are performed. A review can occur before the event (*prospective*), at the time of the event (*concurrent*), or after the event (*retrospective*).

Today, a range of provider-oriented UR approaches exist. One is *preadmission certification*, in which a review organization acting as proxy for the insurer grants permission for a patient to be hospitalized; if permission is not granted, then payment may be denied. Another is *concurrent review*, in which the review organization monitors a hospitalized patient's progress to determine if continued inpatient care is medically necessary. A similar approach, though not technically a review program, is to pay for certain surgical procedures only if they are performed on an outpatient basis (also known as *same day* or *ambulatory surgery*). As mentioned earlier, the Medicare program has an extensive list of such procedures, including small skin grafts, rectal polypectomy, tubal ligation, and gynecologic laparoscopy. Payment can be denied even after the service has been performed and billed, for example, if a physican hospitalizes a patient to perform a skin graft and cannot prove that unusual circumstances required inpatient treatment. The patient is also usually exempt from responsibility for payment in such cases.

To the extent that feedback from UR induces outlying or nonconforming physicians to modify their clinical decisions, it can be used as a mechanism for quality assurance as well. In fact, UR was first developed in the 1930s as part of an effort to improve the quality of care. However, by stiffening criteria and disallowing reimbursements when established standards are not met, UR becomes a cost-control measure; to date, UR programs have concentrated on limiting "unnecessary" use of health care resources rather than on improving the outcome of care. (New trends in this direction, known as "outcome management," will be explored in Chapter 8.) These two purposes may in fact be consistent: a reasonably solid argument can be made that limiting unneeded care will have a positive effect on the patient's clinical outcome; however, at some point, further reductions will clearly have the opposite effect.

Utilization review became prominent as a cost control tool after the enactment of Medicare and Medicaid, when federal law mandated a review of both hospital and physician reimbursement "to avert overservicing in the Medicare and Medicaid programs—e.g., unjustified surgery, which might be both harmful and costly" (Roemer 1981, p. 33). Hospitals were at first put in charge of their own reviews, but this self-regulation was ineffective and replaced in 1972 by *Professional Standards Review Organizations* (PSROs). PSROs, composed of local physicians, were founded in 187 geographic areas and were supported by the federal government to review hospital admissions and lengths of stay for beneficiaries of the Medicare, Medicaid, and Maternal and Child Health programs. They were to identify unnecessary admissions and inpatient days, for which reimbursement would be denied. Given that PSRO actions were mainly retrospective, the provider alone was at financial risk, (because the patient had already received the care). They could also recommend sanctions against individual physicians.

As the first major program to monitor the actual delivery of care, PSROs were a harbinger of future trends. PSRO legislation was promoted to physicians as a way of improving the quality of care and to Congress as a means of controlling costs (both motives in Roemer's quote in the previous paragraph). The potential divergence of these goals, however, created confusion from the start, and the program was also plagued by administrative difficulties, was inadequately supported by practitioners, and showed no clear signs of effectiveness. For these reasons and others, PSROs were terminated in 1982 and replaced by similar entities termed *Peer Review Organizations* (PROs).

In the PRO system, one independent group in each state— often a reborn PSRO—was awarded a contract to do the review work. To qualify, these groups were required to show either sponsorship or support by physicians, and they could not be associated with a health care facility or a third-party payer. PROs review only the care provided to Medicare beneficiaries; Medicaid reviews are no longer supported by the federal program, though many PROs do have separate state contracts for this purpose.

Like their predecessors, PROs were given a mixture of cost and quality goals. Some of their major objectives were to encourage a shift of care from inpatient to outpatient settings, to decrease the number of invasive procedures and of complications from such procedures, to cut down on patient readmissions, and to improve the accuracy of both diagnostic reporting and coding on medical records.

The PRO program is considered by many to be an improvement over its predecessor, but other difficulties remain. These include, notably, the possibility that inaccurate data will lead to inaccurate conclusions, the focus on case-by-case retrospective review rather than on broader patterns of practice, emphasis on identifying the "bad apples" at the bottom of the distribution curve rather than moving the entire curve upward, concern that reputations may suffer unjustly from the 20/20 hindsight that retrospective review fosters, and the lack of an adequate mechanism to deal with disagreements between reviewers and practitioners regarding the management of a case. Despite these drawbacks, however, PRO programs seem likely to serve as the principal public sector UR and quality assurance method for the near future.

When private health insurance companies began to operate in the 1930s, they did not monitor the use of resources by either hospitals or physicians. This began to change with the advent of Medicare, when many private insurers became the *fiscal intermediaries* for the federal government. Not only did they now provide administrative services such as handling claim forms and making payments to beneficiaries and providers, but more generally, they acted as conduits between the government, consumers, and providers. They were also responsible for monitoring both claims and payments and acting on the findings of the PSROs and PROs.

Many insurance companies adopted the Medicare review methods for their own policyholders, and because of pressures from self-insured employers (who used insurers only as third-party administrators) and the insurance companies' own drives to contain costs, UR took on increased importance over time. This surveillance has increased over the years to the point where most insurance companies are now involved in aggressive UR activities, questioning physicians' decisions, and even specifying the norms of current practice. Some term this *the managed-care phenomenon*, involving as it does the managing of physicians' behavior and of health care resources. (See also Chapter 4.)

As discussed previously with regard to patient-oriented cost controls, businesses are also using UR programs to control the costs of health benefits. Many employers now require their insurance carriers to set up UR programs, and others contract with independent review or medical management organizations, which became a booming business for many defunded PSROs. Still other corporations have opted to operate such UR programs themselves.

Regulatory Approaches to Reimbursement

Because it is clear that methods of reimbursement can influence clinical decisions, modifying the reimbursement process is another approach used by third parties to affect medical decision-making.

Resolute policymakers now consider the redesign of payment mechanisms as a means to induce providers to incorporate an awareness of cost into their clinical decision-making.

Rate-setting of one sort or another has been tried several times by government during the cost-containment era. Unlike CON and other regulations that were designed to control providers' investments, rate-setting directly controls the prices that providers may charge. Price freezes and payment caps have been the principal strategies of this type.

From 1971 to 1974, the Nixon Administration attempted to control rampant, economy-wide inflation with the Economic Stabilization Act, which included a 90-day wage and price freeze on all providers. This worked reasonably well during the existence of the program: per-day and per-admission hospital costs decreased, and the annual rate of increase in physicians' fees fell from 7.4 percent to 2.4 percent. When the program was discontinued, however, inflation in these prices resumed at its previous steep rate. A decade later, a 15-month freeze declared in 1984 was extended several times, into 1986.

Congress has legislated adjustments in physician payment through other formulas as well. For example, since 1972, yearly increases in Medicare Part B prevailing charges have been determined on the basis of the *Medicare Economic Index* (MEI), which is a complex formula that considers a variety of economic factors, including practice costs and general wage levels. In some years, Congress has voted to allow no increase at all. Starting in 1987, the prevailing-charge increases of nonparticipating physicians lagged 1 year behind those of participating physicians. Another formula, the *Maximum Allowable Actual Charge* (MAAC), is used to limit the amount of balance billing that is permitted by nonparticipating physicians, and still other formulas, such as fee-schedule conversion factors, are now used to regulate the reimbursement levels of providers.

Many practitioners have responded to these fee freezes by "gaming the system" in various ways, notably, reclassifying services into higher-paying categories, unbundling a single-charge service into separate billable units, and providing more units of service. One controversial argument that some economists have put forth is that physicians have a so-called *target income* and simply modify their behavior as necessary to assure that this income is reached. However accurate this may be, analysts generally agree that both freezes and caps have been ineffective methods of cost control.

Capitation

As noted earlier, President Nixon's advisers were convinced of the cost-saving potential of capitation plans, and they supported their development. The HMO Act, passed in 1973, specified federal qualifications for HMOs, including a minimum benefit package, a quality-of-care review process, and regulations to ensure sound financial backing. Employers with more than 25 employees were required to offer an HMO option if there was a federally qualified plan in their area; this legislation was intended to encourage competition among HMO plans and between HMOs and traditional insurance plans.

In response to fears that HMOs might provide inferior medical care because of their financing structure, HMO regulations were tightened. HMOs were also required to offer far more comprehensive benefits than most traditional insurance policies of the time. This increased their costs, and the resulting higher premiums probably hindered the growth of HMO plans. Businesses did begin to offer such plans to their employees, but their high premiums dissuaded many from signing up. Initially, there was no dramatic increase of the aggregate enrollment in capitated plans.

Since then, however, continued increases in medical costs have stimulated enrollment in HMOs, and more corporate employers now offer such plans as an option. Many seek the financial benefit of enrollment, as some HMOs now are less expensive to join than are traditional indemnity plans. Public attitude toward HMOs also has improved; over time, these alternative-care settings have become more acceptable. Some younger people have grown up receiving all of their care from such organizations and feel quite comfortable with them, even though HMOs still are not used by a majority of the population.

Price Discounting

In this era of cost control, third-party payers have become "prudent buyers," demanding discounts or looking for new providers who are willing to accept lower fees. The surplus of physicians and hospital beds, which created a buyer's market for health care, has facilitated this approach. The resulting contracts benefit not only payers but also providers, who in return for their discount are guaranteed a certain volume of patients at a time when many hospitals and physicians are competing to attract new patients. As part of a discount deal, many payers also agree to expedite payment, which otherwise is rarely swift. Because patients are excluded from this negotiation, however, market forces apply only indirectly to them.

Discounts can be arranged in many ways. Payer and provider may negotiate a contract stipulating discounted fees; the Blues have traditionally negotiated such contracts with hospitals. Providers also may submit competitive bids to serve a given patient population; thus, payers accepting the lowest bid have, in effect, been offered a discount. Some employers have purchased plans for their employees that incorporate discounts negotiated by insurance companies, and still others have negotiated their own discounts. In the public sector, as of 1989, four state Medicaid programs were reimbursing hospitals on the basis of negotiated or competitive bids.

Discounting is the basis of arrangements known as *preferred provider organizations* (PPOs). In a PPO, employers or insurers offer their beneficiaries significant incentives to use "preferred" sources of care, and these providers in turn offer discounts (often 20 percent) from their conventional fees. The PPO entity agrees to accept a degree of accountability by establishing a strong UR program, but because providers under PPO arrangements receive FFS payment, they do not bear the financial risk that is associated with an HMO arrangement.

Patients enrolled in PPOs are usually not *required* to obtain care from the preferred group, but they are rewarded for doing so. In general, the incentives for enrollees involve extra services (such as preventive care) or waived co-payments and deductibles. Enrollees remain free to consult other providers who do not offer such incentives, but they must pay the difference out-of-pocket. In a variant of the PPO, known as the *exclusive provider organization* (EPO), the patient's costs are reimbursed only when care is rendered within the PPO system.

The Medicare Prospective Payment System

In 1983, Congress introduced the Prospective Payment System (PPS) which radically restructured the financing of Medicare Part A. Under PPS, each hospital is paid a prospectively determined, fixed amount per patient admission; this is regardless of how many services that patient receives. This legislation represents the most significant departure in the financing (and consequently in the delivery) of U.S. health care since the inception of the Medicare program itself.

Under PPS, each patient admission is assigned to a category via a system termed *Diagnosis Related Groups* (DRGs); hence, PPS is often termed *the DRG System*. DRGs are based on the *International Classification of Diseases, 9th Revision* (ICD-9), a taxonomy of approximately 10,000 diagnoses and 5000 procedure codes. In the early 1970s, researchers at Yale University classified hospital patients into groups on the basis of diagnoses, procedures, and age as a way of explaining variations in their use of resources and length of stay in the hospital; the outcome was approximately 390 DRGs. This classification was later revised and currently includes 467 categories. Figure 15 depicts how patients with primary conditions related to blood and blood formation are grouped into one of eight DRGs based on their diagnoses, procedures, and age.

Under PPS, each DRG is assigned a coefficient representing the resource intensity deemed necessary to care for a patient assigned that DRG. This coefficient is multiplied by a dollar amount to convert it into a price, and this is the fee paid to a hospital for each patient in that DRG. Patients receive only one DRG assignment no matter how many diagnoses he or she has or procedures he or she undergoes during a given admission. If the hospital's costs for that patient exceed the fee, then the hospital will lose money on the admission; if the fee exceeds the hospital's costs, then the hospital will make a profit. Because a particular hospital is paid on the basis of its entire mix of cases, the DRG payment scheme is sometimes known as a *case-mix* or *per-case* reimbursement system.

The prospective payment rate to a particular hospital for a patient in any given DRG is determined by several factors, including the cost of a typical Medicare inpatient day (based on accounting audits) and the relative resource requirements for that DRG (figured

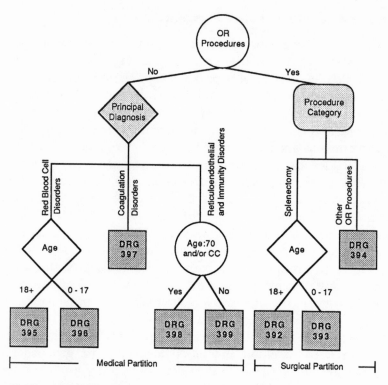

CC = Cormorbidity and/or Complication

Figure 15. A major diagnostic category (MDC) of the diagnosis-related group (DRG) case-mix system: diseases and disorders of the blood and blood-forming organs and immunological disorders. (Source: Health Care Financing Administration 1983.)

in terms of the length of stay in the hospital). Additional reimbursement for *outlier patients,* so named when their hospital bill reaches 150 percent of (or $12,000 more than) the DRG prospective price, has also been incorporated into the system. Medicare pays 60 percent of the hospital bill above the outlier cutoff amount.

The Prospective Payment System applies to inpatient services only. This was the chosen starting point, because inpatient services are the single most expensive component (at over 50 percent) of aggregate federal spending for health care. In its first year, PPS reimbursement was designed to be a *budget-neutral* method: it was not intended to reduce expenditures. The program's designated purpose, however, was to keep the costs of Medicare down by setting in advance the annual level of spending for U.S. acute-care hospitals. The PPS system does make tight control possible, because if spending in year X exceeds accepted levels, then the dollar multiplier can be decreased for year $X + 1$. This downward-ratcheting mechanism has been applied by Medicare program administrators.

The Prospective Payment System was phased in gradually. In its initial stages, local variations in charges were incorporated into payments as a further refinement of separate urban and rural rates. Adjustments were made for sole community hospitals, regional referral centers, and cancer hospitals, but these adjustments were gradually phased out. By 1988, hospitals were paid national rates, which were adjusted only for differences in average area-wage levels, teaching status, and the degree to which hospitals disproportionately care for the indigent.

As part of the initial reimbursement arrangement, Medicare also pays a hospital for a portion of that facility's capital costs. This payment is based on the number of hospital-days that were spent treating Medicare patients. This additional payment may be eliminated, however, and replaced by a standard payment per discharge that would include adjustments for case-mix, geographic area, and the proportion of patients who were indigent. Psychiatric, childrens', and chronic hospitals were excluded from the original plan, and this exclusion has remained in effect.

Several state Medicaid programs have introduced PPS, and in 1989, 17 states were using diagnosis-based, case-mix systems like DRGs. Twenty-one other states were using some variation on this method of reimbursement. In that same year, only nine states were using any type of traditional, retrospective method for hospital reimbursment under Medicaid. Some Blues plans also use PPS (with and without DRGs), but as of 1991, the great majority of privately insured hospital patients were not admitted under a prospective payment plan.

The Future Expansion of Prospective Payment beyond Hospitals

Inpatient services were targeted first for cost containment, because they consume the largest portion of expenditures for health care.

Inflation in other parts of the health care sector has contributed to budget problems as well, however, and to bring the alarming increases in Medicare Part B expenditures under control, federal policymakers are now exploring (and in some cases mandating) new methods of reimbursement to physicians.

DRG-based prospective payment currently applies only to the facility's portion of a hospital charge, but just as hospital services have been bundled for payment purposes, there has been a trend toward looking at the patient or an episode of illness as a "package." In capitation systems, for example, 1 year's worth of patient care is bundled into one prepaid fee.

Services other than hospital admissions could potentially be bundled, so other PPS schemes are in the planning stages or have been introduced on a limited basis. One such scheme is a case-mix approach for ambulatory visits that was designed by several of the developers of the DRGs, known first as *Ambulatory Visit Groups* and now as *Ambulatory Patient Groups* (APGs). This system is based on ICD-9 diagnosis codes and on the Current Procedural Terminology (CPT) codes that the AMA developed. Given the growing importance of ambulatory care, such a system may appear necessary to both payers and policymakers in the future. It is under consideration by HCFA for the reimbursement of hospital-based outpatient care, but it has not yet been applied by any major payer.

Bundling of the costs for long-term care has been explored as well. As the percentage of elderly persons in the U.S. population increases, so does the importance of effectively controlling the costs of long-term care. The Medicare and Medicaid programs together pay for approximately half of all nursing home costs, which amounts to billions of dollars per year. Government analysts have worked on a prospective reimbursement method for nursing home care that would pay the facility a preset fee based on the patient case-mix. This method has not yet been implemented, but it is likely that something similar will gain favor in both the Medicare and Medicaid programs.

No inherent obstacle to prospective bundling of physicians' services for inpatient, ambulatory care or nursing home care appears to exist. Surgeons and obstetricians already are paid for some of their services by the bundle; for example, both pre- and postoperative visits usually are included in the surgical fee, and all charges for a pregnancy are often subsumed under a single fee. Medicare has introduced demonstration projects bundling reimbursement for cardiac bypass surgery, and the program plans to do the same for cataract surgery. Other specialists do not bundle their services, however, and equitable methods of payment for them under such a system are still undetermined. HCFA officials perceive that the bundling of reimbursement in this way would replace government micromanagement (such as per-case utilization review) with a structure to help health care providers decide how best to economize.

Some experts have recommended a per-case approach, known as *MD-DRGs*, whereby the admitting physician would receive a flat fee to provide all of that patient's hospital-based care. A variation on the MD-DRG bundling approach would move beyond the admitting physician to encompass *all* physician services that are provided during an admission, including radiology, anesthesia and pathology (often termed *the "RAP" services*), as well as surgery, any consultations by specialists, and hospital visits by the attending physician. Such a package fee could be paid to the hospital, which then would negotiate a payment arrangement with the physicians. It could also be paid to the medical staff, which would apportion it, or to the attending physician, who would pay the specialists used in that case.

Another issue is whether bundled fees could cover the spectrum from outpatient to inpatient to long-term care, thus preventing practitioners from shifting treatment locations to collect extra fees. Mitchell appears to perceive no difference between medical and business decisions: "Packaging physician services restores much of the burden to the physician making the decision, *as with any entrepreneur.* Under a physician DRG system, the decision to bring in a consultant carries with it specific cost consequences for the physician since these additional costs must come out of a fixed case payment" (1985b, p. 10) (italics added). Apportioning a single fee among a number of providers, however, is potentially inequitable for some physicians. Would specialists on a case be paid more than generalists? Would physicians be less likely to include their patients in treatment decisions? These and other hurdles to implemention of an MD-DRG system make it likely that HCFA will not implement such a method of reimbursement nationally in the near future. Instead, policymakers decided to pursue cost containment through the implementation of physician-fee schedules.

New Approaches to Physician Reimbursement

To address the issue of physician reimbursement, Congress in 1987 created a multidisciplinary Physician Payment Review Commission (PPRC). Two years later, this influential commission recommended a number of changes in Medicare Part B; these included limits on balance billing, the development of clinical practice guidelines, more federal money for research on the effectiveness of care, and most important, the development of a Medicare Fee Schedule.

Acting on these recommendations, Congress enacted legislation in 1989 that will fundamentally change the way that Medicare Part B reimburses physician providers, replacing the UCR–CPR historical payments with a physician-fee schedule. HCFA was assigned the task of developing the fee schedule, which has been termed the *Resource-Based Relative Value System* (RBRVS), and HCFA funded Hsiao and colleagues at Harvard to perform the preliminary research necessary to develop weights for each service so as to assign it a value relative to the other services. Hence, this type of system is termed a *relative value scale* (RVS). (Chapter 5 discusses RVSs further.) The AMA was initially also involved in developing this scale.

"Resource-based" indicates that the relative values of services in this fee schedule are determined by the input of resources that they require (contrasting with historical charge levels CPR used). Resources that are considered in the calculation of RBRVS weights include physician time, mental effort and judgment, technical skill, physician effort, stress, practice expenses, and the costs of malpractice premiums. The system is intended to correct the pricing distortions that heavily reward procedure-oriented care compared with cognitive services, specialists more than generalists, and urban more than rural physicians. Over 4000 procedures were included in the initial RVS.

Once the relative value (or weight) has been determined, each procedure is multiplied by a dollar-conversion factor to create a fee schedule; thus, procedures with a higher relative value receive higher payments. A geographic adjustment (to account for differing business expenses across regions) is also applied through an additional conversion factor. During its 5-year phase-in period (which commenced in 1992), Medicare Part B reimbursements to physicians will be paid on the basis of a blending of the RBRVS-based rates and the historical CPR payments.

The formula in Figure 16 illustrates how the RBRVS reimbursement for the excision of a brain tumor is calculated. Total RVUs (68.44), based on the three subcomponents noted, are multiplied by the conversion factor ($31.001 in 1992). For 1993, 25 percent of the payment is based on this amount and 75 percent on neurosurgeons' historical CPR levels. (The proportion blended from the CPR versus the RVS systems will change each year until 1996, when all Medicare payments are expected to be based 100 percent on the RBRVS fee schedule.)

EXCISION OF BRAIN TUMOR

(CPT Code #61545)

Work RVUs = 36.35

Practice expense RVUs = 27.04

Malpractice RVUs = 5.05

Total RVUs = 68.44

1992 conversion factor = $31.001 = 1 RVU*

1992 Fee for Brain Tumor Excision = 68.44 Total RVUs X $31.001 = **$2122.32**

*RVU = Relative Value Unit

Figure 16. Components of resource-based relative value scale (RBRVS) for one procedure.

Under the new payment scheme, nonparticipating physicians are paid 5-percent less than participating physicians, and their claims are processed more slowly. Fees for the two groups will increase at the same rate, but the 5-percent differential is expected to remain.

The policymakers' original intent for the RBRVS fee schedule was budget neutrality (i.e., funds were meant to be redistributed among providers), but significant budget control is possible simply by modifying the conversion factors. The status of the federal budget has worsened since this legislation was passed, and as a result, the original intent of neutrality will not be realized completely. This has been a point of heated controversy between policymakers and providers.

Another disagreement between those groups relates to one of the purposes of the RBRVS-based fee schedule, namely, to correct the disparities in reimbursement between generalists and specialists and to reduce what many feel are excessive payments for procedures at the expense of cognitive services. Developers of this scale predicted large increases in the reimbursement for providers of cognitive services, with compensatory reductions for procedure-oriented specialists, but when the initial RVS was released, only family practitioners and GPs were expected to receive overall increases in reimbursement. Other cognitive specialists such as psychiatrists and internists were surprised that their expected Medicare reimbursement would remain the same or decrease under the proposed plan, despite previous assurances by government administrators that the fee schedule was intended to correct long-standing distortions in the levels of reimbursement to these groups. During numerous Congressional hearings on the subject, providers registered their disagreement with the proposed changes and gave voluminous testimony that differed from the calculations made by the scale's developers.

As a consequence of lobbying by physician groups as well as concern by HCFA analysts that errors *were* made in the original RVS development, the scale was modified further before the final figures were established. Current HCFA estimates now predict that GPs and family practitioners will be financial winners under the new system. In addition, internists and psychiatrists, on average, will receive higher Medicare payments using the RBRVS system. The surgical specialties and hospital-based specialists are expected to be the financial losers and receive lower reimbursements than under the CPR system; for example, Medicare payment per service is forecast to decline over 20 percent for ophthalmologists, radiologists, and thoracic surgeons. Table 7 compares selected fees based on the CPR system versus the new fee schedule.

Further complications also surround this program. In the past, physicians have appeared to respond to limitations on their fees by increasing the number of services they provided. HCFA estimates that for each 1-percent cut in physician fees, the volume and intensity of services will increase by 0.5 percent. These increases, concomitant with fee decreases, have been termed the *behavioral offset*. As a result of this expected increase in services, HCFA adjusted the initial rates of reimbursement downward.

The adjustment for behavioral offset is quite controversial. Physician groups and some legislators have objected strongly to this additional reduction, and some—though not all—analysts believe little empirical evidence exists to support this forecast. Furthermore, even if increases in volume and intensity are found, their causes are unclear. While they could arise in response to fee cuts, they could also result from changes in medical practice, new technology, and "relentless patient demand" (Iglehart 1989, p. 1159). Not surprisingly, physicians are incensed that HCFA ana-

Table 7. Selected CPR (Prevailing) Medicare Part B Physician Fees Compared with RBRVS-based fee-schedule

Physician service (CPT code)	Medicare Payments		% change
	CPR*	RVS fee schedule†	
Intermediate office visit, old patient (90050/99213)‡	$28	$31	+11%
Intermediate hospital visit (90260/99231)	30	31	+3
Total hip replacement (27131)	2404	1697	−29
Coronary bypass graft (33712)	3894	2225	−42
Cataract removal (66984)	1467	941	−36
Electrocardiogram (93000)	35	26	−26

Source: Data from Physician Payment Review Commission 1991; Health Care Financing Administration 1992.
   Note: Medicare will pay physicians up to 80 percent of these amounts; the beneficiary pays the remaining 20 percent.
   *From 1989.
   †Using 1992 "conversion" factor.
   ‡CPT system has changed.

lysts have assumed that they will increase the volume of services solely for self-serving, economic reasons.

The PPRC also anticipated a repetition of previous governmental experience with fee freezes and decreases. To control for runaway growth in the volume of services, the commission recommended the creation of a Volume Performance Standard (VPS), which is intended to offer an "emergency brake" of sorts. Based on VPS, the annual fee updates will depend on how successfully providers limited increases in the volume of services during the previous year. As described by Mulvey:

A target is set annually, which takes into account inflation, growth and aging of the population, and changes in technology. Consideration is also given to the relationship between volume and inappropriate utilization of services. Each year's actual expenditures are then compared with the target. If actual expenditures exceed the target based on the above factors, the legislation mandates that the overall level of physician fees decline by this difference. Separate targets are set for surgical and nonsurgical services. If a target is not set, the legislation calls for a default target to be implemented. (1991, p. 11)

Because the VPS (originally and less palatably labeled *expenditure targets*) is based on global physician services, Rice and Bernstein (1990) pointed out that this creates a moral scenario like that Hardin (1968) described in "The Tragedy of the Commons," whereby the incentive facing an *individual* is to maximize volume (and thereby personal revenue) at the expense of the group (whose overall incentive should be to minimize volume). Such an approach to cost containment, which foreshadows a global budgeting approach, has never been tried in the United States.

Despite the controversies that both concepts generated, RBRVS fee schedules and VPS took effect in 1992. It is possible, however, that HCFA analysts (and possibly the politicians) will continue to modify the fee schedule, particularly as they obtain data regarding its effects on Medicare expenditures, patient care, and physician incomes and behavior.

Both RBRVS and VPS represent landmark changes in the U.S. cost-containment movement. Regarding RBRVS, Iglehart commented, "it reflects a movement—by both government and physicians' organizations—away from market principles as the favored method of allocating medical resources and toward government policy as the way to achieve equity among patients, payers, and providers" (1990, p. 1251). This program will be one of the first governmental attempts to control both price and volume simultaneously (Rice 1991). As discussed, fee schedules have great potential for controlling costs, and this potential is augmented considerably by the budgeting-like effects of VPS. However, until the system is fully in place, analysts, policymakers, and providers can only surmise its impact on medical practice. Medicare payments account for only one quarter of U.S. physician income, but HCFA is the most influential payer in America. It is likely that if RBRVS is successful, then both state and private payers will follow suit and fee schedules and VPS-like controls will become ubiquitous.

All-Payer Rate Controls

Third-party efforts at cost control have had several unintended effects on the payers themselves. As discounting, fee schedules, and prospective payment become more important aspects of health care financing, *cost-shifting* among the different types of payers has increased. An estimated 13 percent of a private patient's bill now pays for costs that have been shifted from the bills of patients who are covered by public programs or other discount arrangements; for example, because Medicare's PPS and most state Medicaid programs limit the amount that they will pay, providers have compensated by charging higher prices to nongovernmental payers such as private insurance companies and self-insured employers.

All-payer systems eliminate the cost-shifting problem, because every payer then faces the same charge for a given type of service. Such systems have been used in some states for the reimbursement of hospital care. Maryland, New Jersey, New York, and Massachusetts, which all had above-average hospital charges and length-of-stay figures, instituted all-payer rate controls early; as a result, inflation in the cost of health care was held several points below the national average. For example, in 1977, Maryland's hospital costs were 20 percent higher than the national average, but by 1985, they were only 1 percent higher. In that year, Maryland also recorded greater decreases in hospital admissions and length of hospital stays than the United States as a whole. These trends continued through the 1980s.

When PPS was introduced in 1983, the four states with all-payer systems already in place were exempted from it, and states were allowed to remain exempt as long as their growth of hospital rates did not surpass the national average. New York and Massachusetts decided to drop the exemption rather than try to meet that standard (and because of hospital-group opposition to the resulting stringent regulation of rates). New Jersey remained exempt somewhat longer, but it too relinquished its exemption. In 1992, Maryland was the only remaining state with exemption status, and policymakers there hope to remain exempt; they believe that their system leads to more efficient treatment for all patients, not just those under Medicare. Another important aspect of this Maryland program is that a hospital's costs that are attributable to "bad debt" from charity care are shared equally by all private and public payers, which is not necessarily so in other states.

Cost-shifting benefits some payers at the expense of others. Government payers are able to use legislation and regulation to protect themselves from this phenomenon, so it is usually a problem for private insurers, who are understandably angered by this. As private payers continue to feel its economic effects, cost-shifting has the potential to become a significant policy issue.

Furthermore, cost-shifting highlights a feature of the U.S. health care system that has long been felt to be a drawback, namely, its piecemeal nature. From payment source to payment reform, only one part of the system is affected at a time, and like squeezing a balloon, constriction in one area causes expansion in another. As a result, the elusive goal of overall improvement in the economic health of the system has not been achieved.

The United States now has a ten-year history of private sector and public policy efforts toward cost containment, but these efforts have been without major success. Some analysts feel that global budgeting and all-payer (or single payer) reforms are the only potential solutions to this problem. They note that global budgeting, along with other factors, has successfully controlled the costs of health care in countries with such a system. Whether such reforms will be implemented in the current U.S. sociopolitical environment, however, remains to be seen.

The Prospective Payment System has had a profound effect on both patients and hospitals, and RBRVS-based fee schedules and VPS promise to have a similarly significant effect on practitioners. Present trends indicate that UCR-based FFS will continue to give way to other far-reaching systems of reimbursement, featuring new structures and incentives. The following chapter explores the impact of both these as well as other cost-control measures on the new medical marketplace.

CHAPTER 7

THE CHANGING MEDICAL MARKETPLACE

The 1983 Medicare DRG-based prospective payment legislation as well as other cost-containment measures fueled competitive pressures that had been simmering in the health care industry since the 1970s. This chapter explores some of these factors and describes the new competitive milieu in which today's providers practice.

It has been said that the health care industry was motivated in the 1960s by the "access imperative," grew in the 1970s because of the "technological imperative," and was driven in the 1980s by the "managerial imperative" (Iglehart 1986). If trends to date are any indication, the 1990s, building on influences from previous eras, will be the era of accountability and effectiveness.

Efforts at cost containment have led to significant changes in the organization, management, and ownership of health care facilities; in the relationships between the various participants; and in how care is delivered. A transformation is now under way that rivals the restructuring that followed the publication of the Flexner Report in 1910 and the introduction of Medicare and Medicaid in 1966.

The Issues Involving the Prospective Payment System

Because PPS so profoundly affects hospitals, it is worthwhile to consider some potential pitfalls with this program. Some problems derive from DRGs, others from PPS's reimbursement formulas, and still others from the financial incentives that it creates.

A major difficulty with PPS is its basis in DRGs, which critics have called "Damn-Ridiculous Groups." For example, Guillain-Barré syndrome, having an average length of stay of 40 days, is categorized in the same DRG as migraine headache, which rarely requires hospitalization. The present DRG categorization scheme does not account for most components of the severity of an illness.

Payment under PPS also is based on average use of resources and length of stay, but patients who are severely ill consume more resources than the average. The severity of an illness is affected by whether or not there is an accompanying condition, the timeliness with which the patient seeks care, complications such as drug reactions, and many other factors beyond the control of the provider. PPS reimbursement, however, does not allow for increases in payments for more severely ill patients unless their complications place them into another DRG or their treatment reaches the outlier cutoff (at which point the hospital is paid a portion of the additional costs). A variety of methods to derive *severity-of-illness* scores are now being used on a hospital-by-hospital or a statewide basis, mainly for UR purposes.

Some hospital administrators have discovered ways to maximize their DRG-based payment as well. This strategy, which results in "DRG creep," involves the subtle manipulation of diagnostic coding to make patients appear more ill than they actually are. This can be accomplished by reordering or modifying the listing of the patient's discharge diagnoses and procedures in their medical record. In fact, hospital administration and financing journals are replete with advertisements by firms guaranteeing that their computer software can improve DRG reimbursements by x percent or y dollars by just this type of modification (Fig. 17). Payers have become savvy to this type of gaming, however, and flagrant miscoding may result in financial penalties.

Another major concern of the PPS system relates to the stifling of medical progress. The financial incentives that this method of reimbursement creates discourage spending on costly equipment, but such capital investment is usually required to foster the development of new technology. Consequently, analysts are concerned about the long-term, indirect effects that PPS and other cost-containment strategies may have on emerging medical technologies.

One such example is the cochlear implant, a surgically implanted intra-ear hearing aid. This technology was developed in the 1980s, and for some people, it permits better hearing, speech, and sound discrimination than they would ever achieve by using external

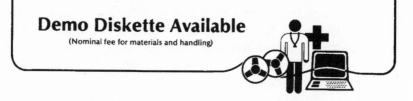
Figure 17. An advertisement from the pages of the *Journal of Health Care Financial Management.*

hearing aids. A number of such devices are under development in major academic centers around the country. Kane and Manoukian (1989) analyzed the effect of PPS on the cochlear implant procedure and found that the DRG-based Medicare payment results in a financial loss to providers for every procedure that is performed on persons over 65. Further development and innovation of this technology subsequently stopped, and some manufacturers ceased producing the device. That this technology targets mainly children makes this phenomenon more disconcerting; if PPS, which affects *Medicare* beneficiaries, was able to influence this technology to such a great extent, then what can we expect with regard to technologies geared more directly to elderly people?

It has been recommended that a budget-neutral set of DRGs be used for emerging technologies. Reimbursement on a costs-incurred basis would give clinicians the financial freedom to develop innovative procedures and therapies to their fullest. Otherwise, medical progress could be inhibited.

The Effects of Cost Containment on the Hospital

A number of changes during the late 1980s transformed the role of the hospital within the health care system. Most of these changes were stimulated by PPS, but other regulatory and competitive approaches also contributed.

First, it was predicted that hospital admissions might *increase* under PPS reimbursement, because hospitals are rewarded financially for maximizing their number of admissions. Financial incentives to the contrary, Medicare admissions actually have *decreased*. This trend began in 1982, before PPS was introduced, and accelerated after its introduction. The rate of decrease peaked from 1983 to 1985, but the decline continues even now. Hospital admissions of Medicare enrollees decreased 11 percent from 1983 to 1989 even though the number of covered beneficiaries increased 13 percent during that period; when this trend is compared to the estimated growth that would have occurred naturally (i.e., from aging of the population and increased technology), the actual decrease in admissions is something over 20 percent.

Next, PPS triggered a decline in the amount of time that patients spend in the hospital. Under PPS, hospitals profit if patients' length of stay is reduced. For the first 3 years after PPS was introduced, the average length of stay in the hospital decreased 17 percent before stabilizing; length of stay decreased 8 percent overall in the 1980s. The decrease of inpatient days attributable to shorter hospital stays peaked from 1983 to 1985, and this factor no longer contributes to the overall reduction in hospital use. The average hospital occupancy rate, which had been steady at approximately 76 percent from 1960 through 1980 showed a marked decline at 1984, and in the late 1980s, it hovered at 66%. From 1985 to

1987, the number of hospital beds decreased almost 4 percent as a result of hospital closures and down-sizings.

Hospital costs increased only 5.3 percent from 1983 to 1984, compared with an average annual increase of 15.7 percent from 1975 to 1983; however, *per-day* costs increased more than 13 percent from 1983 to 1984, indicating that the overall decrease came largely from a decline in the number of days of care. One factor contributing to these increased per-day costs is that end-of-stay days have been largely eliminated, and the shorter hospital stay is more resource intensive. In addition, the percentage of more seriously ill patients in the hospital has increased now that healthier people are so often treated as outpatients and, of course, serious illnesses require more intensive, more costly care.

Several reasons exist for the continuing decline in hospital admissions. Some analysts think it may be due partly to the influence of PROs and other UR agents, because all PPS admissions (as well as most others) come under such scrutiny. As practitioners now must justify their hospital admissions to third-party payers, the decision to admit is likely becoming more conservative. Increases in both the amount and the intensity of care that is delivered in the ambulatory setting also are associated with decreasing admissions, and because admissions have decreased for all payers and not just for Medicare, the general decline likely reflects these other changes in the health care system.

Because a hospital's revenue depends on its number of admissions and the level of services those patients receive while in the hospital, these recent changes potentially have significant financial consequences for U.S. hospitals. In fact, many analysts predicted that PPS reimbursement would cause hospitals severe financial losses. That did not happen across the board, but many hospitals are operating in the red. In contrast, some facilities have earned record profits under PPS, and overall, hospitals have continued to profit, even though margins (i.e., revenue exceeding expenses) have declined from 15 percent in the first year of PPS to 8 percent in its third year.

Hospitals' *patient margins* (revenue in excess of the costs of patient care) have decreased, however, from 1.9 percent in 1984 to the 0 to 0.1 percent range during the 1987–1990 period. Margins for patients under Medicare were approximately 13 percent in 1984 and 1985 and declined to 2.4 percent in 1988. Medicare patient care margins were −3.2 percent in 1989 and −6.0 percent in 1990, thus indicating that, on the whole, hospitals appear to have been losing money by treating patients under Medicare. Cost-shifting has compensated for this, as have revenue from interest income, state tax appropriations, and income from office buildings, private laboratories, real estate holdings, grants, and donations. *Total* margins of American hospitals declined only 1.2 percent during this period (from 6.2 percent to 5.0 percent).

Some hospitals that "closed" reopened under new names or management or merged with other facilities. Of approximately 6900 hospitals, 558 community hospitals as well as 203 hospitals of other types closed, but 120 of these were actually mergers. In fact, the number of employees in the health care industry continues to grow. A shift of emphasis is evident, however; the number of employees in marketing, advertising, and public relations grew 71 percent over 6 years in the mid-1980s while aides, orderlies, and attendants decreased 27 percent during the same period. By 1989, there were 7 percent fewer hospitals than in 1979 and 5 percent fewer beds. In 1990, it was estimated that 12 percent of all hospitals were financially unstable and at continued risk. Moreover, the geographic areas with the greatest need (e.g., inner-city and rural areas) were affected disproportionately by these closures and potential closures.

The Shift toward Ambulatory Care

Because of the pressure from payers to minimize inpatient care, hospitals are once again becoming a place for treating only severe clinical conditions. Lesser problems increasingly are being treated in hospital outpatient departments or at off-site locations.

The Prospective Payment System has encouraged this shift toward ambulatory care, but other forces have contributed as well. As recently as 15 years ago, health insurance policies often excluded ambulatory coverage in favor of the same services but provided in hospitals; patients also seemed to prefer in-hospital care. Once payers discovered that keeping beneficiaries out of the hospital offered the same clinical results while saving them money, however, the payers altered their reimbursement incentives to encourage outpatient care.

Today, both insurers and patients show a preference for outpatient services. In fact, "some have suggested that patients increasingly associate hospitals with death" (Moxley and Roeder 1984, p. 196). This may be a realistic attitude: as in-hospital services become increasingly restricted to major surgery and the treatment of major illnesses, those who are in the hospital are on average much sicker now than a few years ago. (This trend has been documented through the use of severity-of-illness measures.)

Largely resulting from these factors, ambulatory facilities have grown tremendously. Ambulatory surgery is one newly favored type of medical care, now that technologic improvements have made it increasingly feasible. These improvements include better surgical techniques, such as the use of lasers, that minimize cutting and blood loss, and improved anesthetic agents that "can keep patients asleep for 30 minutes to nearly 12 hours and still leave them clear enough to go home shortly after awakening" (ibid., p. 195). An estimated 40 percent of surgical procedures can now be performed safely in an ambulatory setting, and savings have been estimated at 50 percent to 60 percent per procedure, owing primarily to the elimination of the charges associated with the overnight stay in the hospital.

Because no requirement exists that ambulatory surgery take place out of the hospital, many hospitals have responded by creating their own ambulatory surgery facilities, a process that is often termed *same-day surgery*. The patient enters early on the day of the surgery, and the patient leaves later that same day (unless an unexpected complication occurs). Additionally, it is estimated that approximately 1500 independent ambulatory surgery centers (or *surgi-centers*) now compete directly with hospitals.

Other new types of facilities include freestanding emergency-care centers (FECs), urgent-care centers, and convenience-care centers. Offering less expensive care with greater accessibility, these facilities were designed to compete with both hospital emergency rooms and conventional doctors' offices. Those using the word *emergency* in their name (often on a neon marquee) must meet strict regulatory requirements: they must be equipped to provide the same care that is available in a hospital emergency room. There are few true FECs in the United States, and many of these are being recast as urgent-care centers. Those that do exist are usually satellite facilities linked to hospitals, and they usually provide 24-hour care 7 days per week. Many have been built to skirt one or another regulation that applies to hospitals. Little information is known about the quality of care in these facilities, and their role in the health care sector remains controversial.

Centers that are not designed to treat patients who are critically ill are termed *urgent-care* (or "urgi-care") *centers*. These facilities commonly are open 7 days a week for between 12 and 16 hours per day. Most are equipped to do some laboratory and radiologic testing and thus provide episodic care for routine conditions such as sore throats and minor emergencies such as lacerations, sprains, and simple fractures. Many patients view the urgent-care center as a back-up source of care when their family doctor is unavailable.

Because urgent-care centers charge less than hospital emergency rooms, payers have created reimbursement incentives to encourage their use. This helps explain the proliferation of "doc in the boxes" along the major thoroughfares of U.S. suburbs (though doubtless other reasons, such as the accelerating pace of the U.S. lifestyle, also exist). Unlike hospitals, these centers do not maintain expensive standby equipment or specialized, highly trained personnel; patients who are seriously ill are simply transferred to hospitals that can treat them. As a result, urgent-care centers have lower overhead costs and can offer their services at lower prices than hospitals, and to maintain their market share, some hospitals have responded by opening their own lower-priced, urgent-care centers adjacent to their emergency rooms.

Many urgent-care centers now also offer nonurgent, continuing-care services, creating what have been termed *convenience-care centers*. Commonly located in shopping centers and malls, these facilities attract many patients because of their convenient access. Considered together, it is estimated that there were over 2500 FECs, urgent-care centers, and convenience-care facilities in 1990.

Home Care

Home care is another logical extension of the trend toward outpatient care, and home care for certain conditions has become a popular way of saving money. For many years, agencies have provided chronically ill and infirm elderly patients with hygiene and physical therapy in their own homes as a cost-effective alternative to institutional care, and with the aging of the U.S. population, the number of patients who require this level of care can be expected to increase exponentially. Today's technologic sophistication has made it possible to treat additional patients at home, however, as technology-based services have added another dimension to home health care.

One of the most significant advances along these lines is the development of portable equipment for intravenous (IV) therapy that makes it possible to administer antibiotics, chemotherapy, and parenteral nutrition in the patient's home. Outpatient IV therapy was first reported in the medical literature in 1974. Not only is it less expensive than inpatient IV therapy, the rate of complications (such as line infection) has been found to be less than or, at worst, equal to the inpatient rate, particularly compared with hospitals that lack a full-time IV therapy team. The resulting savings for conditions such as osteomyelitis, endocarditis, and cellulitis, which all require long-term IV antibiotic therapy, can be significant.

As expected, payers have perceived the advantages of home health care in such circumstances, and most commercial insurance plans now include home health benefits. Some insurers still pay only 80 percent of home health charges while covering 100 percent of inpatient services, but this policy is in decline.

In the public sector, mandatory Medicaid benefits for home health care (for persons who otherwise would be confined to a nursing home) include nursing services (on a part-time or intermittent basis), services from a home health aide, and medical supplies and equipment. Optional Medicaid benefits include physical therapy, occupational therapy, and speech therapy, as well as private-duty nursing. Medicaid expenditures for home health care have skyrocketed from $25 million in 1973 to $1.35 billion in 1986, comprising a 36 percent annual rate of growth.

Medicare also provides home health care benefits that Congress liberalized in 1981. Medicare provides these services for enrollees who are under a physician's care, confined to the home, and need skilled nursing care. Covered benefits include skilled nursing care, physical therapy, occupational therapy, speech therapy, home health-aide services, and supplies and appliances (excluding drugs). The use of home health care by Medicare beneficiaries has increased, and the program's expenditures for home care have risen dramatically since 1970, when they stood at $61.5 million. In 1986, Medicare spent $1.8 billion, reflecting a 20 percent annual rate of growth during this time.

In response to increasing demand (likely due in significant part to the Medicare legislation, which often establishes the trend for the U.S. health care system), the market for home health care blossomed around 1983. In 1976, there were 2400 Home Health Agencies (HHAs) that met Medicare standards and qualified to receive Medicare reimbursement; by 1986, there were 6000 approved HHAs. These agencies employ some 70,000 home care providers. Many hospitals are entering this market, and some insurance plans now are incorporating home health programs based on the PPO model.

These changes are reflected in a major shift in the work setting for health care employees. A steady decrease in full-time–equivalent hospital employees began in 1983. In 1970, 63 percent of all health care workers were employed by hospitals, but this proportion dropped to 50 percent by 1989 as workers shifted to other settings for the delivery of health care.

Issues Concerning Long-Term Care

Concerns have been raised that patients are discharged from the hospital "sicker and quicker" under PPS. As PPS created financial incentives for the earlier discharge of patients, a new patient category resulted; those who previously would have been kept in the hospital several days longer but who now must leave. National studies have not documented any adverse effects from PPS on the quality of care, but global needs for long-term care have likely increased.

Some patients who are discharged from the hospital earlier are being transferred to skilled nursing facilities for intense rehabilitation. Shaughnessy and Kramer found that in nursing homes with a high percentage of Medicare enrollees, indicators of resource needs increased 15.5 percent from 1982 to 1986. They pointed out that "both the prospective payment system and Medicaid reimbursement and regulatory policies appear to have substantially changed the nature of long-term care at a time when demand for such care is increasing. Physicians and other care givers must recognize that different types of care are now required of long-term care providers. Payers, regulators, and providers alike must understand the need for a careful analysis of the way we pay for long-term care and ensure its quality" (1990, p. 26).

Alternatives to nursing homes are another area of growth, reflecting both the needs and the preferences of patients, families, and payers. Examples include "life-care" communities that provide a continuum of care, supervised housing for infirm elderly people, and adult day-care programs. These programs and facilities proliferated in response to changing societal needs for the care of a growing elderly population.

At present, Medicare does not pay for chronic care in a nursing home. Long-term care coverage for many elderly people is provided by Medicaid, a program not originally intended for this purpose, and policy reforms will likely be needed as a result of these shifts in resource requirements.

For-Profit Medicine

Most hospitals are owned by nonprofit, tax-exempt entities that reinvest surplus revenue into the organization rather than pay it out as dividends to either owners or investors. It is clear from the profit margins reported earlier, however, that a well-run hospital is a potentially profitable investment. As entrepreneurs and Wall Street investors have come to recognize this, the investment in for-profit, investor-owned health care facilities has grown. Three decades ago, a hospital-bed shortage and the passage of both Medicare and Medicaid legislation "created the preconditions for the establishement and growth of the for-profit hospital chains" (Ginzberg 1988, p. 757). In the following decade, nonprofit beds increased 28 percent, while for-profit beds increased 55%. Whereas the number of *nonprofit* hospital beds increased from 446,000 in 1960 to 668,000 in 1988, the number of *proprietary* beds increased from only 37,000 in 1960 to 104,000 in 1988—a much greater proportionate increase.

Some for-profit facilities are owner-operated; others are part of investor-owned multifacility systems. The concerns that most critics have of for-profit medicine focus on the latter: "Because of their size, resources (both economic and political), ambitious growth strategies, and centralized control of multiple institutions, the importance of the investor-owned hospital companies should not be minimized; they are to the old 'doctor's hospitals' what agribusiness is to the family farm" (Gray and McNerney 1986, p. 1525).

Relman coined the label *medical-industrial complex* to describe the for-profit sector of the health care industry, and today, for-profit, investor-owned corporations operate approximately 1000 hospitals, 300 HMOs, 1500 independent convenience-care clinics, more than 14,500 nursing homes (approximately 77 percent of the total), and many other health care facilities. In 1990, more than 15 percent of nongovernmental acute-care hospitals and 50 percent of psychiatric hospitals were proprietary. In addition, numerous home care agencies, diagnostic laboratories, hemodialysis centers, mobile computed tomography (CT) scanners, and other types of delivery organization are part of the for-profit sector. In total, such organization receive approximately 15 percent to 20 percent of all expenditures for health care, and the largest have annual sales in the billions of dollars. It is estimated that the five largest corporations control over two thirds of all investor-owned hospitals. (Part III discusses some concerns about the role of for-profit medicine.)

The growth of for-profit health care facilities as well as heightened competition among hospitals for patients explain why advertising for hospitals now appears on television and billboards. Ginzberg pointed out that investor-owned hospitals did well in the 1970s, but with the changes in reimbursement and the resulting shift toward ambulatory care, the for-profit sector is now downsizing. This is reflected in data from the late 1980s, as the number of for-profit hospitals declined during that time.

The Integration of Providers

Another fairly recent trend is toward corporate consolidation. Given the incentives that cost containment creates, hospital ad-

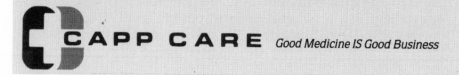

Figure 18. An advertisement from the pages of *Hospitals* seeking institutions to join an integrated "managed-care" network.

ministrators have recognized the advantage of owning a number of facilities. In some cases, medical facilities that are too inefficient or inflexible to survive in the new environment are being acquired by or merged with more successful facilities to form multifacility systems. (Such a trend is evident in the large number of small hospitals that closed in the latter half of the 1980s.) This process, termed *horizontal integration,* occurs in both the for-profit and the nonprofit sectors. The resulting arrangement is analogous to a chain of restaurants: one organization owns a number of facilities that provide the same type of service. In 1990, over one-third of all community hospitals were part of multihospital systems.

To offset the concomitant loss of income as well as to coordinate a variety of services for patients, many hospitals now offer prehospital care (such as ambulatory services) and posthospital care (such as long-term care). As part of this attempt to provide "cradle to grave" services, hospitals are purchasing or merging with nursing homes, psychiatric hospitals, outpatient surgery centers, and other facilities, and they are creating satellite outpatient centers and HMO networks. This type of expansion is known as *vertical integration:* one legal entity operates a group of facilities that together offer a broad range of services. Recently, HCFA has begun to explore a system that would require hospitals to coordinate posthospital treatments and pay for them out of a DRG-like fixed fee. Such a bundling approach, integrating both inpatient and limited posthospital care, would further fuel this trend.

In a further integration of the subsectors within the health care system, some hospitals are selling their own health insurance policies; for example, the Humana Corporation, a large owner of hospitals, has sold group policies to thousands of corporate employers and now insures hundreds of thousands of workers. Conversely, many insurance companies are becoming health care providers either by acquiring or forming their own HMOs and PPOs or by investing in or operating hospital chains. In short, medical providers and insurers—of which many, if not most, are for-profit corporations—increasingly are offering the same services and thus competing with each other.

Some analysts believe that a handful of such integrated companies—termed *Super-Meds* by Ellwood, who also coined the term *health maintenance organization*—in the future may control a majority of U.S. health care delivery. In the extreme outcome, "If current trends continue, the number of major parties involved in the health care enterprise will be reduced to only two. The new first party will be the governmental or business purchaser of health care, and the new second party will be the nationwide suppliers of health care—the megacorporate health care delivery systems" (Freedman 1985, p. 580).

Managed-Care Systems

The two main *managed-care* systems are HMOs and PPOs. In 1991, over 590 HMOs existed, with over 32 million members. Over the last decades, HMOs grew rapidly—over 250 percent since 1983—and became increasingly popular with employers as well as with Medicare and Medicaid officials.

No two HMOs are quite alike, but there are four broad types. In the *Staff Model,* physicians are employed directly by the organization on a salaried basis. Next is the Group Model, in which a large group practice, corporately separate from the HMO, contracts to provide the care. Third, the *Independent Practice Association* (IPA) Model brings together solo practitioners or small groups who agree to see HMO patients in addition to their FFS patients. This is the most common type of HMO, with 40 percent of their total enrollment. Finally, in the *Network Model* (which is similar to an IPA), an HMO contracts with two or more larger group practices to provide care to their patients.

Today, most HMO plans, like indemnity plans, do not cover long-term care; however, as the U.S. population ages, the costs of long-term care will consume an ever-larger proportion of health care expenditures. These facts provided the impetus for HCFA to fund several experiments concerning an interesting new type of HMO, dubbed the *Social HMO* (or S/HMO), which is designed to serve elderly people by integrating the services of a typical HMO with long-term care (notably home care and nursing home care). If current demographic trends continue, then the costs of long-term care will consume an ever-larger proportion of health care expenditures, and there will be increasing pressure to find ways of paying for those costs on a capitation basis.

The rapid growth of HMOs is thought likely to decrease the nation's need for new physicians, at least in the short term, because

HMOs and other types of organized medical care delivery require fewer physicians than FFS arrangements do. As a result, recent projections indicate that even fewer new physicians may be necessary over the next decade or so than experts had previously estimated. (This could exacerbate the apparent oversupply of physicians, but there are other temporizing factors, such as more women physicians and an overall change in preference of practitioners toward shorter work weeks.)

A close cousin of the HMO, termed the *preferred provider organization* (PPO), also is undergoing explosive growth. As of 1990, over 685 plans were offering care to more than 36 million consumers—both figures up by several hundred percent since 1983. PPOs may be operated by insurance companies, independent entrepreneurs, hospitals, physician groups, or by some combination of these sponsors as in the Medical Staff and Hospital (MeSH) PPO, where a hospital and a collection of physicians jointly form a corporate entity. "Meshing," it is claimed, gives both groups incentives to work in tandem to achieve an efficent delivery process. Still uncommon at present, this arrangement may become more prevalent in the future.

Preferred provider organizations have been able to expand rapidly by capitalizing on providers' desires to retain their market share as well as payers' desires to reduce their costs, but the future of such organizations is unclear. Critics not only question whether discounting can go on forever but also fear that in the absence of prepayment or risk-sharing incentives, practitioners will continue to provide more services than are necessary. Some believe that PPOs will take over some of the prepayment market or possibly introduce some risk-sharing provisions, thereby blurring the line between PPOs and IPA-model HMOs.

In the late 1980s, a new variation of the managed-care plan, known as the *open HMO* or *point-of-service plan,* entered the scene. In these hybrid plans, a patient chooses among both HMO and non-HMO providers at the time that medical care is sought. As in PPOs, higher cost-sharing is required for care that is received from non-HMO professionals, but unlike most PPOs, many point-of-service plans use a primary-care gatekeeper.

In the 1980s, several well-known analysts predicted that half of all U.S. citizens could be members of HMOs or PPOs by 1990; statistics reveal that in 1990, approximately 30 percent of the pop-

ulation was enrolled in such plans. PPOs and HMOs did not succeed to the extent predicted, but they have nevertheless dramatically affected both medical practice and insurance. Among other
things, many physicians are either in one of the so-called *three-let-
ter health plans* or competing with one. In either case, an efficient
practice style has become essential.

As a means of retaining their market share against HMOs and
PPOs by improving their own cost efficiency, private indemnity insurance companies have taken to offering *managed indemnity
plans* (MIPs). In these plans, the insurers (or the self-insured employers) have incorporated some characteristics of HMOs. Managed indemnity plans allow the consumer to pick any participating
provider and typically pay hospitals and practitioners on an undis-
counted FFS basis, but for most costly clinical decisions (such as
elective admission to the hospital, nonemergency surgery, psychotherapy, or physical therapy), the practitioner must verify in advance, on pain of nonpayment, that the patient's case meets the
insurer's criteria. Some believe that all FFS insurance plans will
soon have similar provisions. As of 1990, MIPs probably represent
more than 40 percent of all private insurance plans. These plans
can be considered a third major type of managed-care system.
Table 8 shows the probable effect of the major types of health insurance plan on the use of services by patients.

Table 8.   Probable Effects of the Type of Health Insurance Plan on the Delivery of Medical Care

Characteristic of medical care	Expected impact on consumer use/physician practice*				
	Conventional FFS insurance plan	Managed indemnity plan	PPO	IPA/network-model HMO	Staff/group-model HMO
Ability to choose primary–care physician	++	?	–	–	––
Preventive visits	––	––	+	++	++
Illness–related visits to primary–care physician	–	–	+	++	++
Visits to specialists	++	+	+	–	––
Use of diagnostic tests	++	–	–	–	––
Rate of surgery	++	–	–	–	––
Admission to hospital	++	–	–	–	––

Note: ––, should decrease; –, tends to decrease; ?, direction of effect is unclear; +, tends to increase; ++, should increase.
*All else being equal.

Access, 1980s-Style

"Doctors will have to begin appreciating our business and striving to keep it. They'll have to descend to earth." So wrote Jean Lawrence in a 1984 *Washington Post* article that pointed out a trend toward the increasing importance of price, accessibility, and convenience to the patient–physician relationship. Whereas in the 1960s the term *access* denoted the need to make health care available to poor and underserved people, in the 1980s it just as often referred to patients' desire for decreased waiting time and lower costs. Lawrence went on to say, "[consumers] have a right not to wait more than 15 minutes in the doctor's office." The patient-rights movement was in part a reaction to the myriad changes in medicine that affected everything from patients' relationships with their physicians to the settings in which they received their care. This trend continues in the 1990s, tempered only by the financial constraints that patients experience as a result of increased cost-sharing, benefit reduction, and limited choice of provider.

Effective practice management has become very important to physicians, both because patients are demanding convenience and because lower reimbursement necessitates efficiency. Not only have many physicians computerized their record-keeping, billing, and scheduling of appointments, but more and more of them now are using marketing services and advertising (Fig. 19) to attract new patients. Some have gone even further and turned to business management consultants and management-oriented journals to develop skills that will help them in the competition for patients. The best clinicians, however, know that what attracts and keeps patients is knowledge, skill, and caring.

Overall Effects of Cost-Control Measures

It appears that DRGs have led to decreased outlays for health care: expenditures by Medicare Part A per enrollee were estimated to grow just one fourth as fast as the annual rate for Medicare Part B. PPS, however, applies to only inpatient Medicare benefits, which comprise only 10 percent of all U.S. health care costs. Between 1984 and 1987, Medicare's inpatient hospital costs increased 4 percent per year, but outpatient costs increased *20 percent* annu-

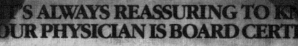
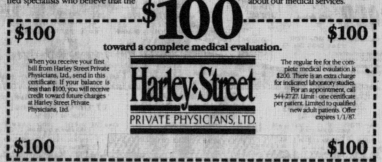
Figure 19.

ally. The costs of posthospital nursing homes also may have increased. The most common analogy is the "squeezed balloon;" as costs of in-hospital care have been squeezed, the costs of ambulatory care have ballooned. Thus, to look at the effect of PPS on costs, it is necessary to look at data regarding the entire spectrum of care settings. The appearance of savings may result not so much from cost control but from cost-shifting. Outpatient services will be targeted next for cost containment.

In 1984, spending on health care increased less than 3 percent in real terms (adjusted for inflation), which was the smallest increase in 20 years. However, overall expenditures have continued their steady increase since then (by approximately 4 percent per year in real terms and 8 percent in dollar amounts), reaching $738 billion in 1991; they continue to constitute a significant portion of national spending (13 percent of GDP in 1991). Moreover, private employer groups are attacking their health care costs with renewed fervor, necessary because in the late 1980s and early 1990s, increases in corporate health insurance premiums (20 percent, on average) were higher than for any other years in recent memory.

How long such increases can go on is unclear. The U.S. government has shown renewed interest in developing a balanced budget, and it is expected that decreases in spending on health care will be part of the balancing process. Meanwhile, adequate health care coverage has become a major political issue as the uninsured population grows and payers intrude more and more boldly into the process of care delivery. It seems unlikely, therefore, that trends in health care expenditures will change greatly until substantial reforms of the system itself are undertaken.

In conclusion, it appears that the new medical marketplace is many things. It is a *vehicle* for cost control, in that many market innovations have been made for that specific reason. It is also a *response* to cost-cutting initiatives, or a way of making them work. But it is more than just a vehicle or a response: it has taken on a life of its own. There is no returning to the fee-for-service and laissez-faire days of the 1960s. The revolution has occurred, and the new medical marketplace not only is established but is self-perpetuating.

PART III

CARE, COST, AND CONSCIENCE

Ideas are clean. They soar in the serene
supernal. I can take them out and look
at them, they fit in books, they lead
me down that narrow way. And in the
morning they are there. Ideas are straight—
But the world is round, and a
messy mortal is my friend.
Come walk with me in the mud. . . .

Hugh Prather

Medical practice occurs within a complex society, of which health care is only one element. As such, the goals of patients, practitioners, payers, and of society at large are not always concordant; conflict may ensue. The chapters that follow examine the relationships between medical practitioners and the other participants in the U.S. system of health care within the context of the broader society.

Part II focused on the payers and policymakers as well as their responses to the crisis in health care costs. In contrast, this section will emphasize the effects of financial and organizational changes on the process of health care delivery and how the new medical marketplace affects both patients and providers. Again, Hammarskjöld's principle applies—this time to payers and policymakers.

Certain problems are inherent in the delivery of health care, and the cost containment era has compounded these difficulties indirectly. The allocation of medical technology provides one example. Before cost containment, some ethical issues surrounding the distribution of scarce high-technology resources were recognized; after cost containment began, expensive technologic care became even more inaccessible to people unable to pay for their medical care. The current emphasis on ethics, the quality of care and resource allocation thus derives from effects of cost containment.

The Elements of Clinical Decision-Making

In the practice of medicine, persons with physical or psychologic complaints seek advice and treatment from trained professionals. *Clinical decisions* are made during these interactions, and those decisions determine how (if possible) the patient's problem will be ameliorated. The patient–physician interaction usually is quite complex. Every meeting is unique, and in the best case, it involves an appropriate combination of both art and sophisticated science. One might argue that such complexity defies analysis.

There are some commonalities across patient–clinician interactions, however. These exist by virtue of the similarity among patients and because standard methods of education are used to teach a somewhat circumscribed body of knowledge. The clinical decision-making process is comprised of three major components: technical, financial, and ethical. Each component has become considerably more complicated since the recent revolution in health care, and in the section that follows, we dissect the clinical decision-making process by sequentially exploring these various factors.

Technical knowledge has contributed to clinical decision-making for the last 100 years, during which time the body of biomedical knowledge has grown exponentially. This progress has affected the nature of medical care and the settings in which it is provided. It has changed both the patient–physician relationship and their expectations about the process of care and its outcomes. Societal goals for the health care system have also evolved. Chapter 8 explores the technical aspect of clinical decision-making in greater detail.

The recent *financial* metamorphosis of the U.S. health care system has superimposed a new dimension onto the clinical decision-making process. Whereas 100 years ago financial transactions between patients and physicians were direct, and 20 years ago third-party payers had a laissez-faire attitude toward clinical decisions, practitioners today are being asked to consider cost as they make decisions about the care of their patients. Chapter 9 explores the influence of financial factors on decision-making.

Ethics has always been a central feature of medical care in that practitioners have been expected to do what is best for their patients, but several developments have served to increase its importance. Scientific progress has altered the provision, the nature, and the quality of medical care, and budget constraints have created questions regarding the optimal use of resources. Social changes have concurrently raised the level of consciousness about patient autonomy and related rights. New ethical issues have developed as a result of these forces, and all reflect a more complex patient–provider relationship. Some of these issues were explored in Chapter 1 from the historical perspective; Chapter 10 explores the evolving roles of ethical considerations and professional standards in today's system.

While we will consider these three relatively distinct aspects of clinical care individually, we recognize that they are fundamentally interwoven in medical practice. They must be considered simultaneously during the process of delivering health care.

The Resistance to Change

Many new elements of the present health care system are here to stay, and clinicians must evolve in response to them. Regarding the financial crisis in the health care system, Lister pointed out that "most clinicians, when presented with these facts, fail to grasp the magnitude of the numbers, dismiss the issue as irrelevant to the care of the suffering, or react defensively as though the honor and integrity of the healing professions were under attack. Once we begin to confuse the willingness of society to continue paying the bill for health care with the legitimacy of our profession's attempts to help people, the possibility of dialogue evaporates" (1991, p. 9).

Physicians and other medical practitioners have generally resisted this type of examination. Surveys have documented that they are more satisfied with the system (Table 9) than are the other key participants. It is understandable to prefer the status quo, but by *reacting* rather than *acting,* clinicians forfeit the opportunity to participate in and influence the process of change. This stance has not gone unnoticed by administrators, patients, policymakers, and payers, who all now perceive clinicians as one of the major barriers to needed change.

It is not only pointless but also counterproductive for physicians to resist the new era, because the interest of all parties is served best by their full participation. Also, because at least some of today's problems were created by practitioners, it can be argued that the primary responsibility for their resolution rests with that same group.

Any change can be perceived either as a constraint or as a possibility for growth and improvement. Whether the process is active or passive, however, change is inevitable, and physicians face choices in

Table 9. Overall Views of the U.S. Health Care System Held by Physicians and Others, 1990

View	201 Physician Leaders	251 Hospital CEOs	1501 Members of the public
On the whole, the health care system works pretty well, and only minor changes are necessary to make it work better	31%	14%	21%
There are some good things in our health care system, but fundamental changes are needed to make it work better	64	80	50
The U.S. health care system has so much wrong with it that we need to completely rebuild it	4	6	25

Source: Adapted from Louis Harris and Associates, Inc. 1990.

how they adapt to the new system and whether to attempt further reform.

Part III highlights current issues and dilemmas in medical practice. We do not expect to provide the answers to these problems, only some ways to consider them. This is a first step, but in itself, it is insufficient. It will be up to individuals and the practitioner groups to attempt workable solutions and compromises to these problems within the numerous professional and political settings that make up the U.S. health care system.

Opening this section with Prather's verse serves both as a warning and invitation. The warning is that the waters we are about to enter are murky. Many of the issues examined are controversial, and some will strike close to home. Complex intellectual and ethical questions abound, and most do not have only one right answer. We hope, however, that an exploration of these complex issues may provide a forum for discussions that could lead toward solutions. Yet even if there is nothing to do but simply muddle on, then a map of the terrain is helpful. What we offer is an invitation to enter the waters.

CHAPTER 8

TECHNICAL KNOWLEDGE AND CLINICAL DECISIONS

C linical decision-making is the process used to determine whether a test or a treatment should be ordered or performed given a specific constellation of patient signs (i.e., the clinicians' findings), symptoms (i.e., the problems reported by the patient), and social circumstances. Observed practice patterns represent the results of such decisions made by medical practitioners. For example, after how many strep throat infections within 1 year will a physician refer patients for tonsillectomy? Or under what circumstances does an internist order a routine chest x-ray for a patient on admission to the hospital?

As discussed in the introduction to this section, clinical decision-making is informed by several factors. The most fundamental of these—technical knowledge of the provider—is discussed in this chapter. First, the strengths and deficiencies in the technical aspects of the medical decision-making process during the present era are explored, and these are followed by a description of the various initiatives now under way to improve the knowledge base that supports clinical decision-making. New methods to evaluate both the process and the outcomes of care also are described.

Variation among Clinicians

It has been known for decades that independent practitioners examining the same patient will often reach differing clinical conclusions. One of the earliest studies of this *practice pattern variation* was carried out in the 1930s with a group of 1000 eleven-year-olds in New York City; of this group, 65 percent had already had their tonsils removed. Those with their tonsils intact were examined by a group of physicians who recommended tonsillectomy for 45 percent of them. Those for whom it was not recommended were sent for examination by another group of physicians, and 46 percent of these children were selected as candidates for tonsillectomy in this round. When this process was repeated again for the remaining children, tonsillectomy was advised for a comparable percentage. At this point, only 65 children remained for whom tonsillectomy had not been recommended, and having exhausted the supply of physicians to whom they could refer the remaining children, the investigators concluded the study.

Such observations are systematized in what are termed *small-area variation* studies, which ascertain the practice patterns within a geographically aggregated population of physicians (or of the patients they treat). According to a landmark work of this type that was carried out by Wennberg and Gittelsohn: "In one area of Vermont the tonsillectomy rate from 1969 through 1971 was such that if it had persisted, 60 percent of all children would have had their tonsils removed by age 20. In a second Vermont area the rate was such that only 8 percent would have had their tonsils removed by age 20" (1982, p. 121).

Wennberg and other investigators have found that some surgical procedures, including hysterectomy, tonsillectomy, and prostatectomy, have consistently shown high variation in incidence (up to 6-fold) across populations or regions. Other procedures, including cholecystectomy, appendectomy, and hernia repair, show lower variation. Significant variation has also been shown in the treatment of several medical conditions, such as congestive heart failure.

Other investigators have replicated these results in both cross-regional and international studies; for example, Leape et al. found that the rate of carotid endarterectomy for Medicare beneficiaries in three areas ranged from 48 to 178 per 100,000. They also found that two variables accounted for most of this variation: "the number of surgeons performing the procedure, and the number of endarterectomies performed by surgeons with high practice volumes" (1989, p. 653).

Differences in Mortality Rate: Another Reflection of Practice Variation?

With the era of cost containment came a general trend toward heightened monitoring of the costs, quality, and outcome of health care delivery. Motivated by concern that the new financial incentives might adversely affect the quality of care, such monitoring increased under Medicare's PPS. The need for monitoring also reflects a heightened interest in evaluating the consumption of health care resources.

The result of both health services research and managed-care oversight has been the generation of more data on health care delivery than in previous eras. Increased assessments have led to some surprising findings. For example, in 1987, HCFA published data indicating that mortality within U.S. hospitals varied widely; also released were lists of hospitals, with their rankings ordered by death rate. Those who provided or received care in hospitals with mortality rates that were high relative to other facilities were justifiably concerned about the meaning of these numbers.

Potential explanations for these results have been considered. For example, variations among hospitals could reflect differences in the severity of their case loads; a high mortality rate for an academic medical center could be considered an inevitable result of caring for patients who were the most ill. Some wondered if the financial incentives of PPS had adversely affected the quality of care (and hence mortality), but the data do not confirm this hypothesis. Some studies indicate that hospital mortality has increased since the introduction of PPS, but most show that PPS has not resulted in an overall reduction in the quality of care. (Furthermore, given the increased severity of illness among inpatients since PPS, the higher mortality rates are probably inevitable.) Because not all of these factors were controlled for in generating the data, however, there is no way to know which combination of potential factors contributed to HCFA's findings.

The HCFA mortality data, which were released with minimal technical interpretation, alarmed the public and generated a firestorm of controversy within the medical community. The level of distress made rational discussion difficult. Surveys indicated that most hospital administrators profoundly distrusted the data, in addition to their uncertainty about the implications; they were, however, called on to justify their facilities' performances. Many perceived in this episode a lesson in the art of public relations. Later analyses have been more sophisticated and have been handled more tactfully as well.

Variations in mortality rates have been confirmed by other studies, including those examining variations in the outcomes of surgery. Researchers have shown that based on the number of procedures performed annually by a given physician or within a given hospital, there are thresholds above which mortality decreases. Studies have been unclear whether such results confirm the hypothesis of a selective referral effect (i.e., certain surgeons operate on the patients who are the most ill) or whether the lower mortality rates result from greater technical proficiency in that "practice makes perfect."

The Sources of Practice Variation

In general, small-area variation appears to be procedure- or treatment-specific, and the variation tends to be stable from year to year. One practical explanation of small-area variation may be that practitioners who have been trained in the same program have been exposed to the same role models and traditions, thus generally adhering to a common philosophy of treatment. This creates what Wennberg (1982) termed an area's *practice signature*. Given the tendency of physicians to practice in the same area where they are trained (or to relocate to facilities where clinicians have similar styles of practice), it is likely that this de facto clustering of similarly trained clinicians contributes to small-area variation.

This still does not explain, however, why physicians in different areas would have such divergent styles of practice. Why these major differences in clinical opinion and practice occur is not at all clear, and attempts to explain small-area variations by documenting underlying differences among patient populations in terms of age, sex, race, and severity of illness have not been completely successful.

One reason that clinical decision-making varies so widely is that *uncertainty* plays such a large role in the process. In addition to the uncertainty that surrounds the usefulness of a given test or treatment, physicians are frequently uncertain whether a disease is present, whether a particular diagnosis is right, what diagnostic tests or procedures to prescribe, and what treatment is the most appropriate in terms of anticipated outcome, patient consent, and compliance. Physicians vary widely in their tolerance for uncer-

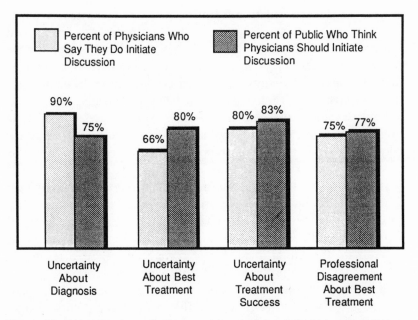

Figure 20. Uncertainty in medical care and the physician–patient interaction. (Source: President's Commission for the Study of Ethical Problems in Medicine and Biomedical and Behavioral Research 1982.)

tainty as well and, as Figure 20 shows, in their willingness to discuss their uncertainty with their patients.

Technology and Uncertainty

A fundamental source of uncertainty in clinical decision-making is the problem of applying medical science and technology to clinical decisions. It has been suggested that small-area variation is influenced by variable technology diffusion; controversial procedures show the highest degree of variability. No standardized process for the evaluation and incorporation of new technology into medical practice exists: it usually occurs in an unscientific, unplanned way. All too often, new medical technologies are applied before their cost, safety, and usefulness are adequately considered and some analysts believe that new medical technologies are proliferating beyond the profession's capacity for assessing them properly. For example, very few treatment modalities (new or otherwise) have been subjected to randomized clinical trials. As a result, "Often in medical practice ... 'the right thing' is simply a matter of opinion because many tests, procedures, and operations have not yet been fully evaluated or scientifically compared with other available measures for cost effectiveness" (Relman 1985, p. 105).

New developments also are usually disseminated through the medical literature, and this is not a value-free process. Authors naturally want to have their work accepted by their profession; thus, they tend to report favorable findings. Researchers are inclined not to report negative results, and if submitted, such reports are rarely published. Peer review mitigates these tendencies, but even this is not an unbiased process. The customary means of reporting adverse effects is the isolated case report, a process that tends to severely underestimate the actual incidence of complications. As a result, the medical literature is probably undercritical of new developments.

An example of this is the process by which the Swan-Ganz catheter (an intracardiac monitoring device that is used in patients who are critically ill or those undergoing major surgery) was adopted. Introduced in 1970, its use was favorably reported in the literature, and information about the catheter spread quickly and informally among clinicians. Its benefits are undeniable in appropriate clinical circumstances, but complications can and do occur. The causes of these complications and their statistical incidence have been examined in a few studies (e.g., Gore et al. 1987), but this procedure has yet to be fully evaluated through random, prospective clinical trials. Robin's opinion is that even though its use "has assumed epidemic proportions" (1985, p. 445), its helpfulness to a given patient or class of patients is uncertain. Much controversy and debate surrounds this issue (see Altschule 1988, Robin 1987 and 1988, Sibbald and Sprung 1988, Spodick 1989).

The opposite problem can also occur, however, whereby clinicians are strongly attached to a traditional method even when the superiority of a newer technique or approach is clearly demonstrated. Staying with the known practice and its known properties seems safer than taking the risks that accompany change, yet the costs that result from such inertia can be high. One example is the use of screening chest x-rays:

The practice of ordering chest films to screen patients admitted to hospitals gained popularity after World War II, when tuberculosis was prevalent in this country . . . However, as the prevalence of tuberculosis decreased, so did the prevalence of abnormalities detected on the chest x-ray film obtained on admission. Later, physicians began to use chest films to screen for lung cancer, hoping that with early detection, more patients would be cured. Several large studies have shown no significant difference in mortality rates between patients in whom lung cancer is detected by chest-film screening and those in whom the disease is detected by other methods, and the American Cancer Society no longer recommends chest-film screening for this disease. (Hubbell et al. 1985, p. 212)

Despite this information, many practitioners who are used to ordering admission chest x-rays resist abandoning this practice. In the mid-1980s, it was estimated that more than $1 billion was spent annually in the United States for routine, preadmission chest x-rays. And this is only one of many costly tests that are either overused or used in an outmoded style. Recently, the Blue Cross/Blue Shield Association and the American College of Physicians jointly published protocols for the appropriate use of simple diagnostic tests; if adhered to (and insurers are attempting to see that they will be), these test-ordering guidelines could save many millions of dollars each year by eliminating unnecessary testing.

The Clinical Consequences of Uncertainty

Uncertainty is an aspect of clinical decision-making that would be impossible to eliminate entirely even with the best technologic advances; however, clinicians usually do attempt to reduce its effects. Ordering tests is one common way. This has been recognized by practitioners and is reflected in several truisms that capture the essence of this approach. In the metaphoric "zebra hunt," the clinician hearing hoofbeats searches for zebras instead of horses; this refers to the tendency—particularly prevalent in academic medicine—to look for unusual conditions even when commonly occurring diseases are far more likely. In a variation on this theme, the motivation is an intolerance for ambiguity. Kassirer (1989) described this tendency to order tests "our stubborn quest for diagnostic certainty." Both the patient and the clinician may be reassured as more tests are ordered, even when further tests cannot resolve a given clinical question.

The impact of this style of practice on clinical care increased with the proliferation of new tests in what Fuchs (1974) termed the *technologic imperative.* The technologic imperative refers to the desire of both clinicians and patients to use available tests not only to reduce their uncertainty but also because of the American tendency to demand "the latest thing." Because more tests are developed as scientific progress continues, this drive only becomes stronger over time.

The epidemic of malpractice litigation has also supported this tendency. Clinicians attempt to resolve doubts about diagnosis or therapy by doing more, and doing more also maximizes the defensibility of their actions in court. As a result, the fear of litigation and this "defensive medicine" significantly influence decision-making. (See also Chapter 11.)

Certain economic influences support expensive clinical decisions as well. Under FFS reimbursement, attempting to resolve uncertainty by doing more coincides with the physician's financial incentives, and today, more than 85 percent of patients receive care under a FFS reimbursement system—for them, the provider is financially rewarded for ordering tests. As Walsh and Egdahl described it, "The Medical Uncertainty Principle states that there is always one more thing that might be done—another consultation, a new drug, a different treatment. Uncertainty is resolved by doing more: the patient asks for more, the doctor orders more. The patient's simple rule for resolving uncertainty is to seek care up to the level of his insurance" (1977, p. 21). Uncertainty may not be reduced, but the possibility that it *could* be is quite salient to both patients and practitioners.

Attempting to resolve uncertainty by doing more, however, can have negative clinical consequences. Iatrogenic damage can occur during the diagnostic process (e.g., internal bleeding from an unnecessary biopsy). Also, if enough tests are ordered, chances are that one will be abnormal, and false-positive results, acting as red herrings, can lead to either inappropriate or unnecessary treatment. Furthermore, positive test results can lead to ethical dilemmas, for example, when a clinically unnecessary sonogram reveals a fetal deformity.

The Quality of Care

In the latter part of the cost-containment era, payers have recognized that cutting costs without assessing the impact of these cuts on patient care is inappropriate. Payers now increasingly focus on the concept of "value," where value is a function of both cost and quality.

The issue of waste in health care is tied closely to the idea of *quality* and it is necessary first to agree on workable definitions of these basic but elusive concepts. Donabedian, a seminal thinker on the quality of care, defined quality as, "the application of medical science and technology in a manner that maximizes its benefits to health without correspondingly increasing its risks. The degree of quality is, therefore, the extent to which the care provided is expected to achieve the most favorable balance of risks and benefits" (1980, p. 4). In later writings, he noted that before the quality of care can be assessed, one must first define quality, health, responsibility for health, and the perspective informing the assessment (1988b). His framework for the comprehensive evaluation of the quality of care includes data on the structure in which care is provided, its process, and also its outcome.

Variables involving structure include facilities, equipment, and training (e.g., is a well-trained surgeon available to perform a bypass operation?). Studies of process evaluate the appropriateness of clinical action (e.g., is the bypass procedure done properly?). Outcome studies focus on the effects of the care on the patient (e.g., does the patient's level of functioning improve as a result of the surgery?).

Recent renewed interest in the quality of care in some ways reflects a general reaction to cutting costs, where both clinicians and consumer groups are saying that the cost-cutting onslaught can go only so far and that quality must be protected. A new trend in this area—borrowed from the manufacturing industry—is termed *Total Quality Management* or *Continuous Quality Improvement,* a comprehensive management approach that is reflected in hospital slogans such as "Quality is Job One" and "Patients First" aimed at employees. Another result is that the difference in goals between utilization review (UR) and quality assurance (QA) has become explicit. QA is no longer always a euphemism for cost containment; in some institutions, QA activities have been clarified to reflect the goal of improving the quality of care, with cost as a secondary concern. Recent changes in the assessment procedures of both PROs and the Joint Commission for the Accreditation of Health-Care Organizations (JCAHO)* reflect this trend.

The "Wasteful" Use of Resources?

The point has been made previously that one's opinion on waste in the health care system depends largely on one's perspective. For payers, increased costs in most instances are the most important consequence of the attempt to reduce uncertainty by doing more. The assumption behind many of today's cost-control measures is that waste can be removed from the system while necessary services are retained. As a result of such measures, fewer new dollars (in adjusted per-capita terms) are now entering the health care sector, and the intention is to spend these dollars first on what is truly necessary. In theory, these reduced funds will be sufficient if the 25 percent or so (some estimates range as high as 40 percent) of all care that is now deemed unnecessary is trimmed from the health care system.

This formulation is deceptively simple, assuming as it does the ability to identify which services are necessary and which are excessive, but it is hardly possible to "trim the fat without cutting into the meat" when no agreement exists on what is the fat and what is the meat. In these circumstances, tradeoffs have inevitably been made, and many have been made uncritically.

It is unclear which rates represent the "best" level of care, but by its very nature, wide variability in decision-making and outcome indicate that some patients are receiving suboptimal care. In the era of cost consciousness, variation in clinical decision-making is not well tolerated by payers. It supports to some extent the contention that some practice patterns cost too much and that costs

*Formerly the Joint Commission on Accreditation of Hospitals.

can be reduced by identifying efficient practice patterns as well as adequate (though not excessive) levels of care.

Cost-conscious payers have several other reasons to distrust the clinical decisions that providers make, including the inflationary incentives of some current methods of reimbursement, the influence of defensive medicine, the increasing incidence of physician ownership of diagnostic facilities, and the often random incorporation of new technology into practice. The growing societal orientation toward patients' rights preceded the publication of the wide variations in clinical decision-making and outcomes, but these data provided empiric support for patients' concerns about the care they receive.

Consequently, the rules of the game have changed. In contrast to only a decade or two ago, patients, payers, and society at large no longer automatically assume that what a physician recommends or does is "correct." In the era of cost containment, a provider who orders too many tests may be penalized for attempting to decrease uncertainty below the point that the payers condone.

Providers resist this type of pressure, which some perceive as an insult to their professionalism. However, for providers to resist questioning of the efficiency of current medical practice requires that they overlook fairly obvious examples of waste, such as excessive diagnostic testing. Clinical decision-making has traditionally been a matter of the practitioner's judgment and preference, but wide variation of both "accepted" practice and clinical outcome undermine the position of physicians who wish to be left alone to set their own standards.

Now is the opportunity for innovation. As Sager pointed out, "demanding more money is the path of least resistance. More money solves...short-term problems. It also obviates thoughtful reform in medical resource allocation. If hospitals and physicians could be encouraged to spend our money more wisely, they could help make equitable access durably affordable" (1988, p. 25).

Furthermore, as Wennberg and others pointed out regarding small-area variation studies, "Unless the medical profession accepts responsibility for the question of 'which rate is right' and addresses these issues within the current cost-containment context, others will see to it that the 'least is always best' theory dominates by default. After all, if physicians can't agree on what is best, why do more?" (1986, p. 311). This possibility should also motivate the profession to assist in the search for ways to reduce variation and, in every way possible, optimize medical care. Practitioners have the skill to accept this challenge as well as to succeed at it.

The involvement of practicing clinicians in this process is critical, because they have technical knowledge to contribute and also because they will be the ones to implement any resulting decisions. There are other advantages to physician leadership in the standardization process as well: "[Protocols] provide a basis for encouraging cost conscious behavior on the part of physicians in hospital settings, but they do so by allowing physicians, as a collectively responsible group, to set their own clinical standards, which effectively constitute financial standards as well" (Young 1985, p. 17). Given the resistance of clinicians to administrative fiat, peer group approaches perhaps are more palatable. It is reassuring that physicians and their professional associations are cooperating now more than ever with epidemiologists, health service researchers, and policymakers to develop practice protocols and guidelines.

As Franklin D. Roosevelt stated in a speech in 1932, "Knowledge—that is, education in its true sense—is our best protection against unreasoning prejudice and panic-making fear, whether engendered by special interest, illiberal minorities, or panic-stricken leaders" (Conlin 1984). This saying is equally applicable to payers, patients, policymakers, and providers in that maximal awareness of both the individual circumstances and societal conditions should inform the use of medical knowledge. Learning about optimal medical practice can help diminish the fire of factional, self-serving debates. Modern approaches must be truly responsive to the cost concerns of managers and payers; this was not always the case in the past. For that reason, *collaboration* among these groups is necessary.

Evaluating the Outcomes of Care

In health care, the product—conceptually speaking—is improved health status and functioning, which are the "outcomes of care." Today, payers, providers, and patients all wonder which style constitutes overtreatment and which undertreatment. Differences in practice style motivate the search for answers to several complex, crucial questions about medical care, answers that can improve the overall quality of care. Recent research trends seek to tease apart the features of successful clinical outcomes, and as the crisis in health care costs permanently changed the attitude of payers toward medical care, the realization that health care could be provided more efficiently and with more thoughtful use of technology resulted in what has been termed the *outcome* and *effectiveness* movements. These movements are likely to change permanently the delivery of medical care (Roper et al. 1988).

Several paths to improved outcomes of care exist. The most simple is to have knowledgeable, technically skilled providers, but while this might seem to be an obvious way to obtain optimal care, the situation in fact is more complex. As indicated by small-area variation, clinical decision-making varies among providers, often without a single "right" way to proceed. Because the application of technology and medical knowledge is not standardized, subtle differences between providers or practice styles may lead to very different results; thus, both *technology assessment* (systematic study of a particular test or treatment) and *medical practice evaluation* (systematic study of the effects of a practice style) have increased in importance. Medical practice evaluation reflects the idea that medical care involves the appropriate application of technology, particularly because the use of available technology is not always beneficial to the patient.

The following approaches potentially provide means toward finding an ethical balance of care, cost, and conscience at the bedside. While the terminology is fairly confusing, the fundamental idea that drives these studies is to optimize the use of resources as well as clinical results.

Types of Studies

Donabedian differentiated between *technology* assessment, or "passing a judgment on the technology itself," and *quality* assessment, which "judges the degree to which available technology is used judiciously, appropriately, and skillfully in the health care of individuals and communities" (1988a, p. 488). Tools for technology assessment and medical practice evaluation include mathematical modeling, systematic observations, experimental trials, meta-analysis, and consensus formulation. These tools can be applied to different classes of studies, three of which are termed *efficacy, effectiveness,* and *efficiency research.*

Efficacy is the study of technology under circumstances that approximate the ideal (e.g., in the laboratory). *Effectiveness* evaluates the technology under everyday circumstances (e.g., actual medical practice), and *efficiency* is the relationship that exists between inputs and outputs or between costs and consequences (ibid., p. 491). For example, when the diagnostic ability of nuclear magnetic resonance imaging (MRI) technology is assessed in major teaching hospitals, that is considered an evaluation of efficacy. An assessment of the sensitivity and specificity of MRI technology today in common practice constitutes an effectiveness analysis. An efficiency analysis would involve a comparison of the costs versus the benefits of MRI technology, either in isolation or compared with other technologies.

Two quantitative approaches that are used to assess the efficiency of treatment alternatives are *cost-benefit analysis* (CBA) and *cost-effectiveness analysis* (CEA). These methods can be applied to any given technology or treatment process. In a CBA, a monetary value is assigned to both the inputs and outcomes (for example, income earned as a result of a year of life saved). After monetary values are assigned to all outcomes, researchers then attempt to determine which of two or more alternative health care services or treatment options—with very different effects—results in the best value to society in terms of the highest monetary outcome. CBA might be used, for example, to decide whether to allocate community resources to a cancer screening program or to a coronary care unit.

In a CEA, no assignment of monetary value is made to the outcomes, and the effects are measured in nonfinancial units, such as years of life saved or morbidity avoided. Because different outcomes are not translated to a common denominator, CEA can be used only to compare programs or treatments that have similar goals (for example, treatment of coronary occlusion with surgical intervention versus medical management). Then, analogous to a CBA, researchers attempt to determine which option would result in the most desirable cost-to-effect ratio.

Table 10. Guidelines for an Economic Analysis of Medical Practice

What are the alternative clinical interventions being compared? Have the most reasonable alternatives been considered?

Is the economic analysis a cost–benefit analysis, a cost-effectiveness analysis, or some other type? Are the alternatives appropriate to the perspective adopted?

Has the effectiveness of each intervention been clearly defined and established? How is outcome being measured?

Are direct, indirect, and intangible costs and benefits explicitly defined and measured? Are both medical and nonmedical costs included? Are both morbidity and mortality costs included?

Are costs and charges differentiated?

Are appropriate adjustments made for the time value of money? For example, are future costs and benefits discounted?

Are uncertainties and biases identified and their potential effects on results measured?

Are ethical issues identified and discussed?

Source: Adapted from Eisenberg 1989.

All practitioners should become familiar with the results of these and other types of economic analysis. "Clinicians who can critically assess data on cost and effectiveness will more likely be able to retain their roles as their patients' advocates while being responsible participants in hospitals, insurance plans, health maintenance organizations, and society at large" (Eisenberg 1989, p. 2886). Table 10 is adapted from Eisenberg's work to assist clinicians in evaluating this type of research.

Data Collection

The first step in any analysis of technology or medical practice is choosing pertinent measurement variables as well as effective methods for collecting data. It is fortuitous, then, that health care analysts are becoming adept at monitoring a wide range of variables that can provide information on quality, efficient use of resources, costs, and other aspects of care.

Given the recent shift in emphasis from inpatient to outpatient care, it will be important that outcome studies collect data on treatment provided in the full spectrum of settings. Different variables will be relevant for different purposes. In some cases, outcome will be most important, and in others, the process of care—what the practitioner does—will take precedence.

Modifications in methods of data collection have been made by several organizations. For example, PROs are being pressured to

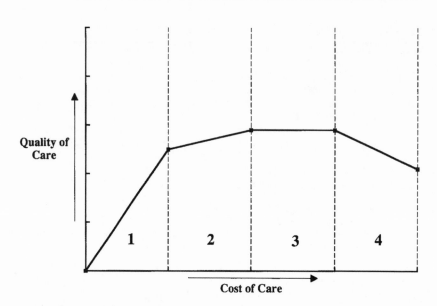

Figure 21. The theoretic relationship between the quality of medical care and the expenditure of resources.

move away from case-by-case reviews to reviewing patterns of practice across time and among patients. The JCAHO is shifting its emphasis from on-site surveys of hospitals to an end-product approach, in which it mandates that hospitals monitor *indicators* that are based on pre-established goals for their facilities.

These changes also reflect a new emphasis among analysts on collecting data regarding quality, whether it relates to an entire population or to an individual patient. Data sources include chart reviews, surveys of patients or providers, and insurance claims. Analysts have recognized that the source of the data as well as the way they are collected affect the conclusions that can be drawn about quality of care. Among the variables used to document "outcome" include morbidity and mortality, patients' functional status, hospital readmissions, and patient satisfaction.

Assessing Marginal Benefits

The concept of marginal benefits can be applied to medical testing (or any other medical technology). Initially, additional investment such as the ordering of tests improves the patient's condition (Fig.

21, Area 1). Eventually, a point of maximum efficiency is reached, where just enough is invested to gain the maximum amount of useful information (Fig. 21, Area 2). Further investment is wasted, however, because it produces no new useful information (Fig. 21, Area 3). Extreme overinvestment (such as unnecessary surgery) leads to a decline in the patient's condition (Fig. 21, Area 4) such as from increased pain or nosocomial infection.

As Donabedian wrote: "Quality costs money, but it is possible by cutting out useless services and by producing services more efficiently to obtain higher quality for the money than is now spent on care, or to have the same quality at lower cost" (1980, p. 7). Thus, improved quality of care can potentially reduce costs as well; however, if increased quality does not reduce costs, then will payers and employers remain interested in it (Geigle and Jones, 1990)? This question remains unanswered.

From the perspective of cost *or* quality, decreasing waste is desirable. But waste is not easily identified: test results are not returned from the lab labeled *useful, useless,* or *questionable.* Some alternative way to define where waste begins is needed, and a logical place to begin is with the economist's concept of marginal benefits. Economists conceptualize an ideal system in which the cost of the latest unit produced (the marginal cost) equals the price that consumers are willing to pay for it (the marginal price). Something like this theoretic point is where clinicians should begin the process of trimming waste: eliminating care that costs more than it is worth.

The following economic analysis of marginal benefits was done 10 years ago, based on the American Cancer Society's recommendation that six guaiac examinations be performed annually on all people over the age of 40. This series of tests would detect approximately 93 percent of all asymptomatic colon cancers, but an analysis of this practice estimated that "the marginal cost of the sixth test—$47.1 million per cancer case detected—was 20,000 times the average cost per case discovered" (Estaugh 1981, p. 33). This analysis raised the following question: "Although six sequential stool guaiacs, followed by barium enemas for all positive guaiacs, will identify virtually all asymptomatic colon cancers, is it worth $47.1 million to detect that one rare case when the resources could be used elsewhere?" (ibid., p. 33). This type of question originated with payers and policymakers, but the medical profession now also is asking such questions. The American Cancer Society's current recommendation has been modified: an annual digital rectal exam for those over 40 years of age, one (not six) annual stool guaiac exam for those over 50, and proctoscopy every 3 to 5 years following two negative annual exams after the age of 50.

Research Efforts

While these techniques have been used for decades, the various forces described earlier have contributed to the outcome or effectiveness movements. These efforts share the common goal of maximizing the potential benefit of medical technology. Significant public and private sector resources have been committed to technology assessment and medical practice evaluation. The public sector effort is spearheaded by the Public Health Services' Agency for Health Care Policy and Research (AHCPR) in collaboration with HCFA (which is providing much of the financial support from a "set-aside" of Medicare funds).

Among AHCPR and HCFA's initiatives is the establishment of "Patient Outcome Research Teams" (PORTs) to collect, analyze, and disseminate information concerning the effectiveness of various medical interventions. PORT activities include monitoring treatment trends within the population as well as individual outcomes following specific interventions. They use Medicare claims data to identify variations in treatment and, if possible, outcome, and once these variations are identified, targeted treatments are analyzed in depth using other sources of data (e.g., medical records, patient surveys) to determine their relative effectiveness. The PORT findings will be disseminated with the intent of promoting widespread change in medical practice.

Responding to the changing socioeconomic atmosphere in which medicine is practiced, a growing number of universities are establishing health services research centers. Also, training programs have been established around the country, and the number of experts in this multidisciplinary field can be expected to grow exponentially during the next few years.

Guidelines, Protocols, and Computers

Technology assessment, clinical trials, and research on the outcomes of care all provide information that can be used with the results of small-area variation studies to create new, empirically based "guidelines" for care. Through the AHCPR, the government is actively promoting the development of such guidelines. It provides a forum for experts from relevant medical specialties, nursing, and consumer groups, and the agency solicits nominations for panel members for each guideline topic from the appropriate organizations and the general public. AHCPR also attempts to select a panel of representatives with diverse opinions and multidisciplinary involvement.

The panel members construct a guideline in accordance with a methodology that was developed with the advice of the National Academy of Science's Institute of Medicine (IOM). This approach gives priority to sound scientific evidence, which is identified through an exhaustive literature review; professional consensus is used as a last resort. Once a complete guideline has been developed, AHCPR publishes and disseminates it in various formats for libraries, practitioners, and consumers. The first guidelines were released in 1992.

The development of clinical care guidelines is not new. For many years, a broad array of organizations, including specialty societies, government committees, pharmaceutical companies, consumer organizations, and individuals, have promoted particular treatment methodologies under given clinical circumstances. Different names have been applied to the recommendations of these various groups (including guidelines, standards of care, practice parameters, and protocols), but all have been intended to guide clinical practice.

Some of these efforts, however, have been criticized as sacrificing quality in favor of proprietary interests; for example, the mammography screening guideline that the American College of Radiology promoted stands virtually alone in recommending routine annual screening of healthy women under the age of 40. Critics charge that adherence to this guideline would result in costly and unnecessary treatment from which the radiologists, not their patients, would profit. This example makes clear that the development of guidelines is not necessarily apolitical. The current federal initiative provides a mechanism to address this concern by bringing together groups that may have competing interests and attempting to unify them under the banner of good-quality care.

Another effort to standardize medical practice is the NIH's Consensus-Development Program. Established in 1977, this program has sponsored numerous conferences at which leading experts discuss the state of knowledge, diagnosis, and treatment of major conditions in their specialty.

Once fiscally responsible, clinically optimal standards have been developed, they can be disseminated by government, specialty societies, hospitals, and other organizations. Protocols of standard practice will increase in importance as more patients move into managed-care systems such as HMOs, where standardization helps administrators control both costs and quality. Given the historical precedence for federal standards to become universal standards, federal recommendations will carry particular weight and potential importance (particularly if HCFA endorses them).

While the potential for improved quality of care exists, there is a countervailing fear that guideline efforts could adversely affect the practice of medicine. Clinical guidelines could also be used by third-party payers to limit reimbursement to only those treatments that fall within the guidelines.

Guidelines could be used to determine standards of care in malpractice litigation as well. A project under way in Maine is exploring the potential impact of guidelines on practitioner liability, and for the purposes of its study, a group of practitioners has agreed to adopt a particular guideline in exchange for a statutory limitation on its application: *adherence* to the guideline provides legislated protection against a negligence claim, but *divergence* from it cannot be used by a patient to prove negligence. The examiners will evaluate the impact of the guideline on the liability experience of practitioners. (See also Chapter 11.)

Some practitioners fear that broad imposition of guidelines will weaken their professional integrity by restricting the role of case-specific judgment. Developers of these guidelines, however, consider their primary motivation as reducing *unnecessary* variation in practice, not to impose absolute uniformity. While vigilance is needed to ensure that the application of guidelines does not exclude medical judgment, it does seem worthwhile to promote uniformity where sound evidence exists to justify it.

Computers have a growing role in medical practice as well. As Morreim pointed out, "One cannot practice good medicine by committee or cookbook or computer" (1985, p. 34), but their large memory and information storage capacity can be used to assist clinicians. In one project, researchers used mathematic modeling to develop "Clinical Prediction Rules" that were based on observed probabilities and clinical experience; in such a system, the patient's symptoms are entered into a computer that estimates the probability that the symptoms are indicative of a particular disease. One system of this sort has been helpful in determining a treatment protocol for patients with pharyngitis (such as whether or not to prescribe antibiotics). Computerized medical information systems have now been used effectively in several hospitals and outpatient settings, and in some of them, this information retrieval capability has been linked with limited treatment or diagnosis-assistance capabilities as described earlier. Such applications, including routine computer-based reminders, can only help improve both the quality and the efficiency of medical practice.

Initially, it might appear paradoxic that impersonal computer programs and financial modeling could assist the art of bedside medicine; similarly, physicians who were active 100 years ago were reluctant to abandon outmoded practices and to adopt such improvements as antiseptic technique. Reticence, however, need not prevent the incorporation of these techniques. When the computer's ability to store and process vast amounts of information is added to human judgment, the best of technology can be combined with the best of the healer's art. Providers with an open mind and a flexible approach can improve professionally through this transitional process. The incorporation of computers, guidelines, practice evaluation, and other innovations is now critical to the effective practice of medicine. Their effect on the outcomes and quality of care, however, will not be known in the near future.

Incorporation into Clinical Practice

The number of both technical and economic analyses in the medical literature is growing, and a strong consensus exists on the importance of this process. As scientists' expertise with this multidisciplinary analysis expands, clinicians can expect ever-improving advice from health services analysts regarding the optimization of clinical decisions, but even when rationally developed standards and other potential improvements are widely disseminated, real change can occur only if the individual practitioners are persuaded to modify their practice. Because *clinicians* implement technical knowledge through medical practice, they are key to this process of change.

Many practitioners understandably see guidelines and other norms of care as serious threats to their independence. They foresee a day when rote, predetermined plans, mandated by payers and hospitals, will be ubiquitous or even exclusive approaches to patient care. Indeed, some hospitals already place explicit restrictions on physicians' practice, and others use economic incentives both to sanction undesired behavior and to reward cost efficiency.

It will never be easy to balance constraints on resources against the patient's best interest, but it has become clear that the process can be made more rational. Whatever the temptations to the contrary, each major clinical decision now more than ever should be arrived at by careful analysis and not by rote. It is also more important than ever for physicians to share with their patients the degree of uncertainty that is present in the clinical situation, and to allow patients to participate as fully as possible in the decision-making process.

Guidelines for Efficient Use of the Hospital

There are fairly simple ways to both decrease costs and increase efficiency while still maintaining quality. Some common sense principles for hospital care have been suggested by seasoned, efficient physicians that would go a long way toward reducing unnecessary medical care. Surprisingly, however, these practices are not followed in a significant proportion of cases:

- Be certain that the patient requires admission by assuring that the services needed cannot be provided outside of the hospital.
- If the patient needs treatment, do it as early in the course of an illness as possible.
- Perform as many tests as possible before admission.
- Do not admit patients electively on a Thursday or Friday if they require tests or procedures that are unavailable on weekends.
- Do not admit patients electively for surgery unless operating room time is scheduled.

- Make sure that those services ordered (tests, procedures, vital signs) are indicated and consistent with the provision of proper care.
- Sequence tests and procedures in a timely manner. Become familiar with radiology and laboratory prep protocols (such as patient preparation for a barium swallow) to avoid delays and assure that the patient gets the most from a test.
- When a consultation is sought, make sure that the question is well defined and the consultation is both necessary and timely.
- Begin planning for discharge on the day of admission by considering the degree of home or institutional support that the patient will require and by involving the discharge planners sooner instead of later.
- Write discharge orders the night before the expected day of departure so that patients may leave early on that day.
- Document why tests and procedures are being performed. Documentation not only is used by utilization reviewers and payers for reimbursement and quality-assurance purposes but also clarifies matters for other physicians, nurses, and hospital staff.

Guidelines for Ordering Diagnostic Tests

Despite the difficulty of developing protocols for ordering tests, some practical guidance can be given. There are several important things to know about any diagnostic test, notably its risk, accuracy, interobserver variability (particularly important for x-rays and EKGs), patient acceptability, cost, and utility compared with other diagnostic modalities. A growing literature provides guidance to clinicians on test ordering.* In general, when ordering or performing a specific test or procedure, a physician should consider the following questions:

- Will the test really provide useful information that will affect the care of the patient? If so, will the result be timely and will someone use it?
- Is the test part of a routine protocol that has been passed down over the years and should be reevaluated? Would another test yield better information?

*Readers interested in current thinking about the utility of common laboratory tests and drug regimens as well as sensible strategies for their use are referred to Friedman and Katt 1991.

- Is a test being ordered quickly ("stat") because speed is medically necessary or will decrease the patient's length of stay and charges, or is it just to have a number to report during rounds? When a large percentage of chemistry and hematology tests are ordered stat, not only are charges higher but it makes the term meaningless; the laboratory staff cannot know which tests actually are needed right away and should be given priority.
- Would the test or procedure be ordered if the physician had to carry it out personally, or pay for it, or had to take it himself or herself or have a close relative take it? (This really is just another version of the Golden Rule.)

In some ways, things seem to be improving. With the stress on holding down costs by using technology efficiently, the "technologic imperative" exerts less influence than it once did. Rather, medical practice is being guided more and more by technology assessment, medical practice evaluation, outcomes assessment, and the other techniques described previously. Such practices have had a particularly dramatic effect on reducing the time that patients spend in the hospital. A growing number of studies suggest that incorporation of this new type of knowledge is possible; for example, over recent years, the average time in the hospital following coronary artery bypass surgery was decreased from 12 to 7 days with no adverse effect on recovery. In another study, surgery rates decreased in one locale when practitioners learned that their rates fell outside the average range in their area.

A controlled, randomized trial showed that displaying cost per test and total cost data on the computer screen while physicians were ordering tests led to a 14 percent reduction in the number of tests ordered compared with the control group. Charges were reduced 13 percent, with a cumulative savings to the clinic of $250,000 for the year. No adverse effect on patient outcome was noted, thus implying that all necessary tests were still ordered during the intervention; unfortunately, this effect did not persist after the intervention was stopped (Tierney et al. 1990).

A survey of the effect of guidelines for cesarean section dissemination to hospitals and obstetricians found that information was not remembered accurately. The guidelines also changed only slightly the cesarean section rate at 1 and 2 years postdissemination. These results suggest that physicians and policymakers must optimize the dissemination process itself, including implementation at the local level (Lomas et al. 1989).

Medical education will be an important means of gaining the profession's acceptance of new methods for clinical decision-making. Traditionally, medical education has generated a "rule-out mentality," a disposition to order every conceivable test in an effort to rule out a range of diseases. Tobin described this as "the 'roundsmanship mentality,' wherein one is criticized for not having ordered the serum cauliflower test" (1980, p. 288). Young practitioners who see their mentors making cost-conscious decisions will be far more likely to use these strategies themselves, and by adopting a fiscally responsible and efficient decision-making style, preceptors will prepare both students and house staff for the hard decisions that they will need to make in today's medical marketplace.

Scientifically derived standards of care have not yet been developed for many conditions, in part because of difficulties at both the scientific and political levels. Many analyses of medical care such as those described earlier are needed before we can be reasonably sure that money spent on health care is being spent in the best possible way. At the moment, we lack not only the information that such studies would give us but also an institutionalized or systemwide method for allocating the resources entering the health care system. However, the system is beginning to move in this direction: as knowledge increases further, the system will reach a new equilibrium.

Meanwhile, most payers will continue to consider low users as their point of reference, arguing that high users should conform unless they can make a strong case to the contrary. Physicians can respond only by doing what is best for their patients given the resources available. This may mean at times agreeing with payers that less is sufficient, but at other times standing firm and insisting that more is in fact necessary. This chapter has described numerous ways to improve clinical decision-making—potentially making this process more efficient, less costly, and maximizing potential clinical outcome.

CHAPTER 9

BALANCING COST WITH CARE

The Health Care System Poised for Change

The U.S. system of health care divides responsibility between those who pay for health care and those who provide it. Until recently, private insurers and government paid essentially whatever the providers charged, in effect endorsing a "more-is-better" approach to health care. Also, medical education engendered the attitude that physicians should be accountable only to the patient and their peers, not to payers—a position that was sanctioned by the population at large. Thus, society, financing mechanisms, and professional tradition mutually reinforced and perpetuated the autonomy of the patient and practitioner.

In effect, the physician has been responsible for the care and the conscience of medicine; payers were responsible for its costs. Because most providers fared quite well financially under this arrangement, not many were motivated to question it. Most physicians were insensitive to the cost consequences of their clinical decisions. Few knew the per-day rates that were charged by the hospitals to which they admitted patients or the costs of common diagnostic and therapeutic procedures, and few were conversant with the workings of their patients' insurance policies.

Change Occurs

As shown previously, inefficient medical practices, inflation, sophisticated technology, and other factors ultimately increased the costs of health care to the point where cost-containment measures became imperative not only to payers but also to society at large. At first, measures to reduce cost focused primarily on the hospital, but they have now expanded to include individual practitioners. Physicians' lack of economic awareness during previous eras is regrettable, but it is now essential that they become sensitive to these aspects of medical practice given today's highly charged, competitive, and often adversarial environment.

As the person who is responsible for most decisions concerning the use of health care resources, the physician serves as the link between the patient and the medical marketplace. This unique role, which requires personal judgment as well as the technical knowledge that is acquired through professional training, is the crux of the patient–physician relationship. Recently, a new set of economic considerations have added still another layer of complexity to the clinical decision-making process. It is clear that cost reduction has affected the patient–physician relationship directly.

Physicians are caught in the middle. They are responsible simultaneously for meeting both societal and managerial cost-control objectives and for the welfare of patients. The new need for this balancing act results from the inevitable fact that reducing costs means that not everything can be done for everyone. Indeed, the current system seems to be moving practitioners inexorably in the direction of making explicit tradeoffs between cost and quality.

In the era of cost control, third parties have displayed a distrust of health care providers, whom they generally see as having abused their autonomy, privilege, and power over the last 30 years or more. As cost containment progresses, providers have argued that as their charges decrease, the quality of care will also decrease, but payers counter with empiric research showing that costs can be reduced considerably without decreasing quality. Thus, they conclude that the true concern of providers lies elsewhere. What is *really* at stake, payers ask: the care of the patient, or the income and status of the physician?

It is obvious that impartial decisions are more difficult to make when they may result in adverse financial consequences to a provider. While indisputably in one of the best-paid professions in the United States, many physicians today are experiencing the financial effects of cost containment. For the first time in recent history, physicians' real (adjusted for inflation) income began to decline in 1983, with a 3 percent decline in that year. This trend reversed from 1985 to 1988, but the decrease resumed between 1988 and 1989.

The causes of this decline include decreasing rates of reimbursement, lower volume of services provided (largely because of utilization controls), increasing supply of physicians, and a shift of physicians into salaried positions. It is too soon to forecast the long-term effects on physicians' earning potential, but it seems clear that both social and economic pressures will continue to wield powerful constraining influences on growth that heretofore had been largely unrestricted. Payers plainly would welcome an even steeper decline. This chapter examines changes that have already occurred and focuses primarily on how cost containment has created or exacerbated conflicting incentives.

Patients Balance Cost with Care

Cost containment not only affects care once patients are in the system but also affects consumers and their potential access to that system. As insurance beneficiaries face increased cost-sharing, they at some point will be less ready to "demand" medical care. As the threshold for seeking care is raised, necessary care may be foregone, and in some cases, adverse health effects may result. The growth of managed-care controls has also altered patients' interactions with the health care system as another layer of clinical decision-makers has been added.

The movement of society to reconsider the way that medical resources presently are used at the end of life reflects another influence of the cost-containment movement on individuals. For example, in the United Kingdom, an individual over the age of 65 with renal failure customarily has not been offered dialysis within the government-sponsored health service; in the United States, even very elderly people with limited prognosis receive this treatment. In current U.S. medical practice, resources are often used very intensively at the end of a patient's life, such that each year, the small percentage of Medicare beneficiaries who die account for a significant percentage of the total expenditures in that program. (It was estimated recently that the 6 percent of Medicare beneficiaries who die annually account for approximately 30 percent of Medicare expenditures in that year.) Adverse financial consequences ensue in addition to what many feel is unnecessary suffering without concomitant benefit. (Chapter 10 discusses the relevant ethical issues.) Some have argued that society should legislate decisions involving the medical care of patients who are dying, and in fact, all states currently have related legislation. Federal law requires Medicare-eligible hospitals to inform every patient they admit of their rights in this area. The provision took effect early in 1992, and it is too early to assess its impact.*

Another approach to legislate cost containment is exemplified by the Oregon Plan, which would allow Oregon to implement explicit rationing of health care based on the predetermined utility of various procedures. The proposed scheme prioritizes procedures by their potential aggregate impact on the population. Medicaid would cover procedures beginning with the highest priority and move as far down the list as the funds of the program allow. No procedures below the priority level at which funds ran out would be covered. Thus, people with high-priority conditions would be covered fully, but those with low-priority conditions would not be covered at all. Oregon's Medicaid-waiver request, required to implement this plan, was denied in 1992. State policymakers intend to resubmit the proposal to the Clinton administration. (This proposal is discussed further in Chapter 12).

Hospitals Balance Cost with Care

The hospital sector's approach to cost–care tradeoffs has been influenced most heavily by Medicare's DRG-based PPS, under which most hospitals are now paid a lump sum for each admission of a Medicare enrollee. The amount of the payment is determined by the patient's primary discharge diagnosis, the procedures performed, and the patient's age. Because of the new financial incentives it offers hospitals, this change in reimbursement has had a major impact on in-hospital medical care.

In many ways, the new era gives short shrift to the intangible (i.e., nonfinancial) rewards of patient care. For example, many hospitals have decreased their labor costs, which account for over 70 percent of the average hospital's budget, by reducing their staff-to-patient ratios. The result is fewer nurses, fewer support staff to care for patients, and more work per employee.

Under PPS, hospitals profit when patients are discharged after the minimal necessary length of stay, and this decreased length of stay has affected inpatient care. Rabkin (1982) pointed out that before the implementation of PPS, the early days of hospitalization were anxious ones for both the patient and the provider. The

*The Patient Self-Determination Act.

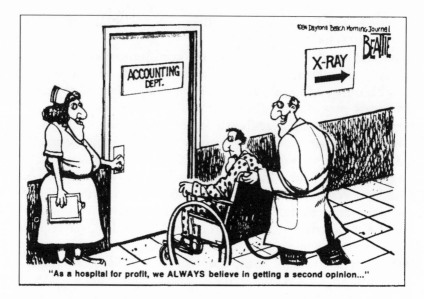

"As a hospital for profit, we ALWAYS believe in getting a second opinion..."

Courtesy of Bruce Beattie and Copley News Service

patient was sick, and the provider was working to diagnose the condition and initiate treatment. In contrast, the last days of the hospital stay were relatively gratifying, as therapy took effect and the patient's condition improved. Under the new system, however, patients leave the hospital just as the days of gratification begin, with both the patient and the provider often feeling pressure for discharge before they feel the patient is quite stable. Concurrent with fewer employees per patient, this has increased the stress and intensity of the in-hospital experience. The physician loses in two ways: the overall intensity of in-hospital care increases, and there is no balancing gratification from observing the patient's return to health.

As a consequence of the decreasing length of stay, hospital workloads have increased. The general atmosphere of most hospitals also has become more emotionally intense and anxious. These changes have affected severely the hospital's frontline professional, the floor nurse, thus leading to a critical exodus of nurses who find their workloads have increased drastically while their compensation has not. House officers have been affected as well, and needless to say, these changes have put added strains on patient–provider relationships.

Because hospitals lose money under PPS on patients who are severely ill, their incentive is that physicians treat the least severely ill. Hospitals could profit under PPS by discriminating—for example, with selective admissions or transfer policies—among patients based on their medical condition. Federal data indicate that this has not yet occurred, but monitoring for such trends will continue. Alternatively, hospital administrators can develop programs and recruit staff to care for patients in lucrative DRGs.

Other profit-maximizing changes require new styles of clinical practice. For example, the diagnostic laboratory before PPS was a *profit center* for most hospitals; by inflating the charges for tests relative to their costs, hospitals could subsidize *loss leaders* such as the emergency room. Under PPS, diagnostic tests are no longer a major source of profit. In fact, the reverse is now true: the fewer the tests ordered, the larger the hospital's profit. Hospital revenue also increases under PPS when a physician readmits a patient for a second procedure that could have been provided during the original admission; when this happens, a hospital is paid twice for what previously would have been a single hospitalization.

As hospital managers struggle to modify their organizational operations to survive the economic straits of the cost-containment era, more stringent ways to cut corners have been necessary. Regulatory bodies such as federally sponsored PROs attempt to monitor hospitals for readmissions, "DRG creep," and inappropriate transfers, all of which work against the intent of PPS by raising costs. The PROs' task is difficult, however, because no payment system is completely immune to manipulation that is intended to benefit those who provide the service.

It is important to note that despite the potential for adverse consequences of PPS on the quality of care, empiric studies generally have not shown such a decline. Researchers have found evidence suggesting the process of care, which began to improve before PPS, continued to improve after its implementation; thus, to some extent, these concerns remain more potential than real. Gail Wilensky (then head of HCFA), commenting forcefully on these findings, stated: "In short, the more aggressive cost-containing atmosphere of the PPS was not accompanied by a cost-quality trade-off. These reports place the burden of proof on those who doubt that we can provide better care at lower cost today" (1990, p. 1997).

Some analysts are not sure that enough information is available yet to make a definite determination regarding the effect of PPS on quality. Several changes that have occurred concurrently with PPS also could have contributed to the improved quality of care during the mid-1980s. These changes include the increased oversight authority given to PROs as well as improved medical-record documentation as part of defensive medicine. Nevertheless, if hospital cost-containment measures continue, then concerns regarding the adverse effects on quality of care at some point inevitably will become reality. Ongoing monitoring is therefore essential.

The Changing Hospital–Physician Relationship

As recently as 15 years ago, it would have been difficult to imagine that the hospital environment could change so radically. This transformation is definitely under way, however, and it continues to progress. For example, most hospital administrators feel compelled to implement strategies that are intended to "game the system" and increase reimbursements. As part of strategic planning efforts, most managers consider the financial implications not only of the insurance status of potential patients but also of the patient's *diagnosis* and its profitability. Staff reductions have been made so that patients, providers, and hospital employees are at times all uncomfortable in the hospital atmosphere.

Administrators only have a limited ability to implement profitable strategies that involve clinical decisions. In such matters, managers are attempting to influence the clinical staff to change their practices. Thus, even though PPS to date has affected hospital management most directly, it has also indirectly affected physicians by altering their working arrangement with hospital management.

Relationships between hospitals and their medical staffs sometimes are strained by the fact that while hospitals receive much of their reimbursement via prospective payment, U.S. physicians are reimbursed almost universally for hospital care on an FFS basis. The financial incentives under PPS are different from the incentives under FFS. FFS reimbursement encourages treatments and procedures, theoretically placing patients at risk for too much care; under PPS, in contrast, because more care can lead to a "loss" for the facility, patients are at risk for receiving less care than they require. Thus, the physician who is financially rewarded for performing a procedure on an inpatient basis in the end penalizes the hospital, which must pay for the institutional costs associated with the procedure out of its fixed payment. Currently, PPS is used mainly for patients with Medicare, but aspects of this method have been adopted by some private insurers, HMOs, and Medicaid agencies. In the future, it likely will be applied more widely, thus heightening the effects that are seen currently.

Some hospitals have tried to compensate for the differing sets of incentives under Medicare's PPS and CPR (and now RVS) reimbursements by introducing either penalty or reward systems aimed at making physicians more cost-efficient. Others have initiated "joint venture" corporations, such as the MeSH arrangement that was discussed in Chapter 7, whereby the institution and its staff share any PPS profits. (Potential problems with such cooperation—or as some might say "collusion—" are raised later.)

Because of these changes, hospitals and other health care organizations are no longer merely workshops for practitioners. Today, health care administrators are actively involved not only with monitoring physicians' practices in terms of cost efficiency, but with actively urging the physicians to use preadmission testing, to order fewer expensive diagnostic tests, to perform fewer procedures, and to discharge patients earlier. Physicians also may be asked to increase the number of admissions they make to the hospital, and computer-generated profiles now are commonly used to compare the average length of stay within a DRG by the admitting physicians. Most institutions monitor their use of resources closely, but few take into account clinical outcomes such as morbidity or death rates on a regular basis. (As discussed in Chapter 8, however, this is beginning to change.)

Some hospitals now grant practice privileges partly on the basis of economic performance, thus putting a premium on cost efficiency in locations where gaining such privileges is no easy matter. Given that DRGs have variable profitability, other hospitals now contract directly with practitioners to care for patients, and these institutions choose their specialists carefully, with an eye to maximizing profits. Facilities also may favor family practitioners, whose services generally are less expensive than specialists'. More and more hospitals now grant privileges to non-M.D. providers as well, such as dentists, podiatrists, and midwives as a way of augmenting their volume of patients.

Managed-Care Controls

Both payers and policymakers have an increasing say in practitioners' medical decisions by the application of managed care (utilization) controls. As a result, today's physician practices in an environment with an unprecedented emphasis on the fiscal bottom line. Physicians must justify most major clinical decisions to third-party payers and managers. "The burden of proof about activities in medicine is shifting so that the presumption is no longer that what the physician chooses to do is automatically correct and must be proven wrong. Rather, increasingly the burden of the physician is to justify why he should perform in a 'higher-cost' manner if it does not offer substantial and worthwhile benefit to the patient" (Fineberg 1985, p. 37).

From the cost perspective, this makes sense: payers, including the government, benefit when costs are kept down. From the care perspective, however, this makes considerably less sense. Regulat-

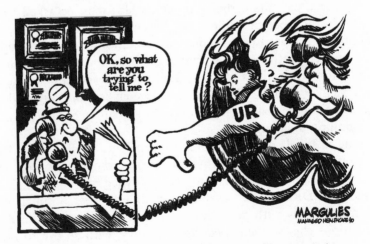

(Source: © 1990 Margulies for Managed Healthcare. Reprinted by permission.)

ing the performance of practitioners may be appropriate for reducing costs, but elimination of the physician's autonomy for clinical decision-making could have catastrophic effects on patient care. The logic of cost-containment strategies—to trim away unnecessary care—is simple; what is not so simple is identifying which services are excessive and which are necessary. The process of clinical decision-making is and always will be replete with uncertainty, and because UR alone is inadequate, professional judgment must remain a key component in this process.

The identification of cost-insensitive decisions provides an opportunity to educate clinicians about more preferable options. The effectiveness movement (discussed in the previous chapter) is also a reaction to this new era in medicine. Research that is planned as part of this initiative potentially will provide empiric evidence as to which practices provide the best balance between care and cost. Treatment protocols and guidelines (based in part on effectiveness research) have similar potential. Clinical decisions by professionals should not be compromised, or overridden however, by financially interested "managers" with varying levels of clinical knowledge and no other stake in the proceedings. Moreover, the outcomes of many decisions can affect patients profoundly, and the ultimate responsibility for these decisions rests with the physician and patient, *not* with the payer or policymaker.

In short, both payers and providers often have conflicting goals and differing perspectives. One would not expect providers to accept fewer dollars and growth restrictions willingly, which is in fact what payers want. Nor would one expect payers to pay more for services that they can obtain for less and that they see as being of equal or even superior quality. The resulting "zero-sum game," in which whatever one side wins the other loses, has hindered effective action toward reasonable compromises.

Nevertheless, payers and policymakers do not bear sole responsibility for the current conditions. It is equally clear that physicians have played a role in the current cost crisis, and they now are bearing the consequences of their practice styles in previous decades. Clinicians finding themselves in untenable situations with regard to managed-care controls may be motivated to change the system, thereby (it is to be hoped) improving it.

Emerging Problems with Managed Care

The original intent of managed-care controls was to reduce the cost of health care, but several problems with UR and other initiatives have emerged. First is the cost of the programs themselves. In 1987, insurers spent an estimated $23.9 billion on administrative costs, with many private insurance companies spending 10 percent to 20 percent of their budgets on such "overhead." In contrast, the administrative expenses of state Medicaid programs have been quite low; in Maryland, for example, it accounts for less than 5 percent of the total budget. The exact level is a point of some debate, but a good proportion of private sector administrative costs are attributable to the new oversight processes that were implemented during the cost-containment era.

Reformers ask whether in an era of fiscal crisis we can afford to spend billions of health care dollars on resources that oversee the process but produce no outputs. Studies suggesting that UR saves less money than it pays to its reviewers provide support for this argument. Reformers wonder whether the fat should be trimmed from insurance company and managed-care payrolls before further reductions in patient benefits and provider reimbursements are made. As Westermeyer pointed out, "[managed-care controls] add further to the cost and complexity of medical care, which is ironic in that the original motivations for changing the status quo ante were to contain costs and reduce complexity" (1991, pp. 1223–4).

In contrast to criteria developed by PROs, many UR and managed-care companies consider their review standards to be "proprietary" and thus unavailable to the public or to the providers who are being scrutinized. In many cases, neither the patient whose care is denied nor that patient's physician are able to find out the reason for a denial; this makes a persuasive argument in the appeal process essentially impossible. This is being changed in many states, however, through enactment of legislation that requires UR firms to release their criteria, particularly in disputed cases. Moreover, an office-based physician may encounter numerous sets of incompatible criteria in the course of dealing with multiple insurers or health plans.

Motivated by problems and deficiencies in the UR system, more sophisticated UR assessment scales and tools are under development, and publication of company criteria and the development of national standards will facilitate rationality in this area. It is hoped that these trends, and guidelines, in tandem with the outcomes and effectiveness movements—intended to improve knowledge regarding the process of clinical care—will improve the UR process.

Firms that perform UR functions solely are a new industry within the health care system. These managed-care companies essentially have been unregulated. This is changing, however, as nearly 80 percent of states have either enacted or proposed legislation to regulate UR firms, and voluntary accreditation groups are forming. It is important not to overlook the fact that oversight *of* an oversight process appears to be necessary. Problems with existing managed-care approaches could further motivate providers to optimize efficiency based on their own initiatives.

Physician Employees

Today, many physicians are hired as outside contractors or employees by large for-profit (and nonprofit) health care corporations. In these circumstances, health care administrators can view clinicians as simply another organizational resource rather than, as in past eras, independent professionals around whom the organization revolves. In some states (notably trend-setting California), more than 50 percent of all physicians contract with one or more HMOs or PPOs. Some anticipate that physician-employees in the future may undergo a "corporate socialization" (Ludmerer 1985) to bring their practice in line with company policy.

Both from their own financial necessity and because so many patients are now enrolled in the new delivery systems, many physicians are entangled in a complex web of legal contracts with HMOs, PPOs, hospital joint ventures, and insurers who to varying extents manage the care and the services provided. In these arrangements, providers usually sign agreements that give payers certain kinds of direct authority over the resources used in patient care, and this indirectly gives the payers some authority over the provider's clinical decisions. Both employed and contracting physicians may encounter conflict between management philosophy

and clinical judgment. It goes without saying that before align-
ing themselves in these arrangements, providers should examine
such contracts carefully to ensure that they anticipate both the
terms and incentives they may face, as well as the ethical issues
that will be raised should these pressures conflict with the patient's
interests.

Traditionally a fiercely independent group, physicians by and
large would rather call their own shots, set their own hours,
choose their own patients, and shape their own practice. [How-
ever], an increasing number of physicians are now employees of
others. Approximately half of all active physicians in the United

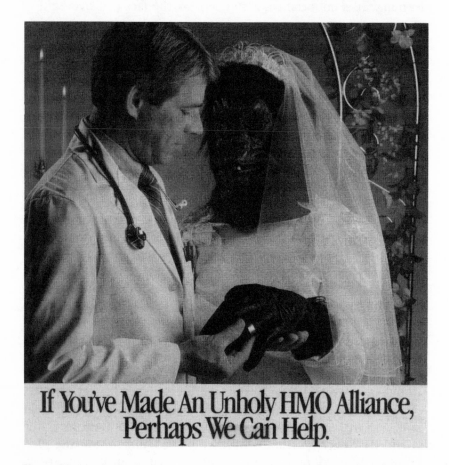

If You've Made An Unholy HMO Alliance,
Perhaps We Can Help.

Figure 22. An advertisement from the pages of the AMA's *American Medical News*.

States now earn at least part of their income as salary. Many group practices pay partners by this method. Another untraditional development that is still too recent to assess is unionization for the purpose of collective bargaining. In the late 1980s, it was estimated that over 40,000 physicians belonged to unions, and the number has grown since then.

A continued shift toward salaried and employee status will be facilitated by the surplus of health care providers in some specialties, which has reduced both the availability of jobs and the physicians' bargaining leverage. Definite benefits to salaried practice or other employee arrangements exist (e.g., guaranteed income and scheduled working hours), but the potential for limited freedom to make clinical decisions is a drawback.

Physician Entrepreneurs

The increasing importance of the "bottom line" in health care has been accompanied by growing competition among providers for both patients and dollars. A new breed of entrepreneurial physician has entered the business of medicine through investment in the corporate delivery of health care. Physician participation in this trend is explained in part by reductions in average physician income, which has motivated some to invest to maintain their income. Recently, it was estimated that 12 percent to 17 percent of physicians who bill Medicare have an ownership interest in the health care entities (e.g., laboratories, imaging centers, nursing homes, proprietary hospitals) to which they refer their patients. Others estimate that as many as 25 percent of physicians now are involved in entrepreneurial arrangements.

For some physicians, management expertise has become necessary for financial survival. Some entrepreneurial physicians have taken to marketing—a classic demand-inducing strategy—despite concerns in some quarters about whether this practice is good for the profession or will lead to improved patient care. Others are raising capital to build facilities that they will own and operate, and still others are key investors in existing for-profit enterprises.

Because of the physician's role as the patient's agent, the balance between professionalism and entrepreneurialism is delicate.

Moreover, because the interests of the investor and the patient may not coincide, the arrangement is complicated further when the physician is an investor in the health care facility.

Consumer, payer, and professional organizations now worry that profit motives are influencing a significant number of physicians, sometimes to the point of reducing their dedication to patients' needs. Indeed, a recent survey in Florida found that on average, doctors involved in joint-venture laboratories ordered almost twice as many tests per patient (at over twice the cost) when compared with physicians who were not affiliated with laboratories.

The problem is not only ethical but, to some extent, political. According to Relman, "the medical profession would be in a stronger position, and its voice would carry more moral authority with the public and the government, if it adopted the principle that practicing physicians should derive no financial benefit from the health-care market except from their own professional services" (1980, p. 967). In 1991, the Department of Health and Human Services issued regulations for physician business deals and patient referral arrangements. These regulations create "safe harbors" for entrepreneurial involvement outside of which physicians would be subject to criminal prosecution. Violators are subject to fines of up to $25,000 or imprisonment for up to 5 years. Any physician who is involved in an entrepreneurial arrangement should consult a lawyer to assure that he or she conforms to these regulations.

A respectable argument also can be made the other way, namely, that a physician who invests in a medical facility has more influence in its operation and can use that influence to improve the balance between care and cost. Because it probably is easier for a physician to grasp cost issues than for a nonphysician manager or entrepreneur to understand medical issues, physician managers arguably are the better qualified to strike the right balance.

On a more practical level, however, the financial solvency of many physicians depends on their investment in for-profit arrangements, so despite the misgivings of Relman and others, such investments will not disappear. The important thing is that they be used, so far as possible, to assure that the patients' needs remain paramount.

Clinicians Balance Cost and Care

Professionals who are trained to put a patient's medical welfare above all else now find themselves obligated to balance clinical considerations not only against patients' financial and personal welfare but also against society's apparent judgment that health care expenditures in general are too high. Therefore, it is not surprising that so many clinicians feel caught between these new economic conditions and their responsibility to uphold their professional code of ethics. Practitioners have seen some changes compromise the quality of medical care and alter their professional relationships with patients, and traditional medical education has left most physicians woefully unprepared to confront the demands of the current system.

Medical education is intended to prepare the physician to make the hard calls, the life-or-death decisions. Clinical experience reinforces this aspect of education, but the era of cost containment has complicated this role by adding a financial dimension to clinical decision-making. After raising a number of potential problems for the clinician in striking a balance between cost and care, we unfortunately have no guaranteed recipe to offer for optimizing this process. As Eisenberg stated: "For the individual physician and individual patient, the need for trade-offs becomes a matter of social responsibility to be weighed against the individual's gain" (1989, p. 2886). Patient-specific circumstances are too variable to invoke simple rule-making principles, and practitioners should be wary of them. By pointing out potential pitfalls, we hope that "forewarned is forearmed."

In an environment that is characterized by strong incentives to minimize care, physicians increasingly find themselves arguing with third-party payers over the existence of extenuating circumstances for a patient's hospitalization or need for a specific type of care. Unwelcome as such arguments are, they now are a part of the role and responsibility of the modern practitioner as the patient's agent. (See definition of agent, p. 193.) At times, the physician will have to accept lower reimbursement—or no reimbursement—for providing care that is deemed to be in the patient's best interest.

Clinical decisions often are context dependent, and at times, physicians will find themselves making decisions that society should make. The economist Uwe Reinhardt described the difficulty of this task: "While detached policy analysts may find it easy to discourse upon the value of life from a safe distance, no one has yet given the individual physician a publicly sanctioned set of guidelines under which to make cost–quality trade-offs at the patient's bedside. So far, society has delicately preferred to leave that matter to the physician's own judgment. . . . The providers of health care must reckon with the prospect that society will increasingly both flagellate them over health care costs and saddle them with ethical dilemmas no politician (and possibly not even most economists) would have the courage to face in the trenches" (1985, p. 57C). In fact, such issues now are addressed more frequently in the public forum. (The Oregon Plan for rationing medical resources under that state's Medicaid program is discussed in Chapter 12.)

To the extent that payers and policymakers have been successful in their cost-containment efforts, physicians must not only balance clinical acumen, cost concerns, and conscience, but they must do so under the scrutiny of powerful third parties to whom costs are the main issue. Some wonder how long this can continue before the pendulum reaches the end of its trajectory, but it is today's reality. (Some see the rise of interest in both quality and outcomes as the rebound in the other direction.)

Not many physicians enjoy this balancing act, especially in the atmosphere existing at present. However, "a small but growing group of clinicians is embracing the administrative challenges and attendant entrepreneurial opportunities by attempting to meld patient advocacy, clinical wisdom, and fiscal imperatives. This is obviously not an easy task. Such clinicians are often looked upon as 'turncoats,' a posture that further discourages dialogue" (Lister 1991, pp. 9–10). Yet the profession as a whole, and physicians as individuals, have a stake in making the new system work and, thus, a responsibility to speak while it is still in a state of flux. Far from turncoats, these visionaries will shape the health care of the future.

CHAPTER 10

ETHICS AND NEW INTERPRETATIONS OF PROFESSIONALISM

Edmund Pellegrino, a noted ethicist and physician, believes that medical practice is more than the application of biological knowledge to the diagnosis and treatment of disease; indeed, "medicine is a moral enterprise" (1987, p. 8). Consideration of the "ethical" component of "professional" behavior has become more important as both the technical complexity of and the financial influences on medical practice have grown. As a result, the interpretation of medical professionalism will continue to change as the new medical marketplace evolves. The concept of "professionalism," including the roles and responsibilities that define the profession, is influenced by ethical, social, legal, economic, and political forces. Changing concepts of professionalism can be seen in the trends toward patients' increasing expectations of clinicians as well as the development of physician employees and entrepreneurs. This chapter explores the ethical component of professional behavior in health care, and it emphasizes the relationship that exists between ethics and current socioeconomic issues in health care. Aspects that are considered include the interests and obligations of the physician as an individual, of the profession as a whole, and of the medical code of ethics.

Popular definitions of ethics include personal beliefs about what is right and wrong, professional codes, and judgments concerning a person's moral behavior. People commonly confuse the concept of ethics with related but distinct notions such as morality, law, or religion. Hard choices are often mistaken for ethical dilemmas as well, and both "ethics" and "ethic" often are incorrectly used interchangeably. Different parties often mean different things when using the same terms, so to resolve conflicts, it is important that the participants speak the same language. This chapter attempts to elucidate the difference between ethical reasoning and the professional ethic and to clarify some of these confusions in terminology.*

The Role of Ethical Principles

Because today's physicians frequently face difficult moral dilemmas, ethical reasoning has become more important than ever. Some physicians might argue that because they themselves are "ethical," medical ethics as a subject of study may be left to academic philosophers, but medical ethics is not a purely academic pursuit. It provides tools that are necessary for clinicians to explore their own values and whether their behavior is consistent with those. Physicians with unimpeachable values and morals still may *behave* unethically by making clinical decisions that ignore either societal considerations or the patient's wishes.

To provide a framework for our discussion, we must first define the major relevant *ethical* or *moral principles.* Ideally, delivery of health care involves a delicate balancing of three primary principles: beneficence, autonomy, and justice.

The principle of *beneficence,* which focuses on promoting the welfare of others, has been described as involving four elements: avoiding the infliction of harm,† preventing harm, removing existing harm, and the affirmative promotion of good (Faden et al. 1991). The application of beneficence to medical care is:

"The alleviation of disease, disability, and injury if there is a reasonable hope of cure or improvement. The harms to be prevented, removed, or minimized are the pain, suffering, and disability of injury and disease. In addition, the health professional is enjoined from *doing* harm, such as when interventions inflict unnecessary pain and suffering." (ibid., p. 15)

---

*The discussion of terminology excludes the language of "rights." We cannot provide a comprehensive discussion of this concept here; suffice it to say that a *right* is a claim that demands respect. For example, many people refer to the right to health care, though others feel this is framed more appropriately as a societal *obligation* to provide health care. (See Chapter 13.)

It is important to recognize the distinction between "rights" and "acting rightly." Many moral controversies in both medicine and public policy involve debates about rights such as a right to die, to life, to reproduce, or to privacy. For example, one can affirm a right to die but not agree to perform euthanasia.

†Some theorists argue that avoiding the infliction of harm constitutes a separate principle that is termed *nonmaleficence.*

The next principle, respect for *autonomy,* relates to a person's right to self-determination. In moral philosophy, autonomy itself refers to "personal rule of the self by adequate understanding while remaining free from controlling interference by others and from personal limitations that prevent choice" (ibid, p. 17). Autonomy is the principle on which both the legal right to privacy and the process of informed consent are based.

Paternalism on the part of clinicians, whereby they assume knowledge of what is best for the patient, overlooks the importance of respect for autonomy in deference to the principle of beneficence. Paternalism is a double-edged sword that highlights the importance of balancing ethical principles: it is motivated by one ethical principle (beneficence) but has adverse effects on another (autonomy). Medical care traditionally has been quite paternalistic in style. Although many professionals are now emphasizing respect for autonomy, it is not clear where on the spectrum the pendulum ultimately will stop.

The third principle, *justice,* refers to the proper distribution of benefits as well as burdens. This principle is particularly relevant in determining the distribution of limited resources on a societal level. "A person has been treated in accordance with the principle of justice if treated according to what is fair, due, or owed. . . . Judgments of what is fair, due, or owed are . . . concerned with the comparative treatment of members of a group when benefits and burdens are distributed" (ibid., p. 18).

Three main theories of distributive justice exist. According to *egalitarianism,* everybody receives an equal share of scarce resources. Egalitarianism can be interpreted as either equality of outcome or equality of opportunity, whereby resources are distributed without the imposition of value judgments about the relative worth of recipients. Under the theory of *utilitarianism,* resources would be distributed so as to do the greatest good for the greatest number. This theory requires a determination of which members of society would benefit most from access to scarce resources and which would suffer least from the denial of such access. According to *libertarianism,* distributions of health care services and goods are best left to the marketplace, which operates on the principle of the ability to pay. Under this theory, the rich can subsidize the poor through charity (if they so choose), but society has no moral obligation to take resources from the rich by taxing them.

It is important not to confuse the terms *just* (as in morally right), *justified*, and *justice*. Many complaints of *injustice* can be linked to violations of the principles of beneficence or of respect for autonomy (e.g., when confidentiality is breached, the principle of respect for autonomy is "unjustly" violated). Apart from the allocation of scarce resources, to which the principles of distributive justice are relevant, the principles that are most likely to be important to physicians dealing with specific cases are beneficence and autonomy—and "justifying" the balance between them.

Moral Dilemmas Versus Hard Choices

Some theorists support a hierarchical ordering of ethical principles; others believe that each principle should have equal weight. The challenge is often to weigh one principle against another and then strike the right balance between them. *Moral dilemmas* arise when a conflict exists between moral principles that generate conflicting demands, but there is a difference between a moral dilemma and a *hard choice*. In a moral dilemma, there are reasons to follow one course of action and equally compelling reasons *not* to follow that course (or to follow another) (Beauchamp and Childress, 1989). If the physician acts on either set of reasons, then those actions will be desirable in some respects but undesirable in others.

The classic example of a moral dilemma is whether physicians have a duty to warn third parties of potential danger (e.g., telling a spouse that a patient has tested positive for the human immune deficiency virus [HIV]) when that information was obtained in the context of a confidential encounter with a patient. If physicians decide they have a duty to warn, then they are deciding that, in this case, beneficence is more important than patient autonomy.

By contrast, "a conflict between a moral obligation on the one hand and self-interest on the other is not a moral dilemma" (ibid., p. 5). This is a hard choice. Hard choices involve self-interest and can often have tragic consequences, but not all consequences are *moral* consequences. The financial transformation of the health care system has created the potential for hard choices in the professional dimension of medical care; however, the dilemma of which path is most beneficial to the provider (financially or otherwise) is *not* a moral dilemma.

We exclude the case of geniune conflict of interest between physicians' role obligations. Sometimes providers seem to be motivated by self-interest (e.g., when research takes priority over patient care), when in fact they are facing a true moral dilemma about how to balance their obligations to research subjects versus individual patients.

The Role of the Professional Ethic

Relman believes that what physicians now face "is basically an internal moral crisis" (1983, p. 19). As he sees it, physicians "are inherently no different from other citizens. They have the same strengths and weaknesses of character and are susceptible to the same economic temptations as anyone else. What gives physicians special influence is the trust reposed in them by the public and the responsibility for the care of their patients invested in them by law. This trust and responsibility, in turn, are based on the assumption that the medical profession has unique technical competence, which it is committed to employ primarily for the benefit of the sick" (1985, p. 104).

Relman's statement highlights the potential conflict—between financial incentives and clinical considerations—in providing medical care under the present health care system. This conflict provides a good example of a hard choice for the provider, *not* a moral dilemma; the salience of this potential conflict in a given situation depends on a number of factors, including practice setting, insurance coverage, and patient needs. Financial conflicts become moral dilemmas when they involve issues of justice that affect access to care or the quality of care (such as whom to assign to an intensive care unit bed or other types of resource rationing).

Relman points out that with medical training also comes an inherent responsibility to apply that training ethically. During medical training, the individual undergoes a professional socialization, adopting the accepted standards of practice in his or her professional behavior. Once training is completed, it is expected that every clinician be acquainted with the rules that the profession has established collectively. In their professional life, clinicians are subject to a certain ongoing ethical tutelage, both from peer pressures and from new rulings of the AMA and specialty societies. Some of these expectations are explicit and codified, but other aspects are more flexible and subject to individual interpretation.

As a point of departure, we can examine one of the most important ethical traditions of medicine—the Hippocratic Oath—to set the framework for modern modifications. Historically, all physicians took this oath on graduation from medical school, a tradition that continues in many schools today.

THE HIPPOCRATIC OATH

I swear by Apollo Physician and Asclepius and Hygieia and Panaceia and all the gods and goddesses, making them my witnesses, that I will fulfill according to my ability and judgment this oath and this covenant:

To hold him who has taught me this art as equal to my parents and to live my life in partnership with him, and if he is in need of money to give him a share of mine, and to regard his offspring as equal to my brothers in male lineage and to teach them this art—if they desire to learn it—without fee and covenant; to give a share of precepts and oral instruction and all the other learning to my sons and to the sons of him who has instructed me and to pupils who have signed the covenant and have taken an oath according to the medical law, but to no one else. I will apply dietetic measures for the benefit of the sick according to my ability and judgment; I will keep them from harm and injustice.

I will neither give a deadly drug to anybody if asked for it, nor will I make a suggestion to this effect. Similarly I will not give to a woman an abortive remedy. In purity and holiness I will guard my life and my art. I will not use the knife, not even on sufferers from stone, but will withdraw in favor of such men as are engaged in this work.

Whatever houses I may visit, I will come for the benefit of the sick, remaining free of all intentional injustice, of all mischief and in particular of sexual relations with both female and male persons, be they free or slaves.

What I may see or hear in the course of the treatment or even outside of the treatment in regard to the life of men, which on no account one must spread abroad, I will keep to myself, holding such things shameful to be spoken about.

If I fulfill this oath and do not violate it, may it be granted to me to enjoy life and art, being honored with fame among all men for all time to come; if I transgress it and swear falsely, may the opposite of all this be my lot.

Physicians who abide by the Hippocratic Oath have made a formal covenant with patients to do their best for them. This is the main intent of the code, part of a centuries-old tradition in medicine. It provides an example of an ethical principle, beneficence, that informs the professional ethic.

Most people think the intent of the Hippocratic Oath is upheld fairly well, on the whole, but society has changed and medicine has progressed. In the process, the expectations of both patient and society have evolved; for example, the code mentions nothing about patient rights or autonomy.* These new expectations call for new interpretations of some parts of the code. The oath also proscribes abortion and euthanasia. As a result, it has had to be modified in some ways to conform to modern times. Many schools have modified the oath that their graduates take, while others have abandoned the Hippocratic framework altogether.

Other codes that inform the professional ethic have also evolved over time. For example, the AMA Code of Ethics no longer proscribes abortion, and many believe that someday it may no longer proscribe euthanasia. Some might perceive the very evolution of the AMA Code as raising questions about what is "ethical," however, and the evolution of codes over time, responding to society at large, might seem to indicate that the core of belief at the heart of the medical ethic is mutable. This would be an oversimplified interpretation of the process, however. Ethical principles are immutable, but the professional ethic and standards of professionalism do evolve as perceptions change regarding how best to balance these principles. This flexibility is necessary for medical practice to conform to the changing societal needs of its health care system.

The Clinician: Responsible to the Patient, the Payer, or Society?

The new medical marketplace creates a fundamental conflict for clinicians as they try to determine whom they are to serve as agent. (*Agent* is defined for these purposes as one who acts as an

---

*Except as it alludes to respect for confidentiality.

advocate in the interest of another.) The object of professional responsibility has been called into question in this new era; as stated by Eisenberg, "For the individual physician and individual patient, the need for trade-offs becomes a matter of social responsibility to be weighed against the individual's gain. The ethical dilemma of how society's resources are distributed and the physician's role as both the patient's agent and a responsible member of society thus becomes explicit ... the biomedical and economic considerations of clinical practice come together" (1989, p. 2886). Is the physician responsible to the patient alone? To the payer? To society? Answers to these questions will likely require redefining the professional ethic, including an explicit definition of *agency*. Solutions will also be influenced by a number of ethical principles, including beneficence, autonomy, and justice.

Clinicians now must wear many hats. Sometimes they are called on to think of the patient's best interest, as when a resource decision involves an identified patient. Sometimes the clinician is asked to think of a hospital's best interest, when capital investment or program development is under discussion. At other times, clinicians are called on to think of themselves as society's agents and to take a global perspective on the health care system. While in many cases the perspective that is required by these various roles seems obvious, distinguishing which hat to wear, and when (particularly when these decisions are confounded by considerations of the physician's self-interest) is not always a trivial matter. Facility at discerning the appropriate response to a given situation will become even more important as resource rationing becomes ever more explicit.

These ideas are relevant for clinicians, whether they are engaged in clinical duties or in assisting the formation of public policy. Redelmeier and Tversky noted that, "Physicians and policy makers may wish to examine problems from both perspectives to ensure that treatment decisions are appropriate whether applied to one or to many patients. An awareness of the two perspectives may enhance clinical judgment and enrich health policy" (1990, p. 1164). Now more than ever, it is important that well-intentioned people whose primary concern is patients' best interests be involved in clinical decision-making. Patients also need advocates beyond the examining room, and in many cases, physicians' authority makes it easier for them rather than their patients to influence policy decisions.

Role of Patients and Families

Decisions about medical care either are governed by patients' wishes or are influenced by input from patients and their families. The ethical principle of patient autonomy, which was defined earlier as a patient's right to self-determination, operates in this aspect of clinical decision-making. The physician's duty to act according to beneficence must be balanced by his or her duty to respect the patient's autonomy; ideally, clinical decisions are made on the basis of discussion among the providers, patients, and families.

Through a new sensitivity to patients' rights, heightened or increased respect for patient autonomy has improved the quality of care, but financial changes in the system now threaten that concern for autonomy. The economic priorities of society, which are embodied in managed care, cost-sharing, and new reimbursement incentives, may significantly constrain the decisions arrived at by patients and physicians.

As might be expected, patients are becoming increasingly concerned with whether the system is working to their advantage or whether (like poor Mrs. Fitch in the cartoon) they are merely pawns in some financial chess game. Today's patients may come to feel that they have no true advocate within the health care system. There is no easy answer here. Patients now have more say in the decisions that are made about their care, and they probably will have even more in the future. Tradeoffs must occur, however, because even with the patient as the first priority, societal objectives will exact their due.

Maximizing the involvement of patients in the clinical decision-making process will mitigate the effects of the marketplace on medical care. Jay Katz, a psychiatrist, proposed a process of *shared* decision-making, requiring conversation between patients and providers to bring out the motivations of each (1984). For example, Katz claimed that physicians are afraid of losing their power;

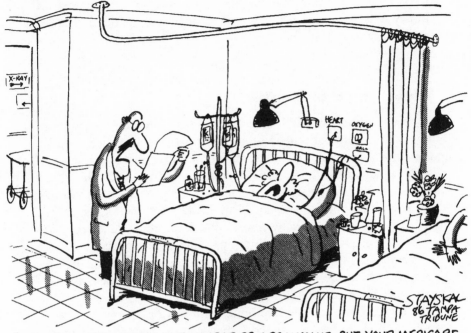

"YOUR BLOOD PRESSURE AND TEMPERATURE ARE WAY UP, BUT YOUR MEDICARE COVERAGE IS WAY DOWN. LOOKS AS IF YOU CAN GO HOME TODAY, MRS. FITCH!"

this fear, which manifests itself as an unwillingness or inability to acknowledge uncertainty, reflects physicians' denial of their fallibility. With habitual denial and suppression of uncertainty, physicians may become unable to share ambiguity and uncertainty with their patients. Thus, while the very existence of uncertainty imposes burdens on physicians, the greater burden is the obligation to keep these uncertainties in mind and to acknowledge them to patients. Katz believes that patients' choices deserve to be honored in the absence of substantial evidence of patient incompetence.*

Several new resources to assist clinicians, patients, and families with ethical dilemmas are becoming an intrinsic part of modern

---

*A legal term referring to an inability to understand the nature and/or consequences of a clinical issue.

medical practice. These include hospital ethics committees that are composed of parties neutral to the conundrum at hand; such committees may include clinicians, hospital administrators or trustees, ethicists, patient representatives, clergy, lawyers, and others. Ethics committees usually do not offer answers (depending on the context of the problem) but instead assist the patient, family, and clinician in resolving their problem by providing new ways of viewing the situation.

Payers and managers often are involved in making policy decisions about the use of resources, but usually not at the individual patient level. Our admitted bias is that physicians and other practitioners alone have the technical knowledge and professional socialization that are necessary to participate in informed, individual clinical decisions. It is incumbent on all parties to learn to make decisions cooperatively, thus optimizing the process for the good of the patients.

The Role of Social Influences

The influence of societal priorities on the health care system is the focus of Part IV, but for the purposes of this discussion, it is necessary to note that societal norms and priorities inevitably affect clinical decision-making. This assertion may appear obvious today, but it by no means has always been so. Historically, no significant conflict existed between the goals of patients and clinicians and the goals of society, the latter playing an essentially invisible role in the process. Apart from some influence (as seen in the modification of the Hippocratic Oath and AMA Code), these aims until recently have come from only the practitioner's individual conscience or the profession as a whole.

The cost crisis and social changes such as the rising importance of patient autonomy, however, have irrevocably changed the dynamic that exists between society and the health care system. Today, societal influences have a definite impact on medical care, which is affected by new rules, and these rules of the new medical marketplace have the potential for both positive and adverse impacts on the quality of medical care.

The first step in modernizing society's influence on clinical decision-making is to identify clearly the desired objectives of all the parties involved, including public and private third-party payers, patients, and providers. Once these objectives are prioritized (a process that may be facilitated by the application of ethical principles), goals for the system will be more clear to all participants. Decision-making for patients and providers will be easier once these goals are explicit and the system has reached a new equilibrium.

Changing Concepts of Professionalism

To accommodate the changing priorities of the new medical marketplace, some aspects of the professional ethic must evolve, and others must be preserved intact. The responsibilities that define the professional's roles will also evolve. This change is already under way in some respects, as ethics committees and administrators have been admitted to the clinical decision-making process in some cases. Case managers and gatekeepers (often clinicians whose major goal is utilization control) are involved in other situations. During previous eras, no one apart from the patient and the hands-on provider was involved to this extent in the process of care delivery.

The growing number of physicians with entrepreneurial involvement in the health care system, as well as the growing number of physician employees, have also sparked debate about the meaning of professionalism. Consensus has not been reached on these issues within the profession itself yet, let alone within society.

The process of modifying the definition of professionalism will likely be difficult, and physician resistance is in some sense understandable. Our hope is that clinicians not only contribute to this process but that they influence it positively, in a nonself-serving way that is consistent with their consciences, professional ethics, and the desires of both patients and society.

Medical Education

Ethical behavior is not only a matter of following the codes that the profession or society delineates. Physicians bring their individuality to professional training and to some degree interpret right and wrong behavior uniquely. Because the clinician's opinion is one of the important aspects of clinical decision-making, there is undeniably a personal, intellectual component to ethical considerations and the interpretation of professional behavior.

This has several implications for medical education. Experienced clinicians will always be vital to the process, but technical knowledge and clinical wisdom are no longer the only goals of medical education. Development of a professional attitude that is consonant with the demands of today's health care system requires education about these issues and socialization to them during the training process. Changes are occurring so quickly that role models may not always be available, and appropriate mentors will likely be found among the younger practitioners. This places more responsibility on the student to sense the complexity of a given situation and his or her proper role within it. Given the conflicts that are inherent in medical practice today, the provider's *conscience,* while always important, is now more important than ever. For all of these reasons, the selection and preparation of appropriate trainees has taken on added importance.

We would like to believe that FDR was right—that education is our best protection against fear and prejudice. This assumes that the education is not limited simply to acquisition of knowledge, however. It should include the social and ethical aspects of health care as well as interpersonal communication skills. This is particularly relevant for the growing number of patients' problems today (e.g., acquired immune deficiency syndrome, substance abuse) that are extremely complex; in such cases, medical education can assist physicians in accepting their inability to solve singlehandedly the social problems that contribute to patients' medical problems and in acknowledging any negative attitudes toward such patients (which stem largely from their own fears and prejudices).

Broadening our notion of education to highlight the importance of self-awareness of one's own idiosyncrasies and motivations, either rational or irrational, would further enable practitioners to keep pace with the changing world. The same approach would benefit payers and policymakers as well; the opportunity to create fair and equitable fiscal and regulatory policies is optimized when personal prejudices are kept to a minimum.

As new approaches to decision-making become more prevalent, the role of biomedical ethics and the professional ethic will continue to increase in importance. While physicians work toward incorporating economic considerations into their practice, beneficence, patient autonomy, and justice must remain central to patient care. Ethical factors and the professional ethic are, as we feel they should be, a matter of increasing discussion, from legislative chambers, to clinical conferences, to the patient's bedside.

PART IV

SOCIETAL ISSUES AND THE NEW MEDICAL MARKETPLACE

Either we all hang together, or we shall certainly all hang separately.

Benjamin Franklin

I n contrast to Part III, which emphasized the provider's perspective, this section focuses more globally, on society in relation to the U.S. health care system. We have included here the issues of malpractice and access to care; while they do involve individual patients and clinicians, they are examined most appropriately at the societal level.

Medical malpractice became a critical issue during the early 1980s. Several factors contributed to the problem. In part, the growth of medical malpractice litigation appears to reflect the patients' rights movement as well as a new mistrust of providers by their patients. This increase in litigation has induced some physicians to alter their clinical decisions in a style termed *defensive medicine,* where marginally necessary tests are performed solely to protect the clinician from potential liability. Defensive medicine has also exacerbated inflation in the costs of health care. Problems within the U.S. legal system contribute significantly to the malpractice problem as well.

Professional liability insurance became prohibitively expensive for many practitioners during this era, forcing some into career changes or early retirement. As a result, the malpractice problem has affected access to medical care. A number of legislative solutions to the malpractice problem have been proposed as well as implemented. This complex issue is explored in Chapter 11.

Because the U.S. health care system has never had a systematic or universal arrangement for providing services to all the members of society, access to care has always been a problem to some extent. Runaway health care expenditures, however, and the resulting cost-containment efforts of the 1970s and 1980s have exacerbated this problem. Today, many Americans face a true crisis in their ability to obtain medical care.

Policy responses to the ever-increasing needs of poor and uninsured people are being mounted in some locales, as in the case of Oregon's proposed Medicaid "rationing" plan. This program as well as a growing awareness of the need for legislative solutions has engendered nationwide debate regarding society's responsibility for assuring publicly financed medical care for all citizens. This controversial issue is explored in Chapter 12.

The final chapter looks at a panoply of other social issues that confront our health care system, both presently and in the years to come. What are individuals and communities willing to do to promote health? How should we use our finite health care resources? Should medical education, technology, and research remain priorities? These choices are explored in Chapter 13.

The issues that Part IV highlights are most contentious, and they reveal great ambivalence toward our health care system. America is among the most heterogeneous of nations; many different value systems operate within it. Because true change usually requires broad societal support for legislative reform, solutions have been elusive.

In the three chapters that follow, we present the issues and some potential solutions from multiple perspectives. Readers can draw their own conclusions, but we believe that certain "facts" are undeniable: the current malpractice climate unnecessarily consumes precious resources, and many Americans face almost insurmountable barriers to needed care.

Unless addressed, the scope of these problems will only expand in the future. Few ideal solutions exist, however, and there inevitably will be disagreement about what is optimal. Still, health care providers, as well as those who bankroll and regulate the system, must respond.

CHAPTER 11

THE MALPRACTICE PROBLEM

It would be a tremendous abrogation of intellectual responsibility to look at a [legal] system with this many problems, that costs this much and serves the public this poorly and say that it is the best we can do.

Daniel Creasey

"**M**edical malpractice** is faulty medical management that injures a patient" (Bovbjerg 1985, p. 38). Plaintiffs must recognize damage to themselves; prove fault on the part of a physician, hospital, or other provider of care; and establish a causal connection between the two (ibid.). Note that *any* action occurring in the course of health care delivery, even one such as helping a patient get out of bed, is considered under the rubric of medical malpractice even if not strictly "medical" in nature.

A legal wrong committed on the person or property of another for which the law gives civil remedy, usually monetary damages for the resulting injury, is termed a *tort*. Common torts are negligence, assault, battery, false imprisonment, libel, slander, and invasion of privacy. Medical malpractice, a negligent tort, occurs if a physician injures a patient through practice that is below acceptable standards. There are four elements to be proved in every negligent tort claim:

- a duty owed by the defendant to the plaintiff
- breach of that duty by the defendant
- harm to the plaintiff
- a causal relationship between the breach and the harm.

Proof that each of these elements is present involves varying degrees of difficulty. Duty is a given in the patient–physician relationship, and harm is usually apparent. Breach and cause are frequently less easy to prove, however. Within the greater legal infrastructure, the tort system serves to determine when, as a matter of law, a tort has been committed. Brennan (1991, p. 1) described three purposes of the tort system:

- compensation of injured parties
- deterrence against further negligent acts on both the individual and systemic levels
- corrective justice in the sense that the person who caused the injury remunerates the injured party in some fashion.

Most would agree that a patient who has been harmed by a physician's unreasonable mistake is due compensation. Ideally, payment is made for claims that are brought in cases where both injury *and* negligence are present, but difficult questions of definition and degree are involved in determining that compensation. These questions have broad ramifications not only in medical practice but throughout society as well. In fact, the system is quite poor in meeting each of the three objectives defined above.

In recent years, a variety of factors—including the structure of the legal system, social attitudes, changes in health care financing, and uncertainty in clinical practice itself—have combined to create further problems in the system. While these issues have been referred to as "the malpractice crisis" this phrase is a misnomer insofar as it implies a single entity. In fact, it is more appropriate to refer to the malpractice *crises*, because distinct aspects of the problems surrounding the application of tort law to medicine affect patients, providers, and payers in different ways. Also, a single solution would not address all of these problems.

Contributors to these malpractice problems are found both within the health care system (providers, ancillary employees, health care organizations, and so on) and without (from patients as individuals to society as a whole). The legal and political systems also play a role in these problems. Similarly, solutions to malpractice problems will require efforts by the health care system, patients, both the legal and political systems, and by the collective society.

Each of the following sections explores a different component of the malpractice problem. A description of the major effects of the malpractice problem follows, and several possible improvements (if not solutions) are proposed.

An Epidemic of Lawsuits

The notion of malpractice has roots in medieval times, but actual lawsuits against physicians were rare until this century. In the past several decades, the number of malpractice suits has increased steadily, and this trend has accelerated in recent years. The AMA reports that before 1981, an average of 3.2 claims per 100 physicians were made annually. Between 1981 and 1984, the rate increased to over 8 claims per 100 physicians, and in 1985, it reached slightly over 10 per 100 physicians. Since 1985, however, the rate has decreased somewhat. In 1988, the average annual rate of malpractice claims was 6.4 per 100 physicians, increasing to 7.4 per 100 in 1989, but despite the decrease, practitioners as well as many lawyers perceive this as too many lawsuits.

Not only has the number of lawsuits increased, judges and juries have increased the amounts that are awarded to successful claimants. Data from a firm specializing in legal case analysis indicate that the average medically related court award increased from $229,000 in 1975 to $888,000 in 1983 and to over $1,000,000 in 1985. (These figures exclude out-of-court settlements.)

Any physician may be sued, but Table 11 illustrates that certain specialties generate a higher percentage of lawsuits, notably obstetrics and gynecology, general surgery, and orthopedic surgery. In contrast, other clinicians, such as family physicians and midwives, are sued relatively infrequently.

What kinds of case are being brought to court? In 1983, the St. Paul Insurance Company reported that the most common reasons among its policyholders for being sued were:

- a bad result, such as complications resulting from allegedly negligent postsurgical care
- falls of all types, including from bed, while walking, and in the bathroom
- delayed or omitted treatment

- injury of a body part adjacent to the treatment site
- wrong diagnosis or incorrect treatment
- infection, contamination, or exposure to an injurious substance.

These remain very common reasons for malpractice lawsuits, and it is apparent that some of the reasons do not result from poor clinical decisions or technical mishaps but from carelessness, such as not supporting patients who are unsteady on their feet. Regarding medical care from its more purely technical aspects, the AMA reported the 10 most frequent allegations of malpractice in the late 1980s:

postoperative surgical complication,

birth-related condition,

failure to diagnose cancer,

inadvertent surgical act,

failure to diagnose fracture or dislocation,

drug side effect,

insufficient treatment,

improper treatment of a fracture or dislocation,

surgically related postoperative death, and

inappropriate surgical procedure.

Table 11.   The Average Incidence of Malpractice Claims by Specialty (1985 and 1989) and the Average Annual Rate of Change

	Annual claims per 100 physicians		Average annual rate of change
	1985	1989	
All physicians*	10.2	7.4	−10.1%
General/Family Practice	5.7	6.6	+5.0
Internal Medicine	6.2	5.9	−1.6
Surgery	16.8	11.2	−12.6
Pediatrics	7.2	5.4	−9.1
Obstetrics/Gynecology	25.8	13.5	−19.4
Radiology	12.8	5.0	−26.9
Psychiatry	2.9	5.1	+20.7
Anesthesiology	7.5	5.9	−7.7

*Also includes physicians in specialties that are not listed separately.
Source: Adapted from the American Medical Association 1991.

An Epidemic of Poor Practice

Some blame the malpractice crisis on a sharp increase in the actual commission of malpractice by practitioners. Some would say this increase is the crisis, and they contend that only a small percentage of the increasing number of injuries caused by physicians' errors ever result in lawsuits.

In fact, data from recent studies support the contention that malpractice occurs quite frequently. Brennan et al. reviewed 31,000 New York State hospital records in 1984 for the incidence of adverse events, which they defined as "an injury that was caused by medical management (rather than the underlying disease) and that prolonged the hospitalization, produced a disability at the time of discharge, or both" (1991, p. 370). Negligence was defined as "care that fell below the standard expected of physicians in their community" (ibid.). The research team estimated the statewide incidence of adverse events as 3.7 percent, with 1 percent of those caused by negligence. Fifty-seven percent of the adverse events led to minor impairment, 14 percent to a 1- to 6-month disability, 26 percent to permanent disability, and 14 percent to death. The rates varied widely by hospital, however, so adverse events may be a better indicator of quality than mortality or readmission rates (discussed in Chapter 8).

Leape et al. (1991), from the same Harvard group, studied the nature of adverse events; they found that 14 percent were wound infections and 13 percent technical complications. Approximately half of the adverse events were surgical. Of the nonsurgical adverse events, 19 percent were drug-related and 8 percent involved a "diagnostic mishap." It is equally important to compare the high incidence of adverse events with the lower rate of lawsuits, and the results of these studies led many to believe that numerous people who would have reason to sue do not. In addition, the Harvard study found that the cases involving negligence were *not* the cases in which a lawsuit was brought.

This is the first time that such a large-scale investigation of medical errors has been performed. The results are striking in that they reveal a significant number of adverse events. As with the first in-depth examination of *any* phenomenon, however, the frequency of clinical errors in previous years is unknown, and this number of problems and complications could be better *or* worse. Thus, it is not known whether the malpractice problem can be attributed to "an epidemic of malpractice." This is not to dismiss the findings—whatever the trend, it is still important that such a high rate of negligence was found.

It was not found that a few physicians are being sued repeatedly; the increased number of lawsuits are widely dispersed among physicians. Thirty-eight percent of all physicians, among them some 60 percent of obstetricians, have been sued at least once in their careers, and Table 12 shows the percentage of physicians (overall and by specialty) who have been sued at least once.

Many cases, however, are dismissed in pretrial hearings because they lack merit. The possibility of an out-of-court settlement also exists. Most cases that reach the trial stage today do so because there is major disagreement among the parties about culpability and the quality of evidence lending merit to the dispute. In cases that eventually do reach the courtroom, plaintiffs are awarded damages less than half the time. Cheney et al. (1989) reviewed approximately 1000 closed claims involving anesthesiologists, and found that standards of care were met in 46 percent of those claims, thus suggesting "that the filing of a lawsuit alleging malpractice does not necessarily imply substandard care as judged by peers" (ibid., p. 1602). Furthermore, payment was made in 42 percent of claims that were peer judged to be either at or above

Table 12.   Physicians' Experience of Lawsuits by Specialty, 1989

Category	Physicians sued at least once during their career
All physicians*	37.8%
General/Family Practice	40.5
Internal Medicine	28.0
Surgery	52.0
Pediatrics	24.9
Obstetrics/Gynecology	60.0
Radiology	35.1
Psychiatry	22.2
Anesthesiology	32.8

*Also includes physicians in specialties that are not listed separately.
Source: Adapted from the American Medical Association 1991, p. 17.

the standard of care; this is compared with payment in 82 percent of cases in which care was peer judged to be below standard. On this point, it is important to remember that the standard of care is judged in the courtroom by a lay jury and not by medical peers.

Crisis of Misunderstanding in the Patient–Physician Relationship

The patient–physician relationship has played a role in malpractice as well. Many patients believe that there is "always" a drug, device, or treatment to cure any condition. To some extent practitioners reinforce this misconception, and a paternalistic bedside manner (see Chapter 10) may reinforce it further. The danger in this belief is that if the patient is not cured, or has a less than ideal outcome, it seems logical to blame the physician. Some feel that physicians are now paying the price (literally, in some cases) for the centuries-old tradition of presenting themselves to patients as infallible. When they *do* fail (as they inevitably do), it is predictable that the trusting patient will be angry; many lawsuits are generated as a result.

During recent years, patients' desire for autonomy has increased, and they have achieved greater discretion over the decisions that are made about their care. As a result, patients are less blindly accepting of physicians' recommendations, and while this wariness serves a protective function for the patient, it also dampens the positive effects (e.g., trust, reassurance) that a clinical encounter should produce. Because the patient–provider relationship has weakened, many patients today do not feel they risk the loss of an important relationship should they file a lawsuit. This situation may be exacerbated by the rise of managed-care plans that preclude patients from choosing individual providers. Because less is at stake for many of today's disgruntled or injured patients, it is easier for them to sue, and this likely is one cause of the increasing number of lawsuits.

Given the number of errors in the provision of health care and the inevitable bad outcomes that result not only from those errors but from diseases themselves, a desire by some patients for compensation is to be expected. Just as a good relationship can prevent lawsuits, however, a bad relationship can promote them (Gutheil et al. 1984). In some ways, this may be more important than whether an adverse event (if not negligence) has occurred. Just as patients do not always know if they need care but do have a subjective experience of dysfunction, they may not know if malpractice has occurred—but they have their subjective experience of the overall manner in which they were treated.

As medical technologies advance, it becomes harder to distinguish between a poor outcome resulting from negligence or error and a poor outcome resulting from natural events. Eventually, all people die, but with high-technology interventions it becomes more difficult to determine when a death is "natural" or inevitable—and when it is preventable, given the extent of scientific knowledge. It may even be difficult to determine whether an intervention has caused benefit or harm, and as a consequence, many lawsuits that are brought against physicians do not involve their negligence but result from events and outcomes that were largely beyond their control.

As previous discussions of small-area variation made clear, uncertainty is inherent in medicine: not only uncertainty about the condition of a particular patient, but uncertainty about the "best" course of treatment. Even experts frequently disagree; for example, two articles in the same issue of the *New England Journal of Medicine* came to conflicting conclusions on the extent to which postmenopausal women increased their risk of cardiovascular disease by using estrogen (Stempfer et al. 1985; Wilson et al. 1985). Some physicians are being sued because bad outcomes resulted from reasonable and unavoidable differences in opinion concerning medical practice.

Patients and practitioners alike wish that medical practice was straightforward, with clearcut solutions to stem disease and suffering. Patients desire the "best" care, and clinicians would like to provide that. As Chapter 8 discussed, however, the denial by both participants that uncertainty and disagreement exist in medical practice breeds problems. A second medical opinion may differ 180 degrees from the first opinion, yet both can be "right"—or at least "not wrong." This is difficult for practitioners to grasp, let alone to convey to society, patients, and lawyers.

Furthermore, there will always be a line below which human error cannot be reduced further. This is termed by Gorovitz and MacIntyre (1986) as *necessary fallibility*. Anderson et al. also included this concept in the interpretation of a large autopsy series that compared diagnoses made both before and after death, noting that "errors may occur as a result of willfulness (intentional injury) or negligence (incompetence or ignorance), but . . . in other cases medical knowledge is inadequate to solve the problem, and furthermore that diagnostic predictions must occasionally fail solely because of . . . 'necessary fallibility'" (1991, p. 1617).

The attribution of error is fundamental to the determination that medical malpractice has occurred. This determination is complicated, however, by the ambiguity that is an undeniable aspect of all clinical decisions. Conflicting expectations from patients, society, and the legal system about uncertainty in medical practice contribute to the malpractice problem, and patients who do not recognize the presence of necessary fallibility may be more likely to sue in cases that have a poor outcome.

Misunderstanding between Professionals

Doctors and lawyers have different standards of evidence and thus, in many instances, fundamentally misunderstand one another. "Scientific evidence must be probable, repeatable, provable. Legal evidence needs merely to be possible, sometimes only remotely possible. Large liability awards for scientifically unprovable but legally possible injuries following alleged acts of malpractice or negligence have become commonplace" (Lee 1986, p. 159).

Many physicians have become cynical toward the legal system, whose premises they see as unrealistic. Lee expressed this disaffection: "For practitioners of liability litigation, a utopian medical world in which all illness is preventable or discoverable and curable by brilliantly empathetic and encyclopedic physicians is indispensable. [They] have created a biologic bill of rights predicated on the notion that illness and injury are unnatural and therefore somebody else's fault. In this non-Darwinian world, the biology of the individual is susceptible only to the actions of other human agents" (1986, p. 159). This attitude contributes to the growing

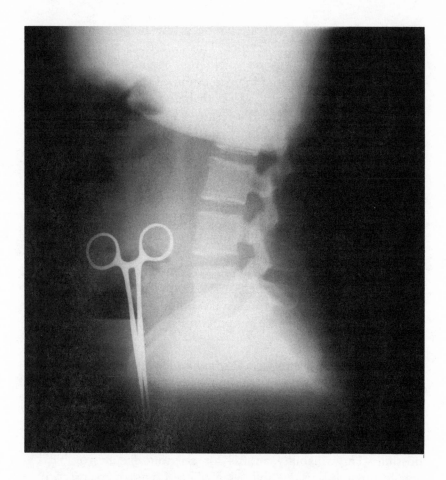

gulf between physicians and lawyers, and while reflecting the feeling of many practitioners about the situation, it is not an accurate
assessment of the legal system.

This is not to say that straightforward mistakes are never made.
The Latin phrase *res ipsa loquitur,* "the thing speaks for itself," is
used in some states when an error is so obvious that no further explanation of it is necessary; the classic example is the proverbial "Kelly in
the belly."* (See photograph above.) The argument that medicine is

---

*Kelly is a type of surgical clamp. This phrase was coined to refer to an x-ray that reveals
a surgical clamp remaining in a patient's abdomen after the surgery was completed and the
incision closed. The phrase is now used more generally, referring to other such obvious
mistakes.

an inexact science is irrelevant if the provider has made such an egregious error, and some causes on the list of the most common reasons for lawsuits do result from such lapses. In such cases, the only issue in a resulting lawsuit is the size of the damage award.

The Structure of the Legal System

The legal system also influences the malpractice problem. The legal system of every society is designed to address societal values; therefore, some problems within this system reflect troublesome societal objectives or problems within society at large. One such major concern is the idea that financial compensation is due when there is a bad outcome, whether or not it resulted from a physician's error. Increasingly, tort law is seen simply as a mechanism to provide compensation for injury, and malpractice lawsuits have evolved into a type of lottery where a big win is possible.

In the United States, an initial outlay of dollars is not required to bring a lawsuit. In most cases, fees for plaintiffs' lawyers are paid as a percentage of the amount awarded (known as a *contingency fee*), while the defendant pays his or her attorney by the hour. Today, a typical contingency fee is 33 percent of the amount awarded. By contrast, citizens in the United Kingdom must pay a lawyer's fee in advance to file a lawsuit, and a claimant who loses a suit must pay the defendant's legal costs. Contingency fees are not permitted. For these reasons, as well as differences between the countries in patient–physician relationships and in the larger societal attitudes, far fewer malpractice lawsuits occur per capita in the United Kingdom, and premiums for malpractice insurance accordingly are much lower. In fact, the United States has, by a considerable margin, the highest per-capita number of medical malpractice lawsuits in the world.

Several different types of award are made to claimants who win malpractice lawsuits. "Compensatory" damages are meant to replace the patient's economic losses. "Pain and suffering" awards are meant to compensate the claimant for the physical and emotional damage that the malpractice caused. "Punitive" damages are meant to punish defendants who are found guilty of willful malpractice.

Juries and judges are poor arbiters for cases that require technical expertise to understand the nuances of the clinical decisions made or the treatment given. In addition, a jury trial is very expensive (one estimate puts the average cost at $250,000). By law, juries are to decide dollar awards by taking into account economic costs, emotional costs (pain and suffering), and lost wages; thus, if two people are similarly injured but were employed in jobs with different wages, the plaintiff with the higher job would receive the higher award. An argument could be made, however, that the plaintiff in the lower-paying job has a greater monetary need.

This relates to another deficiency in the tort system: ineffective deterrence. Many analysts contend that damages and resulting awards are determined arbitrarily, so that similar injuries could result in very different awards. The perception of award determination as arbitrary is one reason that the system does not function well as a deterrent.

The goals of deterrence, as well as that of corrective justice, are further undermined by the availability of malpractice insurance. Practitioners are insulated by their insurance from feeling the financial effect of large awards, but large enough awards, even if erratically given, would deter doctors who were personally liable. This might motivate proper caution in medical practice, and for this reason, more insurers are now basing malpractice premiums on physicians' malpractice experiences.

There are other problems with the legal system as well. Lawyers who are inexperienced in medical malpractice litigation often take such cases and do not give their clients good advice about pursuing claims. The merit (or lack thereof) of a particular claim may be inaccurately recognized, thus, resulting in a massive waste of both time and money for the plaintiff and defendant.

The out-of-court settlement is a solution for many lawsuits. A few are settled out of court, if not because of provider guilt, then at least because the insurance company considered the circumstances as unfavorable for a solid defense. More often, however, the out-of-court settlement is an attempt to avoid the inadequacies of the tort system and the very high cost of mounting a defense. Thus, it is usually cheaper to settle than to defend the physician, regardless of that physician's culpability or innocence: the provider or insurance company saves the cost of legal and court fees. Most such settlements include a proviso that details of the complaint and/or settlement not be released, which may be important to one or both parties. Also, because the civil-suit process can be prolonged, avoiding a lengthy trial by a settlement assures that the patient receives monetary compensation in a timely manner. The length of the process may motivate needy plaintiffs to settle, even if their case is strong; therefore, one cannot necessarily equate settlement with provider wrongdoing.

Effects of the Malpractice Problem

Whatever cause one attributes for the current medical malpractice situation, it has had several undeniable effects. These include the lack of affordable malpractice insurance, defensive medicine, increased costs of health care, and reduced access to care.

The Lack of Affordable Malpractice Insurance

As noted above, providers purchase medical malpractice insurance against the possibility that they will be sued for large sums.

The medical malpractice insurance industry, which for years had been a safe and lucrative business, became financially unpredictable in the mid-1970s with the sharp increase in both the number and the amounts of awards. Several major companies withdrew from the market, leaving many health care providers without protection. "A few others remained, but raised their rates dramatically, in some states by as much as 300 percent in one year. Physicians were faced with the choice of paying exorbitant premiums, 'going bare,' finding other sources of coverage, or limiting or quitting their practice" (Williams 1985, p. 1).

Practitioners who "go bare" do not purchase malpractice insurance; if they are sued, they pay any costs and damages out of pocket. After some insurance companies withdrew from the malpractice business, and the remaining insurers increased their prices sharply, many clinicians could not afford the new premiums and were forced to "go bare." Some states responded to this crisis by limiting the amount of awards, and some for the first time permitted groups of physicians or medical societies to found their own malpractice insurance companies (which are known informally in some quarters as *bedpan mutuals*).

Today, premium prices vary widely depending on specialty (Table 13), geographic area, and other factors. For instance, a neurosurgeon in New York City pays much higher premiums than does a psychiatrist in the rural Midwest. Because of these wide variations, data can be presented selectively to support the argument that malpractice premiums are not becoming unaffordable; indeed, aggregate data indicate that premium payments have remained stable over the past 10 years, at approximately 3 percent to 5 percent of the average physician's yearly gross income, which is not a staggeringly high percentage. Nevertheless, annual increases in premiums during the last half of the 1980s were almost *double* the annual increase in total practice revenues.

Increases in insurance premiums tend to be cyclical; currently, we seem to be at "a soft point" in that cycle. Some see a lull in this aspect of "the malpractice crisis," but experts think that another round of increases is inevitable unless the fundamental problems in the system are addressed (Robert Wood Johnson Foundation 1991, p. 1).

Selective and aggregate figures, however, hide the fact that a crisis of insurance affordability has occurred, especially for specialists

Table 13.   Average Annual Premiums for Professional Liability Insurance of Self-Employed Physicians by Specialty, 1989

Category	Average premium
All physicians*	$15,500
General/Family Practice	9,000
Internal Medicine	8,200
Surgery	25,800
Pediatrics	7,800
Obstetrics/Gynecology	37,000
Radiology	13,300
Psychiatry	6,300
Anesthesiology	21,700

*Also includes physicians in specialties that are not listed separately.
Source: American Medical Association 1991, p. 18

such as neurosurgeons and obstetricians. In 1989, U.S. obstetricians paid an average annual malpractice insurance premium of $37,000; for many, the amount was much higher. In Maryland, the *average* was $42,000. Some New York City neurosurgeons now pay more than $100,000 annually for malpractice insurance coverage, and in Maryland, the average premium price for all physicians has increased 13.9 percent annually since 1985.

The traditional malpractice insurance policy is of the "occurrence" type, which covers care that is provided during the coverage year. If purchased in 1992, this type of coverage would insure the purchaser against all lawsuits involving incidents from that year, even a lawsuit filed 10 years later.

In an effort to lower prices, many companies have now shifted to a new kind of policy, termed *claims-mode*, that insures only against suits that are *filed* during the year for which the premium is paid. Under such a policy, the physician who pays malpractice premiums in 1992 has purchased insurance only against lawsuits filed that same year. Because lawsuits are often filed years after an incident occurs (up to the statute of limitations), this coverage is far more limited than an occurrence policy. It is less expensive, but the premium buys less protection. Some physicians would rather pay more for the extra protection that an occurrence policy affords, but many companies no longer offer this type of policy.

Defensive Medicine

The malpractice crisis has changed the way that medicine is practiced. It has led to defensive medicine, the attitude that a practitioner must provide every possible service because if the patient's outcome is less than ideal, then the practitioner might be sued for negligence. Physicians with this attitude—and there are many—order more tests, refer patients to specialists earlier and more often, and perform fewer high-risk procedures.

Obstetricians are now much more likely to refer high-risk patients to tertiary-care referral centers, and the incidence of cesarean sections is increasing to the point where in 1987 it was estimated that 100,000 unnecessary cesarean sections were being performed each year. Both of these phenomena are due in part to

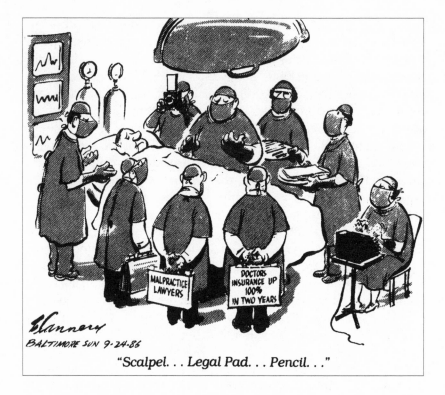

BALTIMORE SUN 9·24·86

"Scalpel. . . Legal Pad. . . Pencil. . ."

the increased fear of complications and subsequent litigation. Malpractice itself has become one of the most common complications, and some obstetricians fear that any child born less than perfect may become the subject of a lawsuit. Cesarean sections and fetal monitoring have become standards of care without adequate medical evidence that they reduce the incidence of adverse events (e.g., brain damage, cerebral palsy). Thus, one must conclude that these costly practices (with their associated adverse effects) are used in many instances for *defensive* purposes and not because they improve patient care. Rostow strongly concluded, in the Institute of Medicine (IOM) committee report on the issue, "Americans have adopted electronic monitoring as standard practice, at considerable added expense to routine obstetrical care, despite the failure of scientific evidence to support its use" (1989, p. 1058).

A defensive practice style may avoid certain harmful procedures, but its disadvantages are many. Because virtually all diagnostic tests carry inherent risks, extensive testing increases the possibility of iatrogenic injury. Moreover, patients and their insurers must pay for these extra tests. These problems escalate as more tests and treatments become available.

The threat of malpractice has also made an impact on the patient–practitioner relationship. People have become more distrustful of the care that they receive; a service even exists in some cities where patients can check a practitioner's lawsuit record. Practitioners, too, have become wary, and in some cities, they subscribe to a new service that identifies patients who sue frequently.

Increased Costs of Health Care

The malpractice problem has significant consequences for society as a whole. Costs of malpractice insurance premiums are estimated to account for at least 2 percent of the dollars spent on health care, because most such costs are passed along to patients and payers in the form of higher charges. Even more costly are the indirect effects of defensive medicine; from 12 percent to 25 percent of the increase in health care costs has been attributed to altered practice patterns, which represent in part the effects of defensive medical practices. Estimates vary, but it appears that some $15 billion to $40 billion annually is spent on defensive and otherwise unnecessary medical care.

Payers are no longer willing to reimburse for care that is meant primarily to protect the physician, so the present high rate of expenditure on medically marginal or unnecessary services cannot be sustained. As reimbursement is ratcheted downward, practitioners will no longer have the option of practicing defensive medicine. Indeed, prepaid and capitated plans actually penalize such behavior, yet the physician remains liable for complications resulting from early discharge or tests that were omitted to save money. Therefore, it is not surprising that today's practitioner "naturally feels caught between the lawyer and the hospital administrator" (Siden et al. 1986, p. 523).

Reduced Access to Care

The availability of medical care is also affected by the high cost of malpractice insurance. Physicians whose expenses are higher because of expensive malpractice premiums are less ready to treat indigent patients, and other inner-city patients are affected as well because young physicians prefer to establish practices in geographic locations with lower premiums. Some medical graduates are now reluctant to train in high-risk specialties such as obstetrics and neurosurgery. Many obstetrician-gynecologists have simply eliminated the obstetric component of their practice; during the 1980s, some 25 percent of those located in Florida limited their practice to gynecology. For these reasons, decreased access to some types of medical care has reached crisis proportions in some areas.

The IOM studied the medical malpractice problem's effect on access to and delivery of obstetric care within the United States. They found that access to obstetric care was affected adversely, particularly "to disadvantaged women, those living in rural areas, and those with high-risk pregnancies" (Rostow et al. 1989, p. 1057). The elimination of care for identified obstetric patients who are at high risk has greater impact on those in the lower socioeconomic classes. Surveys that were conducted by state medical society staffs revealed the extent of this problem: "the percentage of obstetricians and gynecologists who report that they are reducing the provision of care to high-risk women because of concern about professional liability ranges from 16 to 49 percent" (ibid., p. 1057). In some states, reimbursement by Medicaid for delivery of a child is less than the cost of the insurance coverage for the procedure. This was found in eight of 40 states studied, with a $240 per case deficit in Illinois, Missouri, and New Jersey (ibid., p. 1058).

Physicians in other specialties also cite a fear of litigation as a reason to avoid caring for patients in lower socioeconomic classes, including those enrolled in Medicaid. There is a prevailing belief among practitioners that these patients sue more often than others; however, data collected regarding the actual experience of the Maryland Medicaid population contradict this belief, showing that in the mid-1980s, the proportion of nonobstetrical medical malpractice claims filed by persons enrolled in Medicaid was lower than the proportion of the state's population who were enrolled in Medicaid. For obstetrical claims, the proportion filed by Medicaid enrollees matched the percentage of Medicaid obstetric discharges. These findings indicate that "there is no evidence that

Medicaid enrollees injured during obstetric procedures are more likely to litigate when compared with other persons undergoing the same procedures" (Mussman et al. 1991, p. 2994).

Solutions to the Malpractice Problem

No matter what one terms as *the* malpractice crisis, its effects are indisputable, and regardless of where one places the blame, it does not eliminate the responsibility to cooperate in working toward long-term solutions. Changes are urgently needed on several fronts to deal with the malpractice problem.

Legal Reform

Several ways exist to deal with the problems that surround medical malpractice, and one of the most promising is tort-reform legislation. More than 200 organizations have joined together to form the American Tort Reform Association (ATRA). The formation of ATRA was initiated by groups of bus drivers, teachers, manufacturers, sports teams, and others who today must pay expensive malpractice premiums because of the high risk that they will be sued in the course of offering their services to the public. Physicians also have joined these groups to lobby for reform.

It is estimated that only 28 cents to 40 cents of every dollar for insurance premiums goes to the victims of malpractice; the rest goes to insurance companies and lawyers. This is further evidence of how poorly the system meets its objective of corrective justice. Elected federal and state officials could do much to minimize the malpractice crisis by passing laws that would change these proportions.

A number of tort reforms have been proposed to deter claimants from bringing lawsuits with no merit. For example, some states permit countersuits, so that the defendant can sue the plaintiff for bringing a false lawsuit; when the option of countersuit is available to the defendant, persons without valid claims are less likely to sue.

Some states have sought to limit both the types of award and the dollar amounts that can be awarded. Some states have abolished punitive damages completely, arguing that they punish only the insurance company and that more effective ways exist to punish delinquent physicians. In constrast, some states place no financial limit on pain and suffering awards. Others do limit them, on the argument that doing so makes both patients and their lawyers less likely to file a doubtful suit, but after Indiana instituted a cap on awards, payments for claims actually increased (Bovbjerg 1991). Analysts have suggested many possible explanations for this finding, but it suggests that caps are not necessarily effective.

Another proposed tort reform is designed to ensure that expert witnesses-for-hire (who provide services to either side of a case) truly are experts in their fields, so that judges and juries can base their decisions on the most accurate testimony possible. Still another reform that has been adopted by some states is reducing the length of time after an incident during which a person can bring suit (known as the *statute of limitations*). With a decreased amount of time available to file, the number of lawsuits is reduced.

Many other types of tort reform have been proposed as well, among them a no-fault system. In no-fault systems, patients who suffer designated compensable events are paid regardless of whether the physician was negligent; however, the amount of the payment is much lower than a typical jury award. No-fault tort reform for obstetric care has been passed in Florida and Virginia. Under this system, parents of babies who are born with nervous system damage are not allowed to sue for malpractice, instead receiving a set dollar amount that is paid by the obstetrician's or the midwife's insurance company (currently $20,000). Fault is not assigned, thus protecting the provider while compensating the family. In Florida, this reform helps make it financially possible for obstetricians to remain in practice. The no-fault system still might *increase* costs, however, because of the greater number of persons potentially receiving payments.

Because trials are costly and their process prolonged, some "Alternative Dispute Resolution" programs also have been developed. Examples include panels for arbitration, medical screening for cases that merit trial, and neutral evaluation. These proceedings are decided by nonbinding arbitration; if an agreement can be reached, a trial is avoided. Private contracts between providers and patients are another possibility, in that many lawsuits result from inappropriate expectations that in turn arise because of poor or incomplete communications. This problem would be solved, however, if each encounter involved a formal contractual relationship between doctor and patient, with risks and benefits clearly spelled out and a limitation of liability established in advance.

Another potential innovation in the legal system involves the statutory adoption of clinical care guidelines as a *defense*. A doctor who could prove adherence to an accepted guideline would be protected, but a patient would be barred from using nonadherence as evidence of negligence. Maine now has a demonstration project using this type of reform.

More than 35 states have passed laws that are designed to limit malpractice awards and claims. A number of states have not passed any laws to date, and reform has been incomplete in many others. Still, people in the health care industry generally are encouraged by these trends.

A reduction by some lawyers in their quest for malpractice cases would also be helpful. Anecdotes abound of lawyers on medical wards scanning patients' records for evidence of malpractice with little regard for the merit of potential cases. Moreover, as any newspaper reader or TV viewer can attest, some malpractice lawyers advertise aggressively for new clients. In some cases, patients are persuaded to undertake costly legal battles. The legal profession must police such activities within its ranks.

Professional Reform

The medical profession has its own improvements to make. Tort reform and changes in the legal profession alone will not solve the malpractice problem. For one thing, stringent quality assurance programs should be developed to improve the overall quality of medical care; also, as discussed earlier, developing norms of care to assist the decision-making process would not only improve the quality of care but also, by eliminating some of the gray areas of practice where uncertainty and vulnerability are highest, decrease the risk of lawsuits in those areas.

Berwick (1991) pointed out that in this era of frequent lawsuits, it can be dangerous to admit ignorance. Ironically, many improvements in medical care derived in just this way, from providers' admissions of inadequacy in some aspect of care. Examples include incident reports, medication control systems, bed rails, and identification bracelets (Robert Wood Johnson Foundation 1991, p. 2). The informed consent procedure has been improved greatly as well, including a written record of the process and more frequent attempts by practitioners to provide their patients with information about procedures, including their potential risks. (There are also providers, however, who have "admitted" ignorance only after being found repeatedly at fault in malpractice suits.)

It has been suggested that "legal standards" of practice be formulated as a way to support practitioners' arguments in court. Currently, different states have different standards of liability for practitioners' actions. Some states judge such actions by the local standard of care, but in other states, lawyers have argued successfully that given the extent of modern communication through the media as well as the medical literature, physicians should be held liable if they fail to provide the best care that is currently available anywhere in the country (or the world). Lawyers as well as others working in the litigation process support the development of uniform standards of care. Evidence that a practitioner has adhered to accepted standards always helps in their defense.

The effectiveness and outcomes movements potentially could help the situation as researchers continue to document scientifically derived standards of care and the optimal outcomes that can be expected from that care. These results could be adapted on a general basis for use as legal standards of care, as now is occurring in Maine. As noted earlier, however, uncertainty about some aspects of clinical practice will never be eliminated, and it would be a mistake to expect legal standards of care to obviate this aspect of the malpractice problem.

Caution also must be exercised in using uniform standards of care as courtroom evidence. Each medical case is unique. Human judgment not only cannot be replaced by protocols, but it is indispensable in deciding whether a protocol applies to a given case. The danger of uniform standards is that they might be used to convict a physician who made a perfectly appropriate decision not to follow a particular protocol. By contrast, significant ambiguity exists in tort law definitions, with much leeway for interpretation by the court, so each case must be examined on its own merits.

One regulatory measure to oversee physician behavior was mandated by the Health Care Quality Improvement Act of 1986 and implemented in 1990. The goal of this legislation is to track problem practitioners as they move across state lines through mandatory reporting of information about licensing, adverse events, and disciplinary actions to the "National Practitioner Data Bank." For example, hospital administrators must report disciplinary actions, and they must check with the Data Bank during the process of appointing staff. In addition, malpractice insurance companies must report all settlements over a certain threshold, but physicians are permitted to add brief information about a particular claim to the Data Bank file.

Internal policing and disciplinary actions by physicians are important aspects of the solution to the malpractice crisis. The number of practitioners who are censured or have their licenses revoked by state medical societies is astoundingly low; however, the trend is toward an increasing number of disciplinary actions, which in 1990 were up over 9 percent from the previous year. This improvement largely came as a result of changes in state laws that have given the medical boards both more staff and more funding. Most important, these new laws have given the medical boards a greater number of disciplinary tools, allowing them greater flexibility so that intermediate-type offenses can be given appropriate punishment (without having to suspend licenses and so on).

Finally, peer review (like medical boards) must be strengthened and protected from antitrust lawsuits. Stiffer regulations regarding relicensing as well as improved continuing medical education programs are also needed. Such initiatives would diminish the force behind many lawsuits, because then "the public would not regard the courts as the only safeguard against incompetent physicians" (Angell 1985, p. 1207).

Improvements by the Individual Practitioner

While these changes in the system are being made, there are several things the individual provider also can do to minimize the risk of a malpractice lawsuit. One is to keep abreast of new medical developments. Another is to seek help when it is needed. Still another is to involve patients in decisions that regard their own treatment and to be frank with them about the uncertainty of the outcome in medical care. Both patients and family members who participate in a decision will be less quick to challenge it in court—and less likely to succeed if they do.

Another useful move (and one that costs little or nothing) is to be more courteous to patients. Appointments should be scheduled so that a patient's waiting time is kept to a minimum, and office personnel should be given instruction in telephone-answering technique and the importance of respecting the patient's desire for courtesy and privacy in the office and examining room. Even modest improvements along these lines can do much to reduce the frustration that many patients feel in their interactions with the health care system. They also reduce the incidence of lawsuits.

Medical practice has changed in yet another way during the last 10 years. "The chart is not a place for communication, but a tool for audit" (McHugh 1991). Complete, up-to-date medical records are another asset in today's litigious atmosphere, and not only is an accurate record of a patient's visits, tests, and treatments critical to good medical practice, it can serve as a valuable aid to memory in the event of a malpractice lawsuit. The medical record also provides physical evidence of the practitioner's perspective and actions. For all these reasons, physicians should not alter or allow their staff members to alter records. Any necessary changes in the chart should be initialed and dated, and deletions should be made in such a way that the deleted words can still be read. Details of how informed consent was obtained should be documented in a particularly careful fashion; the major points covered in the discussion with the patient and family should be included. Only well-accepted abbreviations should be used, and dictations should be read before they are signed. Last, records should be kept indefinitely (computers and microfilm save space).

The Attitudes of Patients and Society

As the previous discussion made clear, errors inevitably occur in medical practice. Some events are due to negligence, but they are essentially never caused by an outright intentional act. (Sexual misconduct is an exception to this statement; in such cases, intentional, self-serving acts that are unscrupulous and damaging to patients do occur.) Thus, it is important that the patient contemplating a lawsuit against his or her physician carefully examine the reason for the suit. Could the anger or misunderstanding be resolved in a better way? Is a no-fault system available in the state to permit the recovery of economic loss without attempting to prove that the clinician was at fault? It seems apparent that improved communication between patients and their medical practitioners could go a long way to resolving many of the disputes that unfortunately end in court, which for the most part do not satisfy anyone in their resolution.

Poor outcomes and mistakes cannot be prevented entirely. The current atmosphere of extreme litigiousness, mutual distrust, and extravagant dollar awards, however, even in cases where physicians acted competently and in good faith, should be corrected. It is likely that a combination of these potential reforms will be necessary to significantly improve the medical malpractice situation in this country. Such improvements would benefit patients, physicians, medical care, the justice system, and society as a whole.

CHAPTER 12

ACCESS TO MEDICAL CARE

> The American people are entitled to the best medical service which science and art permit, and which they can afford to buy. They are entitled to get it at the lowest price consistent with high quality, or have it given to them if they cannot pay. All the people have a right to medical service on these terms. They are not now getting it.
>
> *James Means*

The attainment of these objectives, written almost 40 years ago by a socially minded physician concerned with problems in the U.S. health care system, still eludes us to this day. As the priorities of society change, the care of patients who are poor and underinsured has resurfaced as one of today's central health policy issues. Many millions of Americans lack health insurance or have inadequate coverage, thereby risking major financial loss in the event of an illness or injury.

The main obstacle to the resolution of this problem is money. Many of the "poor" (defined in 1991 as an annual income below $13,921 for a family of four) are covered by the federal–state Medicaid program, but a sizable group of poor and "near-poor" people also exists, whose income is very low by most standards but not low enough to allow them to qualify for Medicaid coverage. The number of persons in this category is growing substantially as support for governmental programs is reduced; in 1990, it was estimated that Medicaid covered only 47 percent of Americans below the federal poverty level. People in this ineligible group are usually unable to afford either private health insurance premiums or medical bills.

Those with disabilities or major illnesses comprise another class of disadvantaged persons. Such people face significant impediments to employment and, therefore, to eligibility for employer-

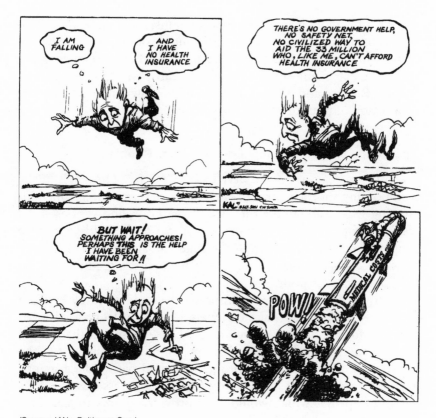

(Source: KAL, *Baltimore Sun.*)

sponsored group health benefits. Furthermore, a pre-existing condition often makes it impossible for an individual to purchase commercial insurance protection; many insurance companies will not sell a policy to someone who already is ill or disabled. This group can only be expected to grow as the HIV epidemic continues.

In 1990, it was estimated that approximately 15 percent of all Americans (approximately 35 million to 37 million people) had no health insurance. This group is primarily composed (75 percent) of persons who are employed in companies that do not offer health insurance benefits and their dependents. Of this employed group, many are marginally employed (i.e., part-time or in low-wage hourly jobs) and can be considered poor, near-poor, or in the so-called *gray area* (i.e., not poor enough for Medicaid, but not wealthy enough to afford their own insurance coverage). People who are unemployed also make up a significant number of those who are uninsured. Surveys indicate that, proportionately, the number of uninsured black Americans, Mexican Americans, Puerto Ricans, and Cuban Americans is much higher than the proportion of uninsured white Americans.

The Policy toward Medical Care for Poor People

A century ago, poor people were treated in charity hospitals; many paid nothing for their care. In later years, government assumed increasing responsibility for the care of the poor, and various social welfare programs were introduced. A national health insurance program, providing universal coverage for all citizens, has been considered for decades as a mechanism to ensure medical care for the poor and near-poor.

The issue of national health insurance was addressed by Franklin Delano Roosevelt, and he envisioned a program to provide medical care for all citizens as well as disability payments that would offset earnings lost because of severe illness. FDR suggested the creation of a state and local program funded with federal grants. The first national health bill introduced in Congress was the Wagner Bill of 1939, which would have provided grants to states for health progams, but this bill was not passed. The Truman Administration in the 1940s also supported the need for a national health program (Means 1953).

Since then, legislative efforts have offered piecemeal solutions to the problem of providing access to medical care for the uninsured. During the mid-1960s, government policymakers attempted to assume full responsibility for the health care of poor people by introducing Medicaid. Some consider the Medicare and Medicaid programs to be a limited and modified form of national health insurance; this legislation was fragmented as a result of political compromises (mainly with powerful health care provider groups). Nevertheless, access to care by poor Americans improved considerably as a direct result of these programs. Table 14 shows that income alone no longer determines the quantity of medical services received; however, compare the obviously income-related disparities in dental care, which is not fully covered by public-sector programs.

Table 14. Visits to Physicians and Dentists and Hospital Discharges and Episodes by Race and Family Income, 1989

Race/ethnicity and family income	Visits to Physicians		Visits to Dentists*		Hospital Episodes	
	Number per person per year	Percentage of persons with 1 or more visits	Number per person per year	Percentage of persons with 1 or more visits	Discharges per 1000 per year	Average days in hospital per episode
Race						
White	5.5	78.2%	2.1	58.4%	92.0	6.9
Black	4.9	77.0	1.3	42.6	105.2	7.6
Income						
Under $14,000	6.3	76.2	1.3	41.0	131.3	7.7
$14,000–$24,999	5.2	76.4	1.3	42.7	91.2	6.6
$25,000–$34,999	5.5	77.1	1.6	49.3	93.0	6.8
$35,000–$49,999	5.2	79.2	2.2	59.0	75.0	6.4
$50,000+	6.0	81.9	2.7	71.8	72.1	6.9
Overall	5.3	77.7	2.0	56.3	92.6	7.0

*Uses 1986 income categories adjusted for inflation.
Source: National Center for Health Statistics 1991

The general trend of U.S. health-related legislation has been to provide coverage for identified groups, such as veterans (through the VA) or elderly people (through Medicare). Some groups have been eligible according to diagnosis (Medicare for ESRD) or income (Medicaid). Notwithstanding this tendency, numerous national health insurance bills have been introduced in Congress over the years, and during the mid-1970s, proposals for national health insurance were supported by Presidents Nixon, Ford, and Carter. None of these proposals, however, passed.

In the 1970s and early 1980s, changes in U.S. health policy in response to economic pressures in fact resulted in decreased public subsidies to health care. Some states did not cut Medicaid spending but simply tried to hold their program budget constant; this was a common approach for local health programs as well. However, because of price inflation both in and out of the health care sector, a constant level of funding effectively meant an 8 percent to 10 percent decrease in real spending.

Government policy grew tougher in the 1980s. The Reagan Administration "called for major cutbacks in entitlement to health care for the poor and elderly" (Davis 1985, p. 51). Some of the more drastic proposals were modified or rejected by Congress, but reductions in spending were still made. Another result of this pol-

icy shift was to lift the requirement that public facilities keep
records of free care provided to patients who were indigent and
report them as part of their continuing Hill-Burton obligation.

Compared with other publicly funded programs, both Medicare
and Medicaid bore a proportionately larger share of the total cuts
that the Reagan Administration made. Expenditures measured in
current dollars continually increased, but the increases have fallen
behind the rate of inflation for health care costs, in effect reducing
public sector support of health care. Many now think it is time for
fundamental reform of the system to provide universal access to
medical care. A recent poll by *The Washington Post* and ABC News
indicated that almost half (44 percent) of those surveyed felt that
it was time for a taxpayer-funded, national health plan to cover all
Americans.

Problems with the Medicaid Program

Medicaid has been touted as the health care "safety net" for poor
people, but recent policy decisions have poked large holes in the
net. Both the absolute number and the percentage of the nation's
poor people who are covered by Medicaid have fallen. This trend
began in the mid-1970s and has continued through the 1980s. In
1980, approximately 10 percent of all Americans under the age of
65 were uninsured for at least some time during the year, and this
grew to 15 percent by the end of the decade. Approximately one
third of those under age 65 without insurance coverage are children, and 35 percent of the uninsured have a family income of less
than $10,000. Among families below the poverty level, 40 percent
of all children had no health insurance coverage in 1990.

Most state Medicaid programs have problems with low physician participation, mainly because of low reimbursement. Variation
in reimbursement levels among states is wide nationally, but Medicaid fees average only 69 percent of Medicare's prevailing charges
(which in turn are lower than private sector prevailing charges).
State programs have attempted to encourage physician participation by streamlining administrative procedures, such as electronic
claims submission, toll-free information lines, and simplified billing; nevertheless, only approximately 34 percent of physicians nationally participate fully in the Medicaid program.

Despite the original legislative intent, Medicaid dollars do not serve exclusively—or even primarily—the poor. In fact, only about one quarter of Medicaid expenditures provide services for those who qualify on the basis of income, with the rest of the budget covering the blind, the disabled, and long-term care and other charges to elderly people not covered by Medicare. "Questions are being raised regarding relative public spending devoted to children versus the elderly, with the term 'intergenerational equity' describing tradeoffs in health and social welfare allocations between the two population groups" (Rice 1990, p. 87).

The New Competitive Industry and Poor People

An age-old problem in the health care field, dating even from before the days of pest-house hospitals and blood-letting, is that physicians and hospitals have difficulty in collecting payments once their services have been supplied. After the enactment of social welfare programs such as Medicaid, providers were reimbursed for more of the care that they previously had donated. Because of this, some argue that the health care industry has benefitted from these programs as much as the poor over the last several decades.

Because public programs have never enrolled 100 percent of those who are unable to afford services, however, uncompensated care has remained a fiscal issue for health care providers. Until recently, this issue had been comparatively insignificant for most hospitals, because the financing system (whether intentionally or not) included sufficient slack to pay for the uninsured. In effect, hospitals used "extra" dollars that were collected from patients and payers via cost-shifting to help cover the expenses incurred by patients receiving charity care.

Times have changed, however. We now have cost-containment measures such as prospective payment, capitation, and managed care whose specific goal is to eliminate these hidden cross-subsidies. With today's price-based competition, payers increasingly negotiate discounts and insist on the reimbursement of costs rather than charges. As a result, discretionary funds that are available to hospitals for noncompensated care have decreased considerably.

It appears that both investor-owned hospitals and not-for-profit hospitals in the same geographic areas provide roughly comparable amounts of charity care, but the majority of for-profit hospitals are located in affluent areas where poor people are not close at hand. As a result of their location as well as their for-profit mission and financial responsibility to investors, these hospitals treat a lower proportion of poor people than do the nonprofits, so the challenge of providing uncompensated care disproportionately affects voluntary (i.e., nonprofit) hospitals.

Poor people generally do not have access to the growing number of independent outpatient facilities. Such facilities can charge significantly lower prices than hospital emergency rooms for comparable services, but because they are primarily investor-sponsored and not mandated to care for poor people, most require payment (or an insurance card) at the time of service. As a result, poor people are further concentrated in the already crowded emergency rooms of inner-city and public hospitals.

Teaching hospitals (often situated in urban ghettos) have traditionally cared for a large proportion of poor people. In 1990, they reportedly provided approximately two thirds of the free care in this country, but they only had 8 percent of the country's acute-care beds. A law passed in 1985 included a PPS formula to increase payments to hospitals caring for a disproportionate percentage of either poor patients or Medicare Part A beneficiaries, the first time that such an adjustment has been made. Ironically, however, the new dollars came from funds that otherwise would have gone to support graduate medical education, thereby canceling any gains that teaching hospitals might have realized.

Effects on the Delivery of Care

As a result of the shifts in government reimbursement policy, today's health care system lacks a mechanism to ensure that providers offer their share of pro-bono charity care. This responsibility has fallen on selected facilities such as teaching hospitals that, because of the very same trends, are now less able to exercise it. Hospitals that want to continue providing care to poor people often cannot afford to do so; in 1988, one source estimated that 250,000 Americans were denied care because of their lack of insurance.

With poorer nutrition, fewer social supports, and the lack of preventive or primary care, persons from lower socioeconomic groups tend to be sicker on admission and to require more resources per hospitalization. Despite these facts, several studies have shown that poor patients now receive fewer tests in-hospital, have a greater chance of dying, and have a shorter average length of stay. A study of Boston-area hospitals found that self-pay patients received 7 percent fewer services and had 7 percent shorter lengths of stay than did insured patients, "[suggesting] that patients who lack insurance may receive unequal treatment even after being hospitalized" (Weissman and Epstein 1989, p. 3572).

Current utilization data indicate that black and white Americans receive comparable amounts of medical care, but the higher levels of disease burden among minority populations suggest that current levels of care received by minorities are inadequate. More black people than white people are uninsured, and many more black Americans receive medical care in emergency rooms. Treating primary health care needs in emergency settings is needlessly expensive. Not only is it cost-ineffective, the emergency room is equipped to handle true emergencies; patients with nonurgent conditions receive suboptimal treatment, "equivalent to tending a rose garden with a bulldozer" (Friedman 1991, p. 2494).

New methods of reimbursement have created additional incentives to transfer poor patients to public hospitals. A Chicago-based study in 1986 found that 87 percent of the patients transferred to the public sector facility, Cook County Hospital, were sent primarily because they lacked adequate third-party medical coverage. The number of reports of patients who are transferred for economic reasons, known as *patient dumping,* has increased continually. Women in labor as well as heart attack and stabbing victims— some with IV lines in place—now regularly arrive on a transfer basis at public hospitals; these patients rarely have a choice in the matter and often are not consulted before the transfer.

Under the old social contract the *cost of indigent care* was the hot potato passed from providers to paying patient. Under the newly emerging contract, the *bodies of the uninsured poor themselves* become the hot potatoes that are being dumped from provider to provider. Politicians ought not to feign surprise at this transformation, nor ought they to remind physicians of the Hippocratic Oath. Indeed, to blame doctors and hospitals for the practice of "patient dumping" all the while refusing to legislate the means of paying for the care rendered to uninsured indigents strikes one as disingenuous. (Reinhardt 1986b, p. 8)

Patient dumping became an especially common occurrence in Texas, with its many for-profit hospitals, high unemployment rate, and a Medicaid program ranked third from the bottom nationally in its level of payments. To stem the flow of indigent patients who were transferred from private to public facilities, Texas passed "anti-dumping" legislation; other states are expected to follow suit.

Critics have charged that government is retrenching without an explicit private sector plan to fill the resulting gap. As one group pointed out, "the moral and economic commitment of private hospitals to provide care is limited to medically necessary emergency treatment" (Kellerman and Ackerman 1988, p. 646). While the negotiations and political maneuvering continue—signs of a

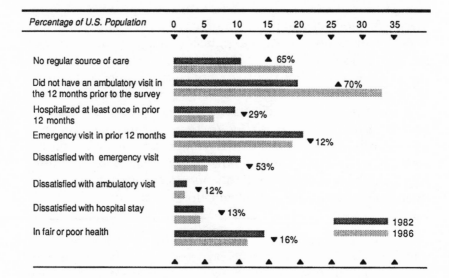

Figure 23. Changes in access to health care, 1982–6. (Source: Robert Wood Johnson Foundation 1987.)

system in flux—increasing numbers of indigent people are being left with little or no medical care; Figure 23 shows changes in the availability of health care to poor people during the 1980s.

From a global cost-versus-benefit perspective, decreasing access to care in this manner makes little sense. People who do not receive timely medical care in the early stages of an illness become seriously ill and may then require resource-intensive hospitalization. When patients who are uninsured are transferred between hospitals, money is squandered on ambulance rides and repeated workups. Apart from the numerous questions of justice that these practices raise, neither patients nor payers benefit.

Effects on Health

Making medical care more accessible to underprivileged people unquestionably helped improve the health of the U.S. population. Whereas the U.S. infant mortality rate remained essentially unchanged in the decade preceding the introduction of the Medicaid program, it decreased during the next 14 years from 25 to 13 deaths per 1000 live births. Death rates for "poverty-related illnesses" such as maternal mortality, influenza, pneumonia, gastrointestinal diseases, and diabetes also declined significantly after Medicaid began (Davis 1985). On a societal level, the average life expectancy of the U.S. population rose steadily from the turn of the century until the mid-1950s, when it leveled off, and began to rise again during the late 1960s following the introduction of Medicaid.

The relationship between dollars spent on health care and improved health is not necessarily one-to-one: other factors, such as nutritional and housing programs and pollution control, have a positive impact on health. Nevertheless, data seem to show that public spending does improve health by increasing people's use of medical services.

As a result of inadequate access to medical care, recent gains in health status may be eroding. A California study compared a group of people whose Medicaid coverage had been terminated 1 year earlier with a control group who had remained in the program; the former group was found to have increased hypertension, higher mortality, less opportunity to obtain care, and less satisfaction with the care they received. Similarly, just as black Americans are less likely to be insured than white Americans, health indicators show that they do not enjoy health status on a par with the white population and have a shorter life expectancy.

Is Access a Societal Problem?

Many Americans undeniably face difficulty in obtaining access to medical care, but one cannot assume automatically that this is a problem of society. If health care is viewed simply as a commodity that is comparable to any other in the U.S. market, distributed on the basis of the ability to pay, then no society-wide dilemma exists. If, by contrast, health care is "a social good of special moral importance" (Daniels 1986, p. 1381), then society would have an obligation to ensure that all its members receive a reasonable level of access to such care. It remains to be seen which notion of medical care the Clinton administration will support.

In the course of crafting (some would say concocting) governmental policy that relates to the uninsured, it has always been very difficult for the interested parties to agree on a definition of what comprises a "basic" level of services. The currently agreed on boundaries for such a definition were described by Welch—the middle ground "between the impossible (covering everything) and the unacceptable (covering nothing)" (1989, p. 1261); he pointed out that to promise too much avoids hard choices and ignores resource limits. As discussed in Chapter 10, theories of distributive justice can be used to systematize this policy debate.

Some improvement in the allocation of resources flows naturally from changes in health care delivery and medical practice that occurred during the 1980s. Both the effectiveness and the outcome movements may improve access indirectly by optimizing the use of resources already within the system. Brown pointed out that some cost-control methods, such as gatekeeping, case management, and UR, improve equity within the system. "These devices apply professional judgment (technical rationality) rather than controlling economic demand (market rationality) in setting priorities for providing care. They also may be more equitable to the extent that access and use are based on need, rather than on ability to pay" (Brown 1988, p. 589). While these developments will likely spread the resources among those who have already entered the health care system, however, they do not help those without access to attain it.

Possible Solutions

Several possible approaches exist to reform the system to increase access. Some legislative approaches build on and otherwise refine the current system; one example of this type involves extending Medicaid coverage to those on the current margins of eligibility (that is, to the near-poor). In fact, Medicaid has been mandated to provide coverage to women who are pregnant and to children under the age of 6 with an annual income of less than 133 percent of the federally defined poverty limit.

Still another proposal is to retain the arrangements whereby higher charges to insured persons help to subsidize the care of the uninsured, thus reversing recent trends that eliminate such cost-shifting. This type of privately sponsored subsidy arrangement already exists in some states.

Insurance Industry Reform

The insurance industry has been targeted for a number of reforms through legislation introduced and, in some states, passed. These initiatives include prohibiting insurance companies from discriminating against a potential client because of a pre-existing condition.

Heightened competition in the health care sector has been seen as a solution to the access problem by some. Insurance companies that base premium prices on an experience rating (i.e., previous costs with their own enrollee groups) charge lower prices than do companies that base premium prices on a community rating (i.e., previous costs of the entire community from which they garner beneficiaries or enrollees). Those companies that target a healthier segment of the population can charge lower premiums, leaving the less-healthy people to community-based policies and creating a cycle that perpetuates this price discrepancy. Proposed insurance reform in some states requires *all* companies to use a community rating; this levels the playing field among companies, but also likely increases the average premiums in the area.

National Health Insurance

Potential solutions on a more global level include the implementation of national health insurance (but even this could be implemented in a piecemeal way). Opinion is divided on whether the passage of national health insurance legislation is imminent or impossible; however, the large number of proposals introduced recently as well as the groundswell of both public and political interest in this area mandate that all clinicians educate themselves regarding the alternatives. Table 15 summarizes these major current proposals.

The terms are often used interchangeably, but *universal* health insurance differs from *national* health insurance. *Universal* health insurance would ensure the coverage of individuals, though not necessarily by the government, in that it could leave intact current public and private plans. In contrast, *national* health insurance would cover *all* people through a single government health plan.

The United States is the only industrialized nation (apart from South Africa) that has not instituted either a national or a universal health insurance program. Many different models exist worldwide. Societal differences between countries do not preclude an examination of other health care systems, but "political, social, and economic contexts are never identical, even in countries that share similar values. Such differences make it difficult to directly apply models of care derived from a health care system in one country to that of another" (Weiner 1987, p. 458). By acknowledging these differences, we can benefit from their experiences and adapt aspects of their systems to our own.

It will likely be difficult for those who benefit from the current system to accept that reform may mean that less is available to each, but if society addresses the issue of access through systemwide reform, certain compromises will be necessary.

Has reliance on competition, freedom of choice, and entrepreneurship provided Americans with the best health care system in the world? Would the impersonality, queuing, and lack of choice inherent in some other countries' health systems be an acceptable trade-off to the American public for more economic efficiency and greater equity? ... perhaps it is time to take a closer look at some of the features of these systems

Table 15. A Comparison of the Alternative Approaches to National Health Insurance Reform in the United States

	Market reform and/or tax incentives only	"Pay-or-play"	Single payer
Brief description of approach	Existing health insurance market would be reformed. Uninsured would receive coverage through tax credits, vouchers, or expansion of Medicaid. Would be financed as presently.	Employers would offer coverage (i.e., "play") or pay special tax to help support government program. Uninsured would obtain coverage from this expanded public sector program.	All persons would be covered by a single government-sponsored program, similar to the Canadian model. Would be financed by taxes.
Role of government	Few changes from today. Federal government would set standards for programs purchased with tax credits. IRS would be involved.	Federal government would set standards for employer plans. Government plan might be administered by DHHS and/or states.	Federal (or possibly state) government would administer.
Consumer coverage/benefits	Near universal coverage. Some plans would offer only basic benefits.	Universal or near-universal coverage. Some plans would mandate only basic benefits.	Universal coverage. Comprehensive benefits.
Approaches to cost containment	Some plans decrease employer/employee tax subsidies to increase cost consciousness. Some plans support managed care models.	Some plans involve price controls and regional expenditure targets. Some plans strongly promote managed-care models.	Fixed budgets. Strong centralized price controls.
Role of private insurers	Possibly increased role as more people are able to purchase private policies.	Similar to today within large employer market. Small-group or individual markets could change drastically.	Industry could be eliminated. Probably would serve as intermediaries for government. Could also sell supplemental policies.
Impact on providers	Few changes from today. Possibly increases in managed care programs.	Probably increased price controls. Possibly increases in managed care program.	Interaction with only single payer. Increased price controls.

Note: This table is intended only as a general summary. The characteristics of the many proposed reform plans within each of the three broad categories vary considerably. DHHS = Department of Health and Human Services.

that have created universal access at lower cost without any demonstrable lower level of quality. (Schieber 1990, p. 167)

In 1946, for example, England established a nationalized health care system, with access to care for all citizens. In terms of the percentage of GDP, England currently spends approximately only half as much per capita on health care as the United States, but English citizens by most indicators are at least as healthy as Americans. The English system is organized on the basis of local areas, each with a predetermined annual budget. Resources are limited within this closed system: funds not spent on one health-related product are spent on another such product. In contrast, the United States has an open system; because dollars in this system are not limited by budgets in the same way as in England, what is not spent on one health-related product may or may not be spent on another.

Recently, a great deal of attention has focused on the Canadian system. Canada adopted a universal health insurance system in 1971. Their single-payer system is administered by the provinces, with annual provincial expenditure caps. For consumers, coverage for hospitalizations and office care is unlimited, but de facto, high-technology treatment is rationed. Physicians are reimbursed under binding fee schedules that are negotiated with the provincial governments; global hospital budgets are set similarly. Problems with this system are emerging, but the Canadian solution has held the costs of health care significantly below those in the United States. If applied to the United States, this type of system is among the most far-reaching of proposed reforms as it would eliminate the need for the private insurance industry. A group of U.S. reformers advocates adoption of a Canadian-type system, but the insurance industry obviously is opposed to the single-payer system.

Some have suggested joint public–private initiatives to make work-related health insurance available to those who are marginally employed at part-time or low-level jobs, because such employees constitute a large proportion of uninsured Americans. These *pay-or-play* proposals would require employers either to provide health insurance for employees or contribute an equivalent amount of money into a fund that would provide this coverage. Employers are concerned about the costs of pay-or-play plans, particularly for small businesses.

A tax-credit–based proposal offering Internal Revenue Service incentives or government vouchers to consumers for the purchase of their own basic, private health insurance policy was proposed by the Bush administration. President Clinton—elected in part because of his health care reform plan—generally supports the pay-or-play approach. His administration appears to support proposals that feature *managed cmpetition* between HMO-like organizations. Proposals based on each of these approaches have been introduced in Congress.

The advantages of a comprehensive national health program are many, but in addition to the problems already described, there are several other concerns that any successful plan must address. First, doubts exist whether any proposal, without strict budgetary limitations, could control costs. Second, U.S. society historically has placed a high value on personal choice, and many of the proposed national health insurance programs would limit the options that are available to consumers. Third, and probably from a practical perspective the most important, the powerful health care provider and insurance industries vehemently oppose the more far-reaching proposals that decrease (or eliminate) their autonomy.

The current political and economic climates make it unlikely that full-scale national health insurance legislation will pass in the near future, but it appears that both political and societal attitudes may be shifting in that direction. Some analysts believe that continued conflicts with numerous unaccountable private payers may lead providers to support a federally based system, with its accountable, publicly elected "board of directors." Others believe that the spread of AIDS (the medical care for which can cost well over $100,000 during its course) will force a unified, nationally sponsored approach to health care financing.

State Initiatives

Most states have proposed plans to improve access in some way. Hawaii is the only state with an operational universal-access program, using employer-mandated coverage and an expanded Medicaid system. Massachusetts passed pay-or-play legislation to be implemented in the future and currently has a program covering the unemployed. Proposals are under consideration in Michigan, Minnesota, California, Maryland, New York, and other states.

Oregon's Basic Health Services Act of 1989 guarantees universal access to basic health care services. Under the proposed structure (disapproved by HCFA) the state would provide care for all persons with incomes below the poverty level through its Medicaid program. It is proposed that resources be rationed on the basis of the type of service, and a government-appointed committee developed a list of treatments ranked on their cost-versus-benefit ratio. For example, immunizations—which cost pennies and prevent potentially serious diseases—are at the top of the list. Relatively ineffective, expensive services to patients who are gravely ill (e.g., liver and lung transplants) are at the bottom. Starting at the top of the list, services will be provided down to a cutoff point that budgetary limits will determine.

The Oregon plan has received a great deal of attention from policy analysts and clinicians alike. The Oregon plan establishes systemwide priorities, identifying the number of persons who are covered as more important than the depth of the coverage that is available to each. By excluding services and not patients, the system explicitly rations resources. Rice added a sobering note to the debate: "this will be the first system in memory to explicitly plan that poor people with treatable illnesses will die if Medicaid runs out of money or does not budget correctly, and providers will be excused from liability for failing to treat them.... It is hardly healthy to establish rules of the game that require such choices" (1991, p. 34). The main criticism is that it rations care only for poor people, not for others. We would like to think that, somehow, the system would find resources to care for those who are not covered, particularly in identified cases, but it is equally likely that some *will* suffer as a result of the plan. Nevertheless, basing these decisions on agreed principles is more equitable than what frequently occurs in today's unstructured system.

Role for Health Care Facilities

While the United States awaits national health reform, hospitals will continue to provide charity care. Precisely what degree of charity care is required is debatable, but judging from the recent average for all U.S. general hospitals, 5 percent annually appears to be a reasonable proportion of hospital revenues designated for charity care. Arguably, a facility with a percentage that is significantly lower should be more involved in providing such care, and physicians using such a facility should be involved in seeing that this happens. While today's hospitals often are run by business-oriented managers, physicians have a responsibility to attempt to influence hospital policy to benefit patients.

For instance, formal protocols for the transfer of indigent patients to public facilities could be developed by clinicians. To be sure, motivations for a transfer often are mixed: some transfers clearly are mandated on medical grounds. An argument can also be made that patients with no insurance should be treated predominantly at taxpayer-sponsored facilities. For once, however, the central issue is simple: the patient's interest and well-being must be the paramount concern. In the words of Annas, a lawyer and health care ethicist, "Physicians cannot and should not permit themselves to be used as financial hatchet-men by profit-maximizing hospital managers. They should act as conscientious objectors to hospital policies that put patients at risk" (1986, p. 76).

Role for the Healing Professions

Physicians have been challenged on their record of providing care to poor and uninsured people. In 1986, David Rogers, a former medical school dean and former head of the influential Robert Wood Johnson Foundation, testified before Congress about the dramatic increase in visits to physicians by poor and by nonwhite people after the establishment of Medicaid. (During the same period, the number of visits by white and nonpoor persons remained fairly steady, at a higher level.) In a similar vein, Reinhardt posed this disquieting question: "Would you interpret the sudden upswing in the physician care received by American's poor since the mid-1960s as (a) a massive attack of unrequited noblesse oblige seizing members of the profession shortly after 1964, or (b) a sudden decrease in the health status of America's hitherto unusually robust and healthy poor, or (c) the emergence of federal financing of physician care for America's poor, many of whom were sick all along?" (Relman and Reinhardt 1986, p. 12).

Both commentaries point out that physicians are more likely to care for poor people when they are receiving financial compensation for that care. Neither the Hippocratic Oath nor the AMA Code explicitly states that practitioners must provide charity care, but this sort of moral obligation is part of what sets medicine apart from other professions. With privileges such as autonomy and status come a degree of social responsibility.

Physicians also can act on their own by providing a certain amount of free or reduced-price care, accepting assignment from Medicare, becoming a Medicaid Participating Physician (which some consider a type of charity service because of the low levels of reimbursement), giving patients with lower incomes more time to pay bills before passing them on to a collection agency, and donating time to free clinics and shelters for homeless people that provide medical services. Free clinics around the country have provided care successfully to indigent people entirely through use of time donated by clinicians. Given the multifaceted nature of the access problem facing many Americans, however, it is likely that a combination of solutions will be necessary.

CHAPTER 13

SOCIETAL EXPECTATIONS AND HEALTH CARE SYSTEM REFORM

> There's one thing I've learned in twenty-five years
> or so of political organizing: People don't like
> to be 'should' upon. They'd rather discover than be told.
>
> *Anonymous*

While the United States faces a number of social problems, health care is becoming one of the most pressing. Despite a number of interventions by both payers and policymakers, a multitude of problems remain. As a result, further health care reform is inevitable.

A large majority of Americans agree that a reform of our health care financing and delivery system is needed, and both individual and societal choices will be necessary. The medical profession is faced with three options: it can react passively and let change happen, stand in the way of change, or take an active part in the process. Each of these responses (including inactivity) is in itself a choice. Broad-based consensus that is reached after a consideration of the facts is preferable, in that it holds the greater potential for long-term acceptance than do reforms that are based on the actions of only a few of the system's participants.

This chapter summarizes some of the reasons that health care issues are so difficult to resolve, followed by a brief exploration of some of the choices that face individuals and society as the future of U.S. health care is reshaped. Finally, potential responses and strategies for health care professionals also are described.

Facing the Problems

Several observers wonder why, despite years of analysis and action, so many fundamental deficiencies remain in the U.S. health care system. The circumstances are most complex, defying easy settlement, but we as a nation clearly have resisted seeking solutions to these problems.

Because our wealth is finite, the system cannot be all things to all people; priorities must be set. We have been reluctant to accept that tradeoffs are inevitable, but we cannot have both "bottom-line repair" and better health care. Money that is spent on medical care is not available for other desirable goods and services. Making difficult choices about the allocation of resources may mean that fewer services are available when we, or our families, are the ones seeking care.

The lack of consensus among the various groups also makes reform elusive. "The American public, in its political inaction, has so far opted for continued temporizing" (Ginzberg 1990, p. 1465). The choice of elected leaders has affected the pace and direction of reform as well. One might wonder at the inconsistency between the American public's desire for increased governmental spending on medical care, simultaneous with their overwhelming support in the 1980s for presidents who were openly committed to reduced governmental spending in this area.

Analysts believe that the Republican health policies during the 1980s did not reflect popular opinion. People liked President Reagan, but they did not agree with his approach to every issue. Health care was one such area. Motivation for change may not have reached critical mass in the 1980s because not enough people had suffered as a result of the current system's deficiencies; as a result, Americans were not ready to compromise. There is evidence, however, that this is changing. The 1991 election of Pennsylvania's political newcomer Harris Wofford to the U.S. Senate over Attorney General and former governor Richard Thornburgh, demonstrated for the first time the strength of health care reform as a political issue. Clinton's presidential election one year later reflected Americans' desire for major reform of the health care system.

Many players are involved, so "progress" depends on one's perspective. What payers see as a solution may create new problems for providers. For example, the managed-care movement and UR industry were created largely in response to inefficient clinical decision-making and suboptimal use of resources. These methods disturb physicians, who are now responding to these pressures with practice guidelines developed by specialty societies as well as other changes from within the profession.

Our government's decentralized structure, pluralistic nature, and large size also account for the slow pace of reform. This often allows multiple governmental programs to work in opposition to one another. More specifically, under the current structure, one unit may be responsible for setting policy, but a new program may be implemented by a separate unit or agency. This arrangement has created inefficiencies in the reform process as administrators interpret policy differently from the way it was intended. Moreover, the track record of government efforts reveals an orientation toward crisis management, which in most cases lacks a unified national agenda or vision. All of these factors, particularly in conjunction with the actions of the massive, status-quo seeking health care industry lobby, have slowed the process of change.

Progress also is slow because what change there has been by and large has been incremental. But to focus on only the remaining problems is to ignore that many changes *have* been made. As in Kuhn's paradigm, the process of evolution is under way, and not all of the changes have been, or will be, pain-free.

Personal Choices and Professional Responses

Eddy made a point of crucial importance regarding society's difficulty in finding a solution to these problems: "A key to resolving our conflicting position on costs is to understand that this is not a debate between different groups that hold different philosophic or economic viewpoints; this is a debate within each of us. Every one of us has two minds when we make a decision about whether health care activity is worth its cost. We have one mind when we are well, sitting in our living rooms, paying taxes, or writing out a check for health insurance. We have another mind when we have a health problem and are sitting in a physician's office" (1990, p. 1737).

In the face of increasingly stringent cost-containment measures, consumers of health care are becoming politically organized to protect their interests, particularly in instances where their positions appear to be at odds with those of providers. "For the first time, health interests have shown signs of forming a broad coalition to battle the administration's budget reductions" (Iglehart 1986, p. 1464). We see this trend in the growth and increased effectiveness of patient advocacy groups such as women's health cooperatives, the AARP, and the National Alliance for the Mentally Ill (NAMI); this trend began in the 1980s and continues today. Such consumer-oriented groups have pointed to many serious deficiencies in our existing delivery system, and they continue to direct tough questions to payers, provider organizations, and members of the healing professions.

On an individual basis, Americans make many lifestyle choices that have health consequences. These choices have both personal and societal effects; for example, during the 1980s, alcohol contributed to thousands of deaths, including a large proportion of those that were linked to cirrhosis of the liver and motor-vehicle accidents. In addition, approximately 30 percent of the population continues to smoke cigarettes, and currently, more than 300,000 deaths per year are attributable to this.

Many ask why physicians—as compared with, say, dentists—have shown only modest interest in activating patients as participants in their own care. As the hazards of cholesterol, smoking, and alcohol abuse became widely known, many Americans changed their eating habits, stopped smoking, and cut down on alcohol. The medical profession, however, while formally advocating and applauding these changes, in actuality has done little to promote them. As a result, health-conscious people rarely turn to conventional practitioners for advice or instruction in how to stay healthy. (Figure 24 shows one example of an attempt to counter this.)

Today's physicians are more responsive to the human dimension of medical care than those of 20 years ago, but they still have a long way to go. Some feel that a major effort to ascertain, publicize, and diminish life-threatening habits may be the next significant step toward improving the human condition, and most physicians at least concede that they can play a significant role before pathology occurs. The ecology movement also reflects this shift in societal attitude; not that technological intervention has become

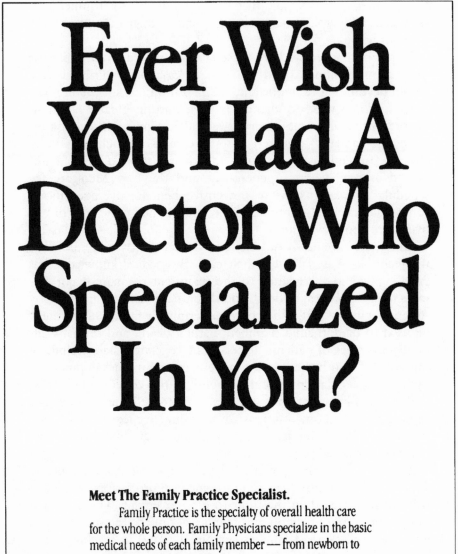

Figure 24. An advertisement from a national campaign sponsored by the American Academy of Family Physicians.

less important, it is simply that lifestyle and the environment are seen increasingly as much more important than they were once thought to be.

To respond aggressively to these changes would require that the medical profession expand the role of *prevention*. Primary care would become more important, specialization less so. Medical education would need to change as well, putting greater emphasis on preventive and ambulatory care and less on high-technology, "once-it's-too-late"–oriented hospital care. Recent changes in financing do reinforce these shifts. Inpatient care is no longer reimbursed as readily or as generously, and the new Medicare fee schedule and expansions in preventive benefit coverage among some insurers are also intended to reinforce the importance of primary care and prevention.

Americans have newly questioned whether they want to use all of the technology available for their care. Biomedical knowledge has been applied so successfully to the treatment of many major diseases that the process of death and dying has been redefined. Many Americans worry that if they become terminally ill, machines might be used to deny them a dignified, natural death, and several well-publicized cases of patients in persistent vegetative states reinforce this concern. Both the hospice movement and the development of right-to-die legislation arose in response to this concern. This view, under which intervention is not presumed to be beneficial, appears to be gathering momentum, as advance directive legislation, growing acceptance of voluntary active euthanasia, and increasing insistence on expanded patient autonomy suggest.

It now is clear that patients' desires in some cases are better served by less intensive care, and the medical profession has several roles to play regarding the right-to-die movement. The physician must counsel both patients and families about the relevant medical issues, as well as assist families (within the law) in reaching decisions about the use of technology at the final stages of life. It is important that physicians remain involved with those patients who choose not to use high-technology care. Also, physicians can and should contribute to the political process that determines the laws that pertain to these matters.

A related issue concerns the differences between providers' and patients' expectations of medical care. A patient consults a physician to rule out the presence of disease and to be reassured that nothing is wrong; this is a different notion of "ruling out" from the physician's. Physicians order tests to eliminate ("rule out") incorrect choices from the differential diagnosis with the goal of identifying ("ruling in") the correct diagnosis.* Detecting a problem in this way reassures the physician that he or she has something concrete to offer the patient. In contrast, patients are reassured primarily when conditions are ruled out. Furthermore, such a "rule-in" mentality among physicians may make patients feel abandoned unless or until disease is "ruled-in" by the detection of pathology (Green 1990).

The goals of both physicians and patients, though different, are not incompatible. Physicians, however, need to become more precise in identifying the conditions that are most likely to explain the patient's problem and attempt to rule those out, thereby providing the reassurance the patient needs. Physicians also need to be careful not to abandon the patient if pathology is *not* detected; this counterbalances the tendency to focus attention on treatable, discernable diagnoses at the expense of ignoring patients' complaints that cannot be delineated readily. Patients treated in this way are more likely to feel satisfied.

Societal Choices

One way that priorities are set in the United States today is by political pressure. As a society, we face myriad questions about our health care system. How much do we want to spend for it? Do we want a public or a private system? The choices that we make today will affect our future circumstances, such as the availability of care, the quality of practitioners, the degree of individual choice of a provider, and the way that we pay for care.

How Should Resources Be Allocated?

This question relates directly to the issue of access to care and national health insurance. If one accepts the premise that society is responsible for the health of its members, then all members have a

---

*Chapter 10 discussed the economic disadvantages and clinical risks accompanying a provider's "rule-out" mindset.

right to at least a basic level of care. How does one determine what is "basic," however? Does each citizen have a right to an annual physical exam and preventive health care, or to the treatment of only life-threatening conditions?

Theories of distributive justice become relevant here. Unfortunately, views about fairness differ widely; well-intentioned people favor different courses of action in a given situation. Even the definition of "fairness" is subject to interpretation. The utilitarian viewpoint asks, how do we use our societal health care resources to provide the greatest good for the greatest number? The egalitarian viewpoint asks, how can limited resources be distributed to provide all with an equal opportunity for health? And the libertarian viewpoint believes that health care resources are best distributed by the free market and that society has no obligation to pay for the care of its citizens.

As people differ in such matters, so do societies. Virtually all developed countries spend a larger percentage of government resources for social programs than does the United States (though in most cases overall levels of spending are lower). As Chapter 12 discussed, given a similar set of public needs, the United States and England have made very different decisions on allocation.

Resources are not infinitely available in any delivery system, thus potentially beneficial care sometimes must be denied. Theoretically, denial occurs when society (or a provider acting on its behalf) judges the marginal cost of a service to be more than its marginal benefit, and the service is therefore withheld. The service may well be one that would benefit the individual, but society may determine that the resources involved could be spent better elsewhere.

England makes explicit tradeoffs between health and other goods (particularly as they relate to resource-intensive services), and for the most part, this decision process treats all people in the system on an equal basis. The U.S. health care system has a different, more implicit set of priorities, but resources are rationed nonetheless: some receive services, others do not. To a large degree, these decisions depend on the characteristics of the individual patient (insurance status, socioeconomic status) or the provider (geographic location, reimbursement incentives), and as a result, "Saying no to beneficial treatments or procedures in the United States is morally hard, because providers cannot appeal to the justice of their denial. In ideally just arrangements, and even in the British system, rationing beneficial care is nevertheless fair to all patients in general. Cost-containment measures in our system carry with them no such justification" (Daniels 1986, p. 1383).

Just as the use of high-technology resources has become an issue for some individuals, it has become a larger issue for society as well. Ethicists have pointed out that medical progress is theoretically limitless, so the concept of "need" is constantly expanding. Costs almost certainly will increase concomitantly, unless we find a successful method to restrain them. At some point, societal choices on this matter will be necessary.

Theoretically, society could decide to openly ration its health care dollars, either by age, diagnosis, an individual's worth to society, or some other parameter. Examples of this already exist on a small-scale or demonstration basis in some areas of the country. Under this set of priorities, available dollars would be rationed to do the most "good." Questions of good are decided by one's system of values, however, and consensus will not be achieved easily. In fact, in today's system, it is difficult if not impossible to imagine society accepting such compromises.

To be sure, U.S. physicians and other practitioners, with the technical knowledge that they possess, can make valuable contributions to the formulation of national policy. What they cannot do ethically is participate in any formal rationing process involving individual patients, because doing so would weaken the physician's responsibility as the patient's agent. In short, the problem of allocating the nation's health care resources requires that the practitioner wear more than one hat—and to decide when and where it is appropriate to wear each hat. These are not easy decisions, but there is no escaping them. Today's physician has a duty to consider the balance between the needs of the individual and those of society.

Is Professional Education Important?

While most Americans desire to be cared for by the best-trained professionals that money can buy, cost controls are having dramatic effects on medical education in this country. For instance, new methods such as PPS reimbursement have had particularly acute effects on university teaching hospitals, not only because they disproportionately care for patients who are severely ill, but also because their "extra" educational and research missions make them less cost-efficient.

When initiated in 1983, PPS allowed for a "graduate medical education add-on" to teaching hospitals amounting to 11.56 percent of the total reimbursement per DRG. As of 1991, this add-on had been reduced to 7.7 percent, significantly decreasing the revenues of academic medical centers. Furthermore, other third-party payers seem likely to follow Medicare's lead and reduce the portion of their reimbursements that subsidizes residency training programs. The issue of how (and whether) payers should reimburse hospitals for their training activities is the subject of considerable debate; should the government subsidize subspecialties in which a surplus of providers already exists or only those with a perceived shortage (e.g., family practitioners, psychiatrists, geriatricians)?

The strained finances of teaching hospitals also have been stretched further by increased competition for patients and the shift toward for-profit health care. Proprietary hospital systems typically select favorable markets for development, such as the Sunbelt region, where they find less regulation, charge-based instead of cost-based reimbursement formulae, and an expanding and comparatively affluent population. As a result, urban academic medical centers often are left to care for the poor and the most severely ill people. Moreover, for-profit hospitals avoid becoming heavily involved in education with its high overhead costs. In a health care industry that is increasingly price-competitive, teaching hospitals risk being squeezed out of the market.

Other legislative changes have made it more difficult to obtain a medical education as well. Because scholarship money is dwindling and the laws pertaining to government-subsidized student loans are getting tougher, medical students now are graduating with significant and growing debt. In 1990, the average medical student debt on graduation was estimated at over $48,000; this figure is expected to increase annually for the foreseeable future. As a consequence, fewer persons from lower socioeconomic backgrounds or members of disadvantaged minority groups will have an opportunity to study medicine. Also, some graduates will base career and specialty decisions on questions of financial necessity instead of academic interest or societal needs.

Are we willing to risk a reduction in the quality of the world's greatest teaching hospitals as a result of cost-containment initiatives? Are we willing to receive care from clinicians who have not received optimal training? Is it acceptable that students of suboptimal academic caliber but strong financial resources become the physicians of tomorrow? What will happen if teaching hospitals cease to be on the cutting edge of technological innovation? These are questions to ponder as the system continues to be reshaped.

Biomedical Research: A Social Priority?

As recently as one generation ago, fear of disease was an everyday experience for Americans. To raise a family without at least one casualty from a communicable disease was the exception rather than the rule. A childhood victim of polio remembers that "each summer, when the epidemics peaked, public swimming pools, camps, and even churches were closed. Children were kept at home, and victims and their families were shunned by many of their neighbors" (Calmes 1984, p. 1273).

In contrast, most citizens today no longer have a personal terror of disease. With very few exceptions, U.S. children no longer are crippled by polio, scarred by smallpox, or incapacitated by rheumatic fever or tuberculosis. Ironically, one result is that the value formerly placed on medical research has declined; at least, that is one way of reading the current all-out emphasis on cutting costs. Some think the AIDS epidemic may reverse this trend, because it has raised fears that are similar to those once engendered by polio.

Strangely enough, problems that scientists have *not* conquered have had a similar effect on social attitudes. Several common diseases remain largely incurable despite today's technologically sophisticated armamentarium. Some result from habits such as smoking and alcohol abuse or from social and environmental problems such as violence and industrial hazards. Such conditions have become the bane of modern existence, analogous to infectious disease in previous eras, and many believe that the medical profession can do little more than treat their victims.

Other chronic diseases of less-clear origin seem to be just as incurable in our present state of knowledge. One problem is that the "half-way technologies" used in treating such diseases—for example, dialysis for ESRD and the artificial heart for terminal cardiac disease—are extremely expensive. Expenditures for this type of high-technology medicine have been blamed as a major cause of runaway inflation in the costs of health care, and with only modest returns in terms of improving the health of the nation's people.

Changes in governmental policy have contributed to the endangerment of technology and research in recent years as well. PPS has erected barriers against the application of new technologies, particularly those that improve care without also improving cost-efficiency. PPS reimbursement regulations currently include an annual increase for purchasing new equipment, but this increase is significantly *lower* than the usual increase was before the institution of DRGs. As Chapter 6 noted, proposed adjustments in PPS reimbursement would jeopardize further a hospital's ability to make the capital expenditures that new technology requires. As a result, the financial ability of most hospitals to introduce technical innovations has decreased.

Another problem is the lack of an adequate DRG for patients who are admitted to a hospital under experimental protocols. Outlier dollars are supposed to subsidize the care of patients participating in research studies, but these funds are inadequate even for the care of patients who are severely ill. "Protocol" patients tend to be still more expensive. To solve this problem, it has been proposed that a new DRG be added expressly for such patients. In the meantime, medical research is hampered by such financial constraints.

For all these reasons—high costs, overzealous application, questionable benefit—some people are uncertain whether society receives a sufficient return on its investment in biomedical research. Both public support for medical research and actual funds (relative to inflation) have decreased, and reductions have been made in both hospital reimbursement and grants to medical-school research centers. Some institutions have cut back significantly on research; others have sought private, sometimes proprietary financing. Many fear that if research funding continues to shift to the private sector, future projects will be chosen more for their potential profitability than for their potential impact on society.

As we have seen, several trends within the current health care system are imposing restrictions. Projects that are designed for potential economic gain as well as projects that are designed to provide results "efficiently" in the face of uncertain sources of funding threaten the quality of research. Still, any tendency toward increasing the "relevance" of research has its dangers, notably that what seems relevant today may not seem so tomorrow. Conversely, what appears to be an unpromising research project today may become a major breakthrough in disease treatment tomorrow.

The direction of medical research is also being questioned in another way. To cure such major epidemics as polio, medical research for many decades has been directed toward exploring pathological mechanisms; some now feel that this path of inquiry is too narrow and that "the turbulence of relentless scientific analysis needs to be stilled" (O'Day 1984, p. 7). They would have the focus of research shift, and the basis of investigation broaden, to include the social, emotional, and psychological aspects of disease; this reflects a wider feeling that the human dimension of medical care is in danger of extinction. Some research projects of this broader sort are under way.

One thing seems certain: a reasonable level of research is needed if there are to be any breakthroughs at all, otherwise the pace of medical progress will inevitably slow. It is important that we find compromises to preserve exploration on the frontiers of research. These issues will have real effects on the medical care that we receive. Are we prepared to pay this price for cost containment? Americans informed on these issues can decide whether these policies reflect their desires for the health care system.

The Future of Medicine as a Profession

Will tomorrow's practitioner be considered a tradesman or a professional? Since 1975, when the exemption of physicians from the antitrust laws was lifted, the law has treated medicine as a trade rather than as a profession. Ten years later, it was suggested that the public is coming to share this perspective. The distinction is more than just a matter of semantics; it will affect directly the ethical responsibilities and the role in society of future physicians. Throughout this century, physicians have been among the most respected members of our society, and deservingly so. To retain that respect, however, they must show very clearly that they are more than tradesmen.

Given these societal attitudes and the present conditions within medicine (from school through established practice), it is unsurprising that demoralization among medical professionals is widespread. The number of applicants to medical school has declined during this era of turmoil in the health care system, and though the numbers are beginning to reverse themselves, the medical profession should ask what is turning away prospective students. American youth have noticed the conflicts. Their impression of physicians may have been adversely affected. Numerous other factors also may play a role, including fear of physician oversupply, greater indebtedness to obtain an education, competition among practitioners, fear of AIDS, and a decline in respect by society for physicians.

Today, many physicians leave practice and discourage others from entering it. Medicine has always been a fast-paced career, but a new, more malignant type of stress has been superimposed on the fatigue from long hours of hard work. Managed care and UR have added mountains of paperwork and several hours to the average physician's work week. Societal, political, and legal threats have also taken their toll on attitudes.

Having believed themselves to be regarded highly by the public and having considered themselves to be exercising professional and economic responsibility in a calling, they now see themselves cast as wrongdoers and incompetents who yearly require new laws, regulations, admonitions, court decisions, and exposés to make them more honest, ethical, competent, corrigible, and contrite. Perhaps it is no wonder if many now look for a change or an exit. (Radovsky 1990, p. 266)

We hope that this overstates the feelings of physicians. The literal use of magic in medical practice is gone, replaced by scientific knowledge, but magic of another kind, deriving from a life of intellectual challenge in the service to others, remains. Physicians remain professionals in every sense of the word. There *is* reason for hope despite the problems and complexities that face the profession today. If the field continues to attract the high quality of students that it has attracted in the past, then the future of medicine will remain bright.

Responses by the Profession

Physicians long have been perceived as being barriers to change within the system of health care. This perception began decades ago based on the profession's initial resistance to public sector involvement in health care financing at the passage of Medicare and Medicaid legislation in the 1960s and continues to today. Both society and politicians see the main goal of organized medicine as self-serving: to protect physicians' financial interests and incomes.

In fact, organized medicine has only recently provided its own proposal for the nation's access problem. An emerging goal within the profession is the optimal use of available resources, and this goal is reflected in the outcomes and effectiveness movements. These practice improvements will not substitute for broad reform, but they do represent a positive response by the profession toward improving the system.

We believe that practitioners should assume direct responsibility for some of today's issues. They should address forthrightly such matters as the ethical and financial aspects of individual clinical decisions and such complex societal problems as access to care and medical malpractice. They should form considered views on the optimal allocation of health care resources and take the necessary steps, whether through writing journal articles, lecturing, consulting, serving as hospital administrators, or serving on appropriate committees, to get those views heard by those who make the decisions. They also should educate their patients on the important effects that their lifestyle has on their health.

Political activity is another means to create change, assuming that it maximizes the role of medical expertise and is not primarily self-serving. A group of physicians representing "organized medicine" and presenting a unified front before legislators on a particular issue not only serves as an appropriate interface between the political system, society, and the medical profession, it also can get things done that the ordinary political process might never accomplish. Organized medicine will need strong leaders and clearly stated goals to make an effective presence.

Compromise likely will be necessary. "Negotiating, we can have an active hand in shaping our own fate. By negotiating, I do not mean being willing to offer everything blindly. All successful negotiators have a 'bottom line' and a sense of what can and cannot be bargained away. If we hold ourselves above negotiation, or lack the perspective to engage in it successfully, we run the risk of inadvertently betraying both our patients and our science" (Lister 1991, p. 10).

Perhaps the most important way to ensure that physicians continue to be awarded professional status is for the profession to establish sensible and believable mechanisms for disciplining delinquent members, licensing, continuing education, and monitoring and improving the quality of care. Such measures are vital if payers, patients, and policymakers are to be convinced that today's physicians take their mission seriously and are willing to be accountable for their own behavior.

Today's health care providers are living through a period of accelerated change. Many issues are on the table that involve not only the health care industry itself but also the legal and political systems. As the financing and organization of U.S. health care are reshaped, the ability to accept change and to adapt to new conditions will be necessary, and the role that practitioners play in resolving these issues will go a long way toward determining the future of the medical profession in the new medical marketplace.

Values that are cherished by all parties now are at stake, and what should be a cooperative enterprise sometimes looks more like a battle. A new equilibrium has yet to be reached, and even its general outlines are not yet as clear as one might wish. Change is everywhere, but some important things will not change. In the words of Harvard's Carola Eisenberg, "The satisfaction of being able to relieve pain and restore function, the intellectual challenge of solving clinical problems, and the variety of human issues we confront in daily clinical practice will remain the essence of doctoring, whatever the changes in the organizational and economic structure of medicine" (1986, p. 114).

LIST OF ACRONYMS

AARP. American Association of Retired Persons.
AHA. American Hospital Association.
AHCPR. Agency for Health Care Policy and Research.
AIDS. Acquired immune deficiency syndrome.
AMA. American Medical Association.
APGs. Ambulatory patient groups.
ATRA. American Tort Reform Association.
CBA. Cost–benefit analysis.
CEA. Cost-effectiveness analysis.
CMP. Competitive medical plan.
CON. Certificate-of-need program.
CPR. Customary-Prevailing-Reasonable.
CPT. Current procedural terminology.
CQI. Continuous quality improvement.
CT. Computed tomography (scanner).
DRGs. Diagnosis-related groups.
EKG. Electrocardiogram.
EPO. Exclusive provider organization.
ESRD. End-stage renal disease.
FASB. Financial Accounting Standards Board.
FEC. Freestanding emergency-care center.
FFS. Fee-for-service reimbursement.
GDP. Gross domestic product (formerly *GNP*, gross national product).
GMENAC. Graduate Medical Education National Advisory Committee.
GP. General practitioner.
HCFA. Health Care Financing Administration.
HHA. Home Health Agency.
HIAA. Health Insurance Association of America.

HIV. Human immunodeficiency virus.

HMO. Health maintenance organization.

HSAs. Health systems agencies.

ICD-9. International Classification of Diseases, 9th Revision.

IOM. National Academy of Science's Institute of Medicine.

IPA. Independent (or individual) practice association.

IV. Intravenous.

JCAHO. Joint Commission for the Accreditation of Health-Care Organizations.

MAAC. Maximum allowable actual charge.

MD-DRGs. Diagnosis-related groups for physician reimbursement.

MEI. Medicare economic index.

MeSH. Medical staff and hospital.

MIP. Managed indemnity plan.

MRI. Magnetic resonance imaging.

NAMI. National Alliance for the Mentally Ill.

NIH. National Institutes of Health.

OEO. Office of Economic Opportunity.

PORTs. Patient outcome research teams.

PPGP. Prepaid group practice.

PPO. Preferred provider organization.

PPRC. Physicians payment review commission.

PPS. Prospective payment system.

PRO. Peer review organization.

PSRO. Professional standards review organization.

QA. Quality assurance (program).

RAP. Radiology, anesthesiology, pathology.

RBRVS. Resource-based relative value scale.

RVS. Relative value scale.

RVU. Relative value unit.

S/HMO. Social health maintenance organization.

TPA. Third-party administrator.

UCR. Usual-Customary-Reasonable.

UR. Utilization review.

VA. Department of Veterans Affairs (formerly Veterans Administration).

VPS. Volume performance standard.

GLOSSARY

accepting assignment. See *assignment.*

access to care. A person's ability to obtain health care when needed. To obtain access, the provider must be available, affordable, appropriate, and acceptable to the patient.

ADS. Alternative delivery system: a generic term for an organization or system that provides health care in an alternative manner to traditional health insurance plans. ADSs usually involve a significant degree of vertical integration and prearranged contracts between insurers and a network of providers. HMOs and PPOs are ADSs. (See *managed care* and *CMP.*)

advance directive. Legally binding document outlining a patient's wishes regarding heroic measures and life-sustaining competent treatment, written by the patient prior to the need for such interventions.

assignment. A provider who accepts assignment submits a bill directly to the insurer and accepts the company's reimbursement as payment in full for the service. The patient may or may not still be responsible for any cost-sharing provisions depending on the insurance plan. A provider who accepts assignment will not "balance-bill." (See *balance billing* and *Participating Physician.*)

autonomy. An ethical principle relating to a person's right to self-determination. (See Chapter 10.)

balance-billing. Direct billing of an insured patient by a provider. The patient then is personally responsible for the payment of any charge exceeding the insurer's allowed reimbursement. (See *assignment.*)

behavioral offset. A term that is applied to expected increases in the volume of physician services in direct response to fee decreases. HCFA estimates that for each 1 percent cut in physician fees under RBRVS, the volume and intensity of services will increase by 0.5 percent.

beneficence. An ethical principle that focuses on promoting the welfare of others. (See Chapter 10.)

capitation. A system of financing in which a provider is paid a per-capita fee for each consumer, which is negotiated before the consumer receives any care.

case manager. A patient's representative who is hired by an insurer or corporate employer to coordinate the care process, especially as it relates to high-cost or long-term care. (See alternative definition under *gatekeeper.*)

CBA. Cost–benefit analysis: an evaluation method in which monetary values are assigned to both the inputs and the outcomes of a health care technology or program. CBA is used to assist in decisions regarding the allocation of resources among alternative technologies or programs.

CEA. Cost-effectiveness analysis: an evaluation method in which the inputs of a health care technology or program are measured in monetary terms but outcomes are measured in nonmonetary units (such as years-of-life saved or morbidity avoided). CEA is used by decision makers to compare programs or treatments having similar effects.

CMP. Competitive medical plan: HCFA's term for HMOs that are not federally qualified. These provide service to Medicare beneficiaries on a "risk-contract," capitated payment basis. The term *CMP* is sometimes also used interchangeably with ADS.

CON. Certificate-of-need program: a program that is coordinated by state planning agencies that requires health care facilities to obtain approval before they make major investments in equipment or services.

cost-plus reimbursement. A FFS payment system where the provider (usually a hospital) is paid retrospectively its actual costs for providing a service plus a preset percentage as "mark-up."

cost-sharing. An insurance arrangement by which insured consumers are required to pay a portion of their medical bills out-of-pocket. Deductibles, co-payments, and co-insurance are all types of cost-sharing. (See Chapter 4.)

cost-shifting. Health care facilities' practice of charging higher prices to patients who pay full price (either because they have no insurance coverage or because their insurance company reimburses the total charge) to compensate for reduced reimbursement from patients who are indigent or covered by public or private insurance or entitlement programs that reimburse less than the amount charged for care.

CPR. Customary-Prevailing-Reasonable: a method formerly used by Medicare for determining the allowable amount to be paid a provider under FFS payment. (See *UCR.*)

CPT. Current procedural terminology: a taxonomy of procedural codes that were developed by the AMA, primarily for billing purposes.

deductible. A type of insurance cost-sharing in which a beneficiary pays a predetermined dollar amount out-of-pocket for medical services before any insurance benefits are reimbursed.

defensive medicine. Clinicians' attempts to resolve doubts about the diagnosis or therapy by doing tests to maximize the defensibility of their actions in court.

demand creation. The ability of medical care providers to initiate demand for their services, such as by scheduling return office visits. When a consumer does not truly require the service, the initiation of the service in considered *inducement.*

DRG creep. Subtle manipulation of diagnostic coding to make patients appear more ill than they actually are. This can be accomplished by reordering or modifying the listing of a patient's discharge diagnoses and procedures in the medical record.

DRGs. Diagnosis-related groups: a set of categories that are based on patient diagnoses, procedures, and age. These are assigned mainly for purposes of PPS hospital reimbursement by the Medicare program.

elasticity of demand. An economic term for the relationship existing between the price of a service and consumers' demand for it.

entitlement program. Public sector programs from which beneficiaries receive benefits without paying into the program.

EPO. Exclusive provider organization: a type of PPO in which patients are required to use providers who participate in the PPO network.

external effect. The value that society in the aggregate derives from the health of its members.

FEC. Freestanding emergency-care center: a nonhospital-based, ambulatory-care facility providing extended-hour emergency services. Similar types of facility providing ambulatory care to nonemergency patients have been termed *urgent-care* (or *urgi-care*) *centers* and *convenience-care centers.*

fee schedule. A system, often based on a RVS, whereby third-party payers reimburse a predetermined amount for a given service regardless of the provider-designated fee. (See *RVS.*)

FFS. Fee-for-service reimbursement: an arrangement in which a provider charges a fee for each separate service. Payment is made after each service is provided. (See Chapter 5.)

for-profit health care. Health care that is provided by a corporation whose surplus income is paid to those who either own or have invested in the corporation. (See also *nonprofit health care.*)

gatekeeper. A primary-care physician who manages the case of an individual patient by coordinating all services. In some health plans, no specialist or hospital care will be reimbursed without the gatekeeper's previous approval. (See *case manager.*)

GMENAC. Graduate Medical Education National Advisory Committee: a blue-ribbon government panel that studied, among other issues, the adequacy of the U.S. health care manpower supply in the 1980s and beyond.

going bare. To forego health insurance or medical malpractice insurance, usually because of its unaffordability or other barriers to purchase (such as a pre-existing condition). (See Chapter 12.)

group model HMO. A type of HMO in which a single, large, multispecialty group practice is the sole (or major) source of care for an HMO's enrollees. (See *HMO.*)

HCFA. U.S. Health Care Financing Administration: the agency that is responsible for Medicare and the federal involvement in Medicaid. This agency is part of the U.S. Department of Health and Human Services.

health insurance. Insurance offering consumer protection against medical expenses in return for a fixed, predetermined premium. Usually covers hospital and professional fees. Insurers may be *nonprofit* or *for-profit,* with the latter also termed the *commercials.* (See Chapter 4.)

HMO. Health maintenance organization: a prepaid health care delivery system in which the organization (and usually its primary-care physicians) assume financial risk for the care that they provide to enrolled members. The HMO is legally committed to provide care to its enrollees, and members must obtain care from within the system if it is to be reimbursed. There are four basic HMO models: staff, group, network, and IPA. (See separate listings and Part II.)

horizontal integration. An arrangement by which a corporation (either for-profit or nonprofit) operates or coordinates a number of health care facilities providing the same level of service (e.g., a chain of hospitals). (See *vertical integration.*)

HSAs. Health systems agencies: regional planning bodies that were created in the 1970s to assess local needs for medical care resources.

ICD-9. International Classification of Diseases, 9th revision: a taxonomy of approximately 10,000 diagnoses and 5000 procedural codes. The DRG system is based on these codes.

IPA. Independent (or individual) practice association: a type of HMO in which independent physicians contract with the HMO corporation to provide care to its enrolled members. (See *HMO.*)

justice. An ethical principle referring to the proper distribution of benefits and burdens. Egalitarianism, libertarianism, and utilitarianism are three approaches to justice. (See Chapter 10.)

MAAC. Maximum allowable actual charge: a mandated cap that is placed on the charge that can be submitted to Medicare by a nonparticipating physician. (See *CPR* and *nonparticipating physician.*)

major medical insurance policy. An insurance policy providing coverage above that provided in a company's core policy, such as outpatient physician visits and reimbursement for hospital bills exceeding the limits of core benefits.

managed care. A term often used generically for all types of ADS (e.g., HMOs and PPOs), implying that they "manage" the care that is received by consumers; the contrast is with traditional FFS care, which is unmanaged. The term also is used to describe a range of utilization controls that are applied to "manage" the practices of physicians and other providers, regardless of whether they are in an ADS. (See *MIP* and *ADS.*)

MD-DRGs. Physician DRGs: a potential reimbursement method in which the admitting physician receives a DRG-based flat fee to provide all hospital-based care during an episode of illness.

Medicaid. A joint federal–state health insurance program (or more correctly, an entitlement program) for poor Americans that is administered mainly by state governments.

Medicare. A national health insurance program for Americans over the age of 65 years and disabled persons. The program is administered by HCFA. Part A of the program covers hospital expenses, Part B covers physicians and other professional services.

medi-gap insurance. Supplemental private insurance that is purchased by most Medicare enrollees to pay for Medicare deductibles and co-insurance charges.

MEI. Medicare economic index: an HCFA formula limiting yearly increases in Medicare Part B reimbusement, based on practice-cost increases and general wage levels.

MeSH. Medical staff and hospital: a "joint venture" in which a hospital and its private-practice medical staff (or other body of independent physicians) form a legal corporation, which then may contract to care for enrollees in an HMO or a PPO or itself become an HMO or PPO.

MIP. Managed indemnity plan: a type of ADS in which a health insurance company, often representing a self-insured employer, mandates standards of practice for providers who wish to be reimbursed via FFS for care that they provide to enrollees. MIPs rely on a range of utilization controls, including prehospital certification, second-opinion surgical programs, and case managers. (See *managed care.*)

moral hazard. An economic term that is applied to the tendency to use, and perhaps overuse, a health insurance policy because of the strong financial incentive to do so. (A misnomer, as it describes what is an economic and not a moral issue.)

national health insurance. A program in which government provides (or certifies) health insurance for all citizens; alternatively, the program may employ providers directly. Such a system is in place in Canada, England, and virtually all other developed countries. (See Chapter 12.)

network model HMO. A type of HMO in which a network of two or more existing group practices contracts to care for the majority of patients who are enrolled in an HMO plan. This type of HMO sometimes also contracts with individual providers in a fashion similar to an IPA.

nonparticipating physician. Physician who does not accept assignment for patients reimbursed under the Medicare program.

nonprofit health care. Health care that is provided by an organization (usually a corporation) whose surplus income is reinvested in the organization itself. (See *for-profit health care.*)

OEO. Office of Economic Opportunity: a governmental unit that was developed during the 1960s to lead the "War on Poverty." This office was responsible for a program of Neighborhood Health Centers.

outlier patient. Under Medicare's PPS, a patient whose bill exceeds the prospective payment for his or her DRG category by 50 percent or $12,000.

participating physician. A provider who agrees to accept assignment from Medicare (or another insurer) for individual patients or all beneficiaries treated during a specified time period. (See *assignment.*)

patient dumping. Transferring a patient to another facility because of his or her lack of ability to pay for care.

per-case payment. A reimbursement method in which the provider receives a flat fee to provide all care for a given patient "case" (i.e., illness episode). The payment amount usually is prenegotiated and independent of the type or amount of services that are provided. The DRG-based PPS system is a per-case payment system.

PPGP. Prepaid group practice: a type of HMO in which a large group (or groups) of physicians provide medical services to the enrollees of the plan. The group usually receives payment on a capitated basis. If the group is incorporated separately from the HMO, then it is considered a group-model HMO; if the physicians practice in a group primarily salaried by the HMO, then it is considered a staff-model HMO. (See *HMO.*)

PPO. Preferred provider organization: a health care plan that acts as a broker between the purchaser and the provider of care. Providers usually receive payment on a discounted FFS basis (e.g., 80 percent of usual fees) without financial risk-sharing. In return for patient referrals, providers agree to managed-care controls. Enrollees are given incentives (e.g., no co-insurance) to use the providers within the PPO, but they may seek covered services from outside the PPO system.

PPS. Prospective Payment System: a hospital reimbursement system for Medicare's Part A in which the provider is reimbursed a prospectively determined, fixed amount per patient admission regardless of the quantity of services that are received by that patient. (See *DRG* and *per-case payment.*)

PRO. Peer review organization: a public sector–funded UR program, composed of independent-contracting physician groups in each state. PROs are charged with monitoring the cost and quality of care that is received by Medicare beneficiaries. To date, PROs review hospital care and Medicare-participating HMOs. (See *UR.*)

PSRO. Professional standards review organization: the predecessors of PROs.

QA. Quality assurance (program): a program that has been implemented in many hospitals and other facilities to ensure a high quality of care. Many QA programs also are responsible for UR. (See *UR.*)

RAP. Radiology, anesthesiology, pathology: an acronym that is used largely in reimbursement negotiations with HCFA.

RBRVS. Resource-based relative value system: a RVS on which the fee schedule for Medicare Part B physician reimbursement is based. The 5-year phase-in period for RBRVS began in January 1992. (See *RVS* and Chapter 6.)

risk-sharing. A payment arrangement in which providers accept at least some risk of decreased reimbursement if their performance is inefficient. Capitation payment systems involve risk-sharing, as do systems in which a certain percentage of the provider's FFS payments (e.g., 20 percent) are placed in escrow pending an evaluation—usually annual—of the financial performance of the physician or the plan. In general, all HMOs incorporate risk-sharing.

RVS. Relative value scale (or system): a methodology for weighting the value of different medical services. A RVS is often used to develop a fee schedule. (See also *RBRVS, fee schedule,* Chapters 5 and 6.)

RVU. Relative value unit: the weighting units used by RVSs.

safe harbors. A legal entrepreneurial investment for health care providers as delineated in recent HCFA regulations.

self-insurance. An arrangement in which an employer acts as a health insurer by paying employees' medical expenses directly rather than by paying their insurance premiums. Most self-insured employers contract out the administration of such plans. Some employees purchase "minimal insurance" to cover catastrophic expenses (e.g., services over $50,000).

S/HMO. Social health maintenance organization: a new type of HMO developed on a demonstration basis with HCFA funding, intended to expand HMO services to provide social support and long-term care to elderly and disabled Medicare enrollees.

small-area variation. The variation in the medical services that are provided in different geographic locales. Such variation is identified by epidemiologic comparisons of the practice patterns of populations of clinicians in different areas.

staff-model HMO. Physicians are employed directly by the organization on a salaried basis, usually with some degree of provider risk-sharing.

technologic imperative. The tendency (and desire) of both clinicians and patients to use available tests not only to reduce uncertainty but because of the U.S. inclination to demand the most up-to-date services.

third-party administrator. A private firm that is hired to serve as an intermediary between a self-insured corporation and its employees' health care providers to provide and facilitate claims processing, case management, and reimbursement.

third-party payers. Those who reimburse providers for health care services, as distinguished from the patient and the provider (the first two parties). In the United States, the major third parties are the U.S. government (which is responsible for Medicare and Medicaid), the non-profit Blue Cross/Blue Shield plans, and the commercial insurers. Through their involvement in self-insured plans, corporations also can be considered an important third party.

tort law. The area of law that concerns legal wrongs committed on the person or property of another for which the law gives civil remedy, usually monetary damages for the resulting injury. Common torts are negligence, assault, battery, false imprisonment, libel, slander, and invasion of privacy. Medical malpractice occurs and tort law is breached if a physician injures a patient through practice that is below acceptable standards.

UCR. Usual-Customary-Reasonable: a method that is used by insurers to determine the amounts paid under FFS reimbursement. (See *CPR.*)

uncompensated care. Medical services that are provided to a patient for which no reimbursement is received. Uncompensated care is provided mainly to uninsured patients.

UR. Utilization review: a case-by-case evaluation of the use of clinical resources in which actual practices are compared to predetermined criteria. (See *QA.*)

vertical integration. An arrangement by which a corporation (either for-profit or nonprofit) operates or coordinates a group of facilities that collectively offer many levels of health care service. A vertically integrated organization usually provides or arranges for the delivery of primary care, specialized ambulatory care, hospital care, and long-term care. HMOs can be viewed as a type of vertically integrated organization. (See *horizontal integration.*)

REFERENCES/BIBLIOGRAPHY

Introduction to Part I

Division of National Cost Estimates, Office of the Actuary. 1987. "National Health Expenditures, 1986–2000." *Health Care Financing Review* 8, 4: 1–36.

Gonzalez, Martin, ed. 1991. *Socioeconomic Characteristics of Medical Practice, 1990/1991.* Chicago: AMA Center for Health Policy Research.

Radovsky, Saul. 1990. "U.S. Medical Practice before Medicare and Now—Differences and Consequences." *New England Journal of Medicine* 322, 4: 263–267.

Tarlov, Alvin. 1983. "The Increasing Supply of Physicians, the Changing Structure of the Health-Services System, and the Future Practice of Medicine." *New England Journal of Medicine* 308, 20: 1235–1244.

Chapter 1

Ackerknecht, Erwin. 1982. *A Short History of Medicine,* rev. ed. Baltimore: Johns Hopkins University Press.

AMA Office of Socioeconomic Research Information. 1991. *Trends in U.S. Health Care 1990.* Chicago: AMA Center for Health Policy Research.

"An Overcrowded Profession—the Cause and the Remedy." 1901. *Journal of the American Medical Association* 37, 12: 775–776.

Anderson, Odin. 1985. *Health Services in the United States: A Growth Enterprise since 1985.* Ann Arbor, Mich.: Health Administration Press.

Bergman, Norman. 1985. "Forerunners of Modern Anesthesiology: Dwarfs and Giants." *The Pharos,* Fall: 8–12.

Berliner, Howard. 1975. "A Larger Perspective on the Flexner Report." *International Journal of Health Services* 5, 4: 573–92.

Bordley, James, and A. McGehee Harvey. 1976. *Two Centuries of American Medicine: 1776–1976.* Philadelphia: W.B. Saunders.

Buhler-Wilkerson, Karen. 1985. "Public Health Nursing: In Sickness or in Health?" *American Journal of Public Health* 75, 10: 1155–61.

Califano, Joseph. 1986. "A Corporate Rx for America: Managing Runaway Health Costs." *Issues in Science and Technology,* Spring: 81–90.

Commission on Hospital Care. 1947. *Hospital Care in the United States.* New York: Commonwealth Fund.

Committee on the Costs of Medical Care. 1932. *Medical Care for the American People.* Chicago: University of Chicago Press.

Corning, Peter. 1969. *The Evolution of Medicare . . . From Idea to Law.* Social Security Administration, Office of Research and Statistics, Research Report 29. Washington, D.C.: Government Printing Office.

Editors of *Fortune.* 1970. *Our Ailing Medical System: It's Time to Operate.* New York: Harper and Row.

Evans, Bergan. 1978. *Dictionary of Quotations.* New York: Avenel Books.

Fein, Rashi. 1962. *The Doctor Shortage: An Economic Diagnosis.* Washington, D.C.: Brookings Institution.

Fleming, Donald. 1954. *William H. Welch and the Rise of Modern Medicine.* Boston: Little, Brown.

Freymann, John. 1974. *The American Health Care System: Its Genesis and Trajectory.* New York: Medcom Press.

Fuchs, Victor. 1974. *Who Shall Live? Health, Economics, and Social Choice.* New York: Basic Books.

Garrison, Fielding. 1929. *An Introduction to the History of Medicine.* Philadelphia: W.B. Saunders.

Gillick, Muriel. 1985. "Common-Sense Models of Health and Disease." *New England Journal of Medicine* 313, 11: 700–3.

Gornick, Marion, Jay Greenberg, Paul Eggers, and Allen Dobson. 1985. "Twenty Years of Medicare and Medicaid: Covered Populations, Use of Benefits, and Program Expenditures." *Health Care Financing Review,* Annual Supplement: 13–59.

Hatfield, Charles. 1920. "Relative Functions of Health Agencies: II. Viewpoint of the Non-Official Agency." *American Journal of Public Health* 10, 12: 948–52.

Health Care Financing Administration. 1991. *Health Care Financing Program Statistics: Medicare and Medical Data Book, 1990.* Pub. 03314. Baltimore: HCFA.

Hearings before the Committee on Education and Labor. 1945. United States Senate. Bill S.191. February and March 1945. Washington, D.C.: Government Printing Office.

HIAA. 1991. *Source Book of Health Insurance Data*. Washington, D.C.: HIAA.

Hirshfield, Daniel. 1970. *The Lost Reform: The Campaign for Compulsory Health Insurance in the United States from 1932 to 1943*. Cambridge, Mass.: Harvard University Press.

Howell, Joel. 1986. "Early Use of X-Ray Machines and Electrocardiographs at the Pennsylvania Hospital: 1897 Through 1927." *Journal of the American Medical Association* 255, 17: 2320–3.

King, Lester. 1984. "The Flexner Report of 1910." *Journal of the American Medical Association* 251, 8: 1079–86.

Kingsdale, Jon. 1981. *The Growth of Hospitals: An Economic History in Baltimore*, vol. 1. Ann Arbor, Mich.: University Microfilms International.

Knowles, John, ed. 1977. *Doing Better and Feeling Worse: Health in the United States*. New York: W.W. Norton.

Kuhn, Thomas. 1962. *The Structure of Scientific Revolutions*. Chicago: University of Chicago Press.

Lewis, Irving, and Cecil Sheps. 1983. *The Sick Citadel*. Cambridge, Mass.: Oelgeschlager, Gunn and Hain.

National Center for Health Statistics. 1987. *Health, United States, 1986*. Hyattsville, Md.: Public Health Service.

National Center for Health Statistics. 1989. *Monthly Vital Statistics Report*. 26 September. Hyattsville, Md.: Public Health Service.

National Center for Health Statistics. 1991. *Health, United States, 1990*. Hyattsville, Md.: Public Health Service.

Pierce, R. V. 1895. *The People's Common Sense Medical Advisor*. Buffalo, N.Y.: World Dispensary Printing Office.

Reed, Louis. 1933. *The Ability to Pay for Medical Care*. Publication of the Committee on the Costs of Medical Care. Chicago: University of Chicago Press.

Reiser, Stanley. 1984. "The Machine at the Bedside: Technological Transformations of Practices and Values." In: Reiser, Stanley, and Michael Anbar, eds. *Machine at the Bedside*. New York: Cambridge University Press.

Relman, Arnold. 1988. "Assessment and Accountability: The Third Revolution in Medical Care." *New England Journal of Medicine* 319, 18: 1220–2.

Ricardo-Campbell, Rita. 1982. *The Economics and Politics of Health*. Chapel Hill, N.C.: University of North Carolina Press.

Roemer, Milton. 1986. *An Introduction to the U.S. Health Care System.* New York: Springer Publishing.

Rosen, George. 1958. *A History of Public Health.* New York: MD Publications.

Sardell, Alice. 1983. "Neighborhood Health Centers and Community-Based Care: Federal Policy from 1965 to 1983." *Journal of Public Health Policy* 4, 4:484–503.

Shorter, Edward. 1985. *Bedside Manners.* New York: Simon and Schuster.

Shyrock, Richard. 1962. *Medicine and Society in America: 1660–1860.* Ithaca, N.Y.: Great Seal Book.

Spingarn, Natalie. 1976. *Heartbeat: The Politics of Health Research.* Washington, D.C.: Robert B. Luce.

Starr, Paul. 1982. *The Social Transformation of American Medicine.* New York: Basic Books.

Tarlov, Alvin. 1983. "The Increasing Supply of Physicians, the Changing Structure of the Health-Services System, and the Future Practice of Medicine." *New England Journal of Medicine* 308, 20:1235–44.

Thomas, Lewis. 1983. *The Youngest Science: Notes of a Medicine-Watcher.* New York: Viking Press.

U.S. Department of Health and Human Services. 1982. *Health Care Financing Program Statistics: The Medicare and Medicaid Data Book, 1981.* Pub. 03128. Washington, D.C.: Government Printing Office.

U.S. General Accounting Office. 1985. *Constraining National Health Care Expenditures: Achieving Quality Care at an Affordable Cost.* Pub. GAO/HRD-85–105. Washington, D.C.: Government Printing Office.

Walsh, Diana, and Richard Egdahl. 1977. *Payer, Provider, Consumer: Industry Confronts Health Care Costs.* New York: Springer-Verlag.

Williams, Greer. 1971. *Kaiser-Permanente Health Plan: Why It Works.* Oakland, Calif.: Kaiser Foundation.

Young, Hugh. 1910. "After Fifteen Years: A Glance at Recent Progress in Medicine and Surgery." In: *History of Surgery.* Charlottesville, Va.: Michie Co.

Ziporyn, Terra. 1985. "The Food and Drug Administration: How 'Those Regulations' Came to Be." *Journal of the American Medical Association* 254, 15: 2037–46.

Chapter 2

AARP. 1991. "A Profile of Older Americans: 1990." Brochure. Washington, D.C.: American Association of Retired Persons.

AMA. 1991a. *Physician Characteristics and Distribution in the United States, 1990.* Chicago, AMA.

AMA. Office of Socioeconomic Research Information. 1991b. *Trends in U.S. Health Care, 1990.* Chicago: AMA.

Altman, Stuart. 1991. "Why Healthcare Executives Should Support a National Cost-Containment Plan." *Healthcare Executive* 6, 4: 21–4.

"AMA Insights." 1985. *Journal of the American Medical Association* 254, 6: 746.

Anderson, Odin. 1985. *Health Services in the United States: A Growth Enterprise Since 1985.* Ann Arbor, Mich.: Health Administration Press.

APHA. 1991. *The Nation's Health.* Washington, D.C.: American Public Health Association.

Blendon, Robert, and David Rogers. 1983. "Cutting Medical Care Costs: *Primum Non Nocere.*" *Journal of the American Medical Association* 250, 14: 1880–5.

Blendon, Robert, and Jennifer Edwards. 1991. *System in Crisis: The Case for Health Care Reform.* Washington, D.C.: Faulkner and Gray.

Blumenthal, David. 1986. "Prescriptions for America's Health Care System." *Washington Post Book World.* 13 April: 1–2.

Califano, Joseph. 1986. "A Corporate Rx for America: Managing Runaway Health Costs." *Issues in Science and Technology.* Spring: 81–90.

Employee Benefit Research Institute. 1986. "Features of Employer Health Plans: Cost Containment, Plan Funding and Coverage Continuation." Washington, D.C.

Enthoven, Alain. 1989. "A 'Cost-Unconscious' Medical System." *New York Times,* 13 July: A23.

Finder, Alan. 1991. "Health Care Costs are New Crux of Contract Talks." *New York Times,* 27 October: 1.

Freedman, Steven. 1985. "Megacorporate Health Care: A Choice for the Future." *New England Journal of Medicine* 312, 9: 579–82.

Fry, John, and John Hasler. 1986. *Primary Health Care 2000.* Edinburgh: Churchill Livingstone.

HCFA, Division of National Cost Estimates. 1987. "National Health Expenditures, 1986–2000." *Health Care Financing Review* 8, 4: 1–36.

HIAA. 1987. *1986–1987 Source Book of Health Insurance Data.* Washington, D.C.: HIAA.

HIAA. 1991. *Source Book of Health Insurance Data.* Washington, D.C.: HIAA.

Iglehart, John. 1985. "The Veterans Administration Medical Care System Faces an Uncertain Future." *New England Journal of Medicine* 313, 18: 1168–72.

Illich, Ivan. 1976. *Medical Nemesis: The Expropriation of Health.* New York: Random House.

Jonas, Steven. 1986. *Health Care Delivery in the United States,* 3rd ed. New York: Springer Publishing.

Levit, Katharine, and Cathy Cowan. 1991. "Business, Households, and Governments: Health Care Costs, 1990." *Health Care Financing Review* 13, 2: 83–93.

Levit, Katharine, Helen Lazenby, Cathy Cowan, and Suzanne Letsch. 1991. "National Health Care Expenditures, 1990." *Health Care Financing Review* 13, 1: 29–54.

Luther, Jim. 1991. "States May Be Forced to Cut Spending More Despite Tax Increases." *Baltimore Sun,* 30 October: 6A.

Maple, Brenda, Cathy Cowan, Carolyn Donham, and Suzanne Letsch. 1991. "Community Hospital Statistics." *Health Care Financing Review* 13, 2: 95–114.

Marder, William, David Emmons, Phillip Kletke, and Richard Willke. 1988. "Physician Employment Patterns: Challenging Conventional Wisdom." *Health Affairs* 7, 4: 137–145.

National Center for Health Statistics. 1991. *Health, United States, 1990.* Hyattsville, Md.: Public Health Service.

Radovsky, Saul. 1990. "U.S. Medical Practice Before Medicare and Now—Differences and Consequences." *New England Journal of Medicine* 322, 4: 263–7.

Reinhardt, Uwe. 1985. "Future Trends in the Economics of Medical Practice and Care." *American Journal of Cardiology* 56, 5: 50C-9C.

Rublee, Dale. 1985. "Self-Funded Health Benefit Plans: Trends, Legal Environment, and Policy Issues." *Journal of the American Medical Association* 255, 6: 787–9.

Sardell, Alice. 1983. "Neighborhood Health Centers and Community-Based Care: Federal Policy from 1965 to 1982." *Journal of Public Health Policy* 4, 4: 484–503.

Sawyer, Kathy. 1991. "Health Care Spending May Reach 14% of GNP." *Washington Post,* 30 December: A6.

Schieber, George. 1990. "Health Expenditures in Major Industrialized Countries, 1960–1987." *Health Care Financing Review* 11, 4: 159–67.

Schieber, George, and J.P. Poullier. 1986. "International Health Care Spending." *Health Affairs* 5, 3: 111–22.

Schramm, Carl. 1983. "The Teaching Hospital and the Future Role of State Government." *New England Journal of Medicine* 308, 1: 41–5.

Sorkin, Alan. 1986. *Health Care and the Changing Economic Environment.* Lexington, Mass.: D.C. Heath and Co.

Starr, Paul. 1982. *The Social Transformation of American Medicine.* New York: Basic Books.

Steinwachs, Donald, Jonathan Weiner, Sam Shapiro, et al. 1986. "A Comparison of the Requirements for Primary Care Physicians in HMOs with Projections Made by the Graduate Education National Advisory Committee." *New England Journal of Medicine* 314, 4: 217–22.

"A Survey of Public Opinion Trends Affecting Government and the Economy." 1982. *Opinion Outlook* 2, #3.

Thurow, Lester. 1984. "Learning to Say No." *New England Journal of Medicine* 311, 24: 1569–72.

U.S. Department of Health and Human Services. 1985. *Health. United States. 1985.* USDHHS (Public Health Service) 86–1232. Washington, D.C.: Government Printing Office.

U.S. Department of Health and Human Services, Bureau of Health Professions. 1990. *Report to the President and to Congress on the Status of Health Personnel in the United States.* Washington, D.C.: General Accounting Office.

U.S. Department of Health and Human Services, Health Resources Administration, Office of Graduate Medical Education. 1980. *Report of the Graduate Medical Education National Advisory Committee to the Secretary, Department of Health and Human Services,* vols. 1–8. Washington, D.C.: Government Printing Office.

U.S. General Accounting Office. 1985. *Constraining National Health Care Expenditures: Achieving Quality Care at an Affordable Cost.* Pub. GAO/HRD-85-105. Washington, D.C.: Government Printing Office.

Waldo, Daniel, Katharine Levit, and Helen Lazenby. 1986. "National Health Expenditures, 1985." *Health Care Financing Review* 8, 1: 1–21.

Walsh, Diana, and Richard Egdahl. 1977. *Payer, Provider, Consumer: Industry Confronts Health Care Costs.* New York: Springer-Verlag.

Chapter 3

Aaron, Henry, and William Schwartz. 1984. *The Painful Prescription.* Washington, D.C.: Brookings Institution.

Bailey, Richard. 1977. "An Economist's View of the Health Services Industry." In: Weeks, Lewis, and Howard Berman, eds. *Economics in Health Care.* Germantown, Md.: Aspen Publication, pp. 22–37.

Commission on Hospital Care. 1947. *Hospital Care in the U.S.* New York: Commonwealth Fund.

Cowan, Belita. 1987. *Health Care Shoppers Guide: 59 Ways to Save Money.* Baltimore: Consumer Protection Division of the Maryland Attorney General's Office.

Eisenberg, John. 1986. *Doctors' Decisions and the Cost of Medical Care.* Ann Arbor, Mich.: Health Administration Press.

Enthoven, Alain. 1978a. "Consumer-Choice Health Plan: Inflation and Inequity in Health Care Today: Alternatives for Cost Control and an Analysis of Proposals for National Health Insurance." *New England Journal of Medicine* 298, 12: 650–8.

Enthoven, Alain. 1978b. "Consumer-Choice Health Plan: A National-Health-Insurance Proposal Based on Regulated Competition in the Private Sector." *New England Journal of Medicine* 298, 13: 709–20.

Feldstein, Paul. 1983. *Health Care Economics,* 2nd ed. New York: John Wiley and Sons.

Gabel, Jon, and Michael Redisch. 1979. "Alternative Physician Payment Methods: Incentives, Efficiency, and National Health Insurance." *Milbank Quarterly* 57, 1: 38–59.

Ginzberg, Eli. 1983a. "The Grand Illusion of Competition in Health Care." *Journal of the American Medical Association* 249, 14: 1857–9.

Ginzberg, Eli. 1983b. "Cost Containment—Imaginary and Real." *New England Journal of Medicine* 308, 20: 1220–4.

Himmelstein, David. 1990. "Will Competition Have a Long-Term Impact on System Reform?" In: Elliot Stone, ed. *The Future of Health Care: Public Concerns and Policy Trends.* Waltham, Mass.: Massachusetts Health Data Consortium, pp. 71–5.

Hsaio, William, and William Stason. 1979. "Toward Developing a Relative Value Scale for Medical and Surgical Services." *Health Care Financing Review* 1, 2: 23–37.

Joseph, Hyman. 1977. "Empirical Research on the Demand for Health Care." In: Weeks, Lewis, and Howard Berman, eds. *Economics in Health Care.* Germantown, Md.: Aspen Publication, pp. 65–75.

"Medicare: Paying the Physician—History, Issues, and Options." 1984. An information paper prepared for use by The Special Committee on Aging of the United States Senate. Washington, D.C.: Government Printing Office.

National Center for Health Statistics. 1985. *Health. United States. 1985.* Department of Health and Human Services Pub. (PHS) 86–1323. Washington, D.C.: Government Printing Office.

Pear, Robert. 1987. "38.5% Rise Asked in 1988 Premiums of Medicare Users." *New York Times,* 15 September: 1.

Reinhardt, Uwe. 1980. *On the Future of the American Economy and Its Impact on the Health Care Sector.* Chicago: University of Chicago Press.

Relman, Arnold. 1983. "The Future of Medical Practice." *Health Affairs* 2, 2: 5–19.

Relman, Arnold. 1985. "Antitrust Law and the Physician Entrepreneur." *New England Journal of Medicine* 313, 14: 884–885.

Relman, Arnold. 1988. "Assessment and Accountability: The Third Revolution in Medical Care." *New England Journal of Medicine* 319, 18: 1220–2.

Rice, Thomas. 1991. *Containing Health Care Costs in the United States.* Washington, D.C.: Public Policy Institute (AARP).

Rosenblum, Robert. 1985. "Medicare Revisited: A Look Through the Past to the Future." *Journal of Health Politics, Policy and Law* 9, 4: 669–81.

Sharfstein, Steven, Anne Stoline, and Howard Goldman. 1993. "Psychiatric Issues and Health Insurance Reform." *American Journal of Psychiatry* 150, 1:7–18.

Somers, Anne. 1987. "Insurance for Long-Term Care: Some Definitions, Problems, and Guidelines for Action." *New England Journal of Medicine* 317, 1: 23–9.

Sorkin, Alan. 1975. *Health Economics: An Introduction.* Lexington, Mass.: D.C. Heath and Co.

U.S. General Accounting Office. 1985. *Constraining National Health Care Expenditures: Achieving Quality Care at an Affordable Cost.* Pub. GAO/HRD-85-105. Washington, D.C.: General Accounting Office.

Wilensky, Gail, and Louis Rossiter. 1983. "The Relative Importance of Physician-Induced Demand in the Demand for Medical Care." *Milbank Quarterly* 61, 2: 252–77.

Introduction to Part II

Hammarskjöld, Dag. 1980. *Markings.* New York: Alfred A. Knopf.

Chapter 4

Aiken, Linda, and Karl Bays. 1984. "The Medicare Debate—Round One." *New England Journal of Medicine* 311, 18: 1196–2000.

Altman, Stuart. 1991. "Why Healthcare Executives Should Support a National Cost-Containment Plan." *Healthcare Executive* 6, 4: 21–4.

AMA. 1986. *Socioeconomic Characteristics of Medical Practice, 1986.* Chicago: AMA.

AMA. 1991. *Socioeconomic Characteristics of Medical Practice, 1990/ 1991.* Chicago: AMA.

Anderson, Gerard, and James Studnicki. 1985. "Insurers Competing with Providers." *Hospitals* 59, 23: 64–6.

Arnett, Ross, and Gordon Tranell. 1984. "Private Health Insurance: New Measures of a Complex and Changing Industry." *Health Care Financing Review* 6, 1: 31–42.

Blumenthal, David, Mark Schleshinger, Pamela Drumheller, and the Harvard Medicare Project. 1986. "The Future of Medicare." *New England Journal of Medicine* 314, 11: 722–8.

Brook, Robert, John Ware, William Rogers, et al. 1983. "Does Free Care Improve Adults' Health?: Results From a Randomized Controlled Trial." *New England Journal of Medicine* 209, 23: 1426–34.

Brown, E. Richard. 1988. "Principles for a National Health Program: A Framework for Analysis and Development." *Milbank Quarterly* 66, 4: 573–617.

David, Karen, and Diane Rowland. 1986. *Medicare Policy: New Directions for Health and Long-Term Care.* Baltimore: Johns Hopkins University Press.

Demkovich, Linda, ed. 1991. *State Health Notes,* #115. Washington, D.C.: George Washington University.

Dowd, Bryan, John Christianson, Roger Feldman, and Cathy Wisner. 1990. "Issues Regarding Health Plan Payments under Medicare and Recommendations for Reform." Unpublished report to HCFA, University of Minnesota.

Ellis, Randall, and Thomas McGuire. 1986. "Cost-Sharing and Patterns of Mental Health Care Utilization." *Journal of Human Resources* 21, 3: 359–79.

Ellwood, Deborah. 1986. "Medicare Risk Contracting: Promises and Problems." *Health Affairs* 5, 1: 183–9.

Enthoven, Alain. 1984. "A New Proposal to Reform the Tax Treatment of Health Insurance." *Health Affairs* 3, 1: 21–39.

Enthoven, Alain. 1989. "A 'Cost-Unconscious' Medical System." *New York Times,* 13 July: A23.

Finder, Alan. 1991. "Health Care Costs are New Crux of Contract Talks." *New York Times,* 27 October: 1.

Findlay, Steven. 1991. "Plugging the Medigap: New Health Plans Should Cut Costs." *U.S. News and World Report,* 1 July: 60–3.

Friedland, Robert. 1991. "Medicare: Meeting the Health Care Needs of the Elderly." *Issue Brief* (AARP), #7.

Gabel, Jon, Steven DiCarlo, Cynthia Sullivan, and Thomas Rice. 1990. "Employer-Sponsored Health Insurance, 1989." *Health Affairs* 9, 3: 161–75.

Gabel, Jon, and Dan Ermann. 1985. "Preferred Provider Organizations: Performance, Problems, and Promise." *Health Affairs* 4, 1: 24–40.

Ginsburg, Jack, and Deborah Prout. 1990. "Access to Health Care." *Annals of Internal Medicine* 112, 9: 641–61.

Ginsburg, Paul, and Glenn Hackbarth. 1986. "Alternative Delivery Systems and Medicare." *Health Affairs* 5, 1: 6–22.

Ginzberg, Eli. 1985. "The Restructuring of U.S. Health Care." *Inquiry* 22, 3: 272–81.

Harris, Seymour. 1975. *The Economics of Health Care: Financing and Delivery.* Berkeley, Calif.: McCutcheon Publishing Corp.

HCFA. 1986. *Medicare and Medicaid Data Book 1984.* Pub. 03210. Baltimore: HCFA.

HCFA. 1987. "National Health Expenditures." *Health Care Financing Review* 8, 4: 1–22.

HCFA. 1991. *Health Care Financing. Program Statistics. Medicare and Medicaid Data Book, 1990.* Pub. 03314. Baltimore: HCFA.

HIAA. 1985. *Survey of Group Health Insurance Programs.* Washington, D.C.: HIAA.

HIAA. 1992. *Source Book of Health Insurance Data.* Washington, D.C.: HIAA.

Holahan, John, and Sheila Zedlewski. 1991. "Expanding Medicaid to Cover Uninsured Americans." *Health Affairs* 10, 1: 45–61.

Iglehart, John. 1985. "The Veterans Administration Medical Care System and the Private Sector." *New England Journal of Medicine* 313, 24: 1552–6.

Interstudy. 1990. *The InterStudy Edge. Managed Care: A Decade in Review, 1980–1990.* Excelsior, Minn.: Interstudy.

Jacobs, Phil. 1980. *The Economics of Health and Medical Care.* Baltimore: University Park Press.

Juba, David. 1985. "Medicare Part B: A Time for Reform." *Business and Health,* November: 5–8.

Kimball, Merit. 1991. "Governors Say Medicare Shifts Strain Medicaid." *Health Week* 5, 3: 1, 34.

Kleinfield, N.R. 1986. "When the Boss Becomes Your Doctor." *New York Times,* 5 January: F1, F3.

LeBlanc, Alex. 1991. "The Future of Retiree Health Plans." *Medical Interface* 4, 4: 31–44.

Lewin, T. 1991. "High Medical Costs Affect Broad Areas of Daily Life." *New York Times,* 28 April: A1, A28–9.

Lohr, Kathleen, Robert Brook, Caren Kamburg, et al. 1986. *Use of Medical Care in the Rand Health Insurance Experiment: Diagnosis-and-Service-Specific Analyses in a Randomized Controlled Trial.* Pub. R-3469-HHS. Santa Monica, Calif.: RAND Corporation.

Luft, Harold. 1978. "How Do Health-Maintenance Organizations Achieve Their 'Savings'?: Rhetoric and Evidence." *New England Journal of Medicine* 298, 24: 1336–43.

Marquis, Susan, and Kathleen Lohr. 1984. "Medicare and Medicaid: Past, Present, and Future." RAND Corporation report for DHHS. Santa Monica, Calif.

McIlrath, Sharon. 1991. "No More Medicare Cuts, Witnesses Say." *American Medical News* 8 April: 1, 26.

Mechanic, David. 1991. "Changing Our Health Care System." *Medical Care Review* 48, 3: 247–60.

Moore, Stephen, Diane Martin, and William Richardson. 1983. "Does the Primary-Care Gatekeeper Control the Costs of Health Care?: Lessons from the SAFECO Experience." *New England Journal of Medicine* 309, 22: 1400–4.

Morris, William, ed. 1978. *American Heritage Dictionary of the English Language.* Boston: Houghton Mifflin Co.

Mulvey, Janemarie. 1991. "Physician Payment Reform under Medicare." *Issue Brief* (AARP), #8.

National Center for Health Statistics. 1992. *Health, United States, 1991.* Hyattsville, Md.: Public Health Service.

Newhouse, Joseph. 1978. "Insurance Benefits, Out-Of-Pocket Payments, and the Demand for Medical Care." *Health and Medical Care Services Review* 1, 4: 1–15.

Newhouse, Joseph, Willard Manning, Carl Morris, et al. 1981. "Some Interim Results from a Controlled Trial of Cost Sharing in Health Insurance." *New England Journal of Medicine* 305, 25: 1501–7.

PPRC. 1991. *Annual Report to Congress 1991.* Washington, D.C.: Government Printing Office.

Reiser, Stanley, and Michael Anbar, eds. 1984. *Machine at the Bedside.* New York: Cambridge University Press.

Rice, Thomas. 1991. "Containing Health Care Costs in the United States." Washington, D.C.: Public Policy Institute (AARP).

Saward, Ernest, and E. K. Gallagher. 1983. "Reflections on Change in Medical Practice: The Current Trend to Large-Scale Medical Organizations." *Journal of the American Medical Association* 250, 20: 2820–5.

Siu, Albert, Frank Sonnenberg, Willard Manning, et al. 1986. "Inappropriate Use of Hospitals in a Randomized Trial of Health Insurance Plans." *New England Journal of Medicine* 315, 20: 1259–66.

Sorkin, Alan. 1975. *Health Economics: An Introduction.* Lexington, Mass.: D.C. Heath and Co.

Sorkin, Alan. 1986. *Health Care and the Changing Economic Environment.* Lexington, Mass.: D.C. Heath and Co.

Tenery, Robert. 1991. "How Far Must Medicine Compromise?" *American Medical News,* 14 January: 21.

U.S. Congress, Office of Technology Assessment. 1986. *Payment for Physician Services: Strategies for Medicare.* OTA-H-294. Washington, D.C.: Government Printing Office.

U.S. Department of Health and Human Services. 1987. *Health. U.S. 1986.* USDHHS (PHS) 87-1232. Washington, D.C.: Government Printing Office.

U.S. Department of Health and Human Services, National Center for Health Services Research. 1982. "Prescribed Medicines, Users, and Expenditures." USDHHS (PHS) 82-3320. Washington, D.C.: Government Printing Office.

U.S. Department of Health and Human Services, National Center for Health Services Research. 1987. "A Summary of Expenditures and Sources of Payment for Personal Health Services." USDHHS (PHS) 87-3411. Washington, D.C.: Government Printing Office.

Chapter 5

Aaron, Henry, and William Schwartz. 1984. *The Painful Prescription: Rationing Hospital Care.* Washington, D.C.: Brookings Institution.

AMA. 1986. *Socioeconomic Characteristics of Medical Practice.* Chicago: AMA.

Bock, Randall. 1988. "The Pressure to Keep Prices High at a Walk-In Clinic." *New England Journal of Medicine* 319, 12: 785–7.

Burney, Ira, George Schieber, Martha Blaxall, and Jon Gabel. 1979. "Medicare and Medicaid Physician Payment Incentives." *Health Care Financing Review* 1, 1: 62–78.

Epstein, Arnold, Colin Begg, and Barbara McNeil. 1986. "The Use of Ambulatory Testing in Prepaid and Fee-for-Service Group Practices: Relation to Perceived Profitability." *New England Journal of Medicine* 314, 17: 1089–94.

Feldstein, Paul. 1983. *Health Care Economics,* 2nd ed. New York: John Wiley and Sons.

Gabel, Jon, and Michael Redisch. 1979. "Alternative Physician Payment Methods: Incentives, Efficiency, and National Health Insurance." *Milbank Quarterly* 57, 1: 38–59.

Ginsburg, Paul, and Frank Sloan. 1984. "Hospital Cost Shifting." *New England Journal of Medicine* 310, 14: 893–8.

Ginsburg, Paul, and Glenn Hackbarth. 1986. "Alternative Delivery Systems and Medicare." *Health Affairs* 5, 1: 6–22.

Gonzalez, Martin, ed. 1991. *Socioeconomic Characteristics of Medical Practice 1990/1991.* Chicago: AMA Center for Health Policy Research.

Harris, Seymour. 1975. *The Economics of Health Care.* Berkeley, Calif.: McCutcheon Publishing Corp.

HCFA. 1991. *Medicare and Medicaid Data Book, 1990.* Pub. 03314. Baltimore: HCFA.

Health Policy Alternatives, Inc. 1986. "Physician Payment Reform Under Medicare: Implications for Emergency Medicine." Report prepared for the American College of Emergency Physicians.

HIAA. 1991. *Source Book of Health Insurance Data.* Washington, D.C.: HIAA.

Hillman, Alan. 1987. "Financial Incentives For Physicians in HMOs: Is There a Conflict of Interest?" *New England Journal of Medicine* 317, 27: 1743–8.

Hillman, Alan, Mark Pauly, and Joseph Kirstein. 1989. "How Do Financial Incentives Affect Physicians' Clinical Decisions and the Financial Performance of Health Maintenance Organizations?" *New England Journal of Medicine* 321, 2: 36–92.

Holoweiko, Mark. 1986. "Non-Surgeons' Earnings: Which Specialties Are Hung Up?" *Medical Economics,* 3 February: 206–25.

Hsaio, William, and William Stason. 1979. "Toward Developing a Relative Value Scale for Medical and Surgical Services." *Health Care Financing Review* 1, 2: 23–38.

Hsaio, William, Peter Braun, Edmund Becker, and Stephen Thomas. 1987. "The Resource-Based Relative Value Scale." *Journal of the American Medical Association* 258, 6: 799–802.

Jencks, Stephen, and Allen Dobson. 1985. "Strategies for Reforming Medicare's Physician Payments." *New England Journal of Medicine* 312, 23: 1492–9.

Juba, David. 1985. "Medicare Part B: A Time for Reform." *Business and Health,* November: 5–8.

Juba, David, and Jack Hadley. 1985. "Relative Value Scales for Physicians' Services." *Health Care Financing Review* 6, 4: 93–101.

Luft, Harold. 1981. *Health Maintenance Organizations: Dimensions of Performance.* New York: John Wiley and Sons.

Manning, Willard, Arleen Leibowitz, George Goldberg, et al. 1984. "Controlled Trial of the Effect of a Prepaid Group Practice on Use of Services." *New England Journal of Medicine* 310, 23: 1505–10.

O'Sullivan, Jennifer, and James Reuter. 1986. "Physician Reimbursement Under Medicare." Report prepared for the Committee on Finance. Washington, D.C.: Government Printing Office.

PPRC. 1991. *Annual Report to Congress 1991.* Washington, D.C.: Government Printing Office.

Reinhardt, Uwe. 1985. "Future Trends in the Economics of Medical Practice and Care." *American Journal of Cardiology* 56, 5: 50C-9C.

Relman, Arnold. 1985. "Cost Control, Doctors' Ethics, and Patient Care." *Issues in Science and Technology,* Winter: 108–11.

Relman, Arnold. 1988. "Salaried Physicians and Economic Incentives." *New England Journal of Medicine* 319, 12: 784.

Roe, Benson. 1981. "The UCR Boondoggle: A Death Knell for Private Practice?" *New England Journal of Medicine* 305, 1: 41–5.

Scovern, Henry. 1988. "Hired Help: A Physician's Experience in a For-Profit Staff-Model HMO." *New England Journal of Medicine* 319, 12: 787–90.

"Third-Party Funds Significant Part of Physicians' Revenues." 1985. *American Medical News,* 4 October: 34.

Udvarhelyi, I. Steven, Kathleen Jennison, Russell Phillips, and Arnold Epstein. 1991. "Comparison of the Quality of Ambulatory Care for Fee-for-Service and Prepaid Patients." *Annals of Internal Medicine* 115, 5: 394–400.

U.S. Congress, Office of Technology Assessment. 1986. *Payment for Physician Services: Strategies for Medicare.* OTA-H-294. Washington, D.C.: Government Printing Office.

U.S. General Accounting Office. 1985. *Constraining National Health Care Expenditures: Achieving Quality Care at an Affordable Cost.* Pub. GAO/HRD-85-105. Washington, D.C.: General Accounting Office.

Chapter 6

Anderson, Gerard, and Earl Steinberg. 1984. "Hospital Readmissions in the Medicare Population." *New England Journal of Medicine* 311, 21: 1249–53.

Comptroller General of the U.S. Charles Bowsher addressing the House Committee on Ways and Means, 17 April 1991. *U.S. Health Care Spending.* GAO/HRD-91-104. Washington, D.C.: General Accounting Office.

Culler, Steven, and David Ehrenfried. 1986. "On the Feasibility and Usefulness of Physician DRGs." *Inquiry* 23, 1: 40–55.

Dans, Peter, Jonathan Weiner, and Sharon Otter. 1985. "Peer Review Organizations: Promises and Potential Pitfalls." *New England Journal of Medicine* 311, 18: 1131–7.

Davis, Karen, Gerard Anderson, Steven Renn, et al. 1985. "Is Cost Containment Working?" *Health Affairs* 4, 3: 81–94.

de Lissovoy, Greg, Thomas Rice, Dan Ermann, and Jon Gabel. 1986. "Preferred Provider Organizations: Today's Models and Tomorrow's Prospects." *Inquiry* 23, 1: 7–15.

Dolenc, Danielle, and Charles Dougherty. 1985. "DRGs: The Counter-revolution in Financing Health Care." *Hastings Center Report* 15, 3: 19–29.

Ellwood, Deborah. 1986. "Medicare Risk Contracting: Promises and Problems." *Health Affairs* 5, 1: 183–9.

Fielding, Jonathan. 1983. "Lessons From Health Care Regulation." *Annual Review of Public Health* 4: 91–130.

Frank, Richard, and Judith Lave. 1986. "Per Case Prospective Payment for Psychiatric Inpatients: An Assessment and Alternatives." *Journal of Health Politics, Policy and Law* 11, 1: 83–96.

Friedland, Robert. 1991. "Medicare: Meeting the Health Care Needs of the Elderly." *Issue Brief* (AARP), #7.

Gabel, Jon. 1989. *Trends in Managed Health Care.* Washington, D.C.: HIAA.

Gabel, Jon, and Thomas Rice. 1985. "Reducing Public Expenditures for Physician Services: The Price of Paying Less." *Journal of Health Politics, Policy and Law* 9, 4: 595–609.

Gapen, Phyllis. 1985. "Empty Beds are Major Problem in Maryland." *American Medical News,* 27 December.

Ginsburg, Paul, and Glenn Hackbarth. 1986. "Alternative Delivery Systems and Medicare." *Health Affairs* 5, 1: 6–22.

Goldfield, Norbert, and Seth Goldsmith. 1987. *Alternative Delivery Systems.* Rockville, Md.: Aspen Publication.

Guterman, Stuart, and Allen Dobson. 1986. "Impact of the Medicare Prospective Payment System for Hospitals." *Health Care Financing Review* 7, 3: 97–114.

Hardin, Garrett. 1968. "The Tragedy of the Commons." *Science* 13, 3859: 1243–8.

HCFA. 1983. *The New ICD-9-CM Diagnosis Related Groups Classification Scheme.* Pub. 03167. Baltimore: HCFA.

HCFA. 1991. *Federal Register* 56. November, 25, #227. Washington, D.C.: HCFA.

HCFA. 1992. *Medicare and Medical Data Book 1991.* Baltimore: HCFA.

Iglehart, John. 1982. "The New Era of Prospective Payment for Hospitals." *New England Journal of Medicine* 307, 20: 1288–92.

Iglehart, John. 1986. "Early Experience with Prospective Payment of Hospitals." *New England Journal of Medicine* 314, 22: 1460–4.

Iglehart, John. 1989. "The Recommendations of the Physician Payment Review Commission." *New England Journal of Medicine* 320, 17: 1156–60.

Iglehart, John. 1990. "The New Law on Medicare's Payment to Physicians." *New England Journal of Medicine* 322, 17: 1247–52.

Iglehart, John. 1991. "The Struggle over Physician-Payment Reform." *New England Journal of Medicine* 325, 11: 823–8.

Jencks, Stephen, and Allen Dobson. 1985. "Strategies for Reforming Medicare's Physician Payments." *New England Journal of Medicine* 312, 23: 1492–9.

"Keep an Open Eye on PRO Criteria." 1991. *American Medical News,* 15 April: 15.

Lee, Philip, and Paul Ginsburg. 1991. "The Trials of Medicare Physician Payment Reform." *Journal of the American Medical Association* 266, 11: 1562–5.

Luft, Harold. 1985. "Competition and Regulation." *Medical Care* 23, 5: 383–99.

Maryland Hospital Association. 1986. *Research and Data Analysis,* #11.

McCormick, Brian. 1991. "Medicare Rules Would Fold Capital Costs Into PPS." *American Medical News,* 8 April: 5.

McIlrath, Sharon. 1991. "Bad News on RBRVS Rules: Regulations Cut Pay More Than Expected." *American Medical News,* 17 June: 1, 32–3.

McIlrath, Sharon. 1991. "Cataract Surgery is New Medicare Pilot." *American Medical News* 1 April: 4.

McIlrath, Sharon. 1991. "Here's How to Get More Information About RBRVS Rules." *American Medical News,* 2 December: 7–8.

McIlrath, Sharon. 1991. "PPRC Ponders All-Payer System, Refines Pay Rules." *American Medical News,* 15 April: 1, 26–7.

Medicare: Paying the Physician—History, Issues, and Options. 1984. Paper prepared for use by The Special Committee on Aging, United States Senate. Washington, D.C.

Meiners, Mark, and Rosemary Coffey. 1985. "Hospital DRGs and the Need for Long-Term Care Services: An Empirical Analysis." *Health Services Research* 20, 3: 359–84.

Mitchell, Janet. 1985a. "Physician DRGs." *New England Journal of Medicine* 313, 11: 670–5.

Mitchell, Janet. 1985b. "Physician DRGs: How Would They Work?" *Business and Health,* November: 10–12.

Mulvey, Janemarie. 1991. "Physician Payment Reform under Medicare." *Issue Brief* (AARP), #8.

PPRC. 1991. *Annual Report to Congress 1991.* Washington, D.C.: Government Printing Office.

Relman, Arnold. 1985. "Cost Control, Doctors' Ethics, and Patient Care." *Issues in Science and Technology,* Winter: 103–11.

Rice, Thomas. 1991. *Containing Health Care Costs in the United States.* Washington, D.C.: Public Policy Institute (AARP).

Rice, Thomas and Jill Bernstein. 1990. "Volume Performance Standards: Can They Control Growth in Medicare Services?" *Milbank Quarterly* 68, 3: 295–319.

Roemer, Milton. 1981. *An Introduction to the U.S. Health Care System.* New York: Springer Publishing.

Roemer, Milton. 1985. "I.S. Falk, the Committee on the Costs of Medical Care, and the Drive for National Health Insurance." *American Journal of Public Health* 75, 8: 841–8.

Schumacher, Dale, M. Jo Namerow, Barbara Parker, et al. 1986. "Prospective Payment for Psychiatry—Feasibility and Impact." *New England Journal of Medicine* 315, 21: 1331–6.

Segal, Mark. 1985. "Diagnosis-Related Groups for Physician Reimbursement?" *Journal of the American Medical Association* 254, 18: 2639–40.

Simpson, James. 1985. "State Certificate-of-Need Programs: The Current Status." *American Journal of Public Health* 75, 10: 1225–9.

Sorkin, Alan. 1986. *Health Care and the Changing Economic Environment.* Lexington, Mass.: D.C. Heath and Co.

Steinwald, Bruce. 1986. "The Impact of New Reimbursement Schemes on Clinical Research in Hospitals: The Case of the Prospective Payment System." *Journal of General Internal Medicine* 1, Supplement: S56-9.

Steinwald, Bruce, and Frank Sloan. 1981. "Regulatory Approaches to Hospital Cost Containment: A Synthesis of the Empirical Evidence." In: Olson, M., ed. *A New Approach to the Economics of Health Care.* Washington, D.C.: American Enterprise Institute for Policy Research.

U.S. Congress, Congressional Budget Office. 1991. *Rising Health Care Costs: Causes, Implications, and Strategies.* Washington, D.C.: Government Printing Office.

U.S. General Accounting Office. 1985. *Constraining National Health Care Expenditures: Achieving Quality Care at an Affordable Cost.* Pub. GAO/HRD-85-105. Washington, D.C.: Government Printing Office.

Walsh, Diana, and Richard Eghald. 1977. *Payer, Provider, Consumer: Industry Confronts Health Care Costs.* New York: Springer-Verlag.

Young, David. 1985. "Physician Accountability for Health Care Costs." *Business and Health,* November: 16–8.

Chapter 7

AHA. 1990. *AHA Guide to the Health Care Field,* 1990 ed. Chicago: AHA.

Anderson, Gerard. 1985. "National Medical Care Spending." *Health Affairs* 4, 3: 100–7.

Anderson, Gerard, and James Studnicki. 1985. "Insurers Competing with Providers." *Hospitals* 59, 23: 64–6.

Arbitman, Deborah. 1986. "A Primer on Patient Classification Systems and Their Relevance to Ambulatory Care." *Journal of Ambulatory Care Management* 9, 1: 58–81.

Blendon, Robert, and Jennifer Edwards. 1991. *System in Crisis: The Case For Health Care Reform.* Washington, D.C.: Faulkner and Gray.

Cassidy, Robert. 1983. "Will the PPO Movement Freeze You Out?" *Medical Economics,* 18 April: 262–74.

Davis, Karen, Gerard Anderson, Steven Renn, et al. 1985. "Is Cost Containment Working?" *Health Affairs* 4, 3: 81–94.

Eisenberg, John, and Deborah Kitz. 1986. "Savings from Outpatient Antibiotic Therapy for Osteomyelitis: Economic Analysis of a Therapeutic Strategy." *Journal of the American Medical Association* 255, 12: 1584–8.

Fitzgerald, John, Leonard Fagan, William Tierney, and Robert Dittus. 1987. "Changing Patterns of Hip Fracture Care Before and After Implementation of the Prospective Payment System." *Journal of the American Medical Association* 258, 2: 218–21.

Folse, Lynn. 1985. "Alternative Sites Offer New Options for Consumers." *Advertising Age,* 24 October.

Freedman, Steven. 1985. "Megacorporate Health Care: A Choice for the Future." *New England Journal of Medicine* 312, 9: 579–82.

Fuchs, Victor. 1986. "Has Cost Containment Gone Too Far?" *Milbank Quarterly* 64, 3: 479–88.

Fuchs, Victor. 1987. "A Hard Look at Cost Containment." *New England Journal of Medicine* 316, 18: 1151–6.

Gabel, Jon, Cindy Jajich-Toth, Karen Williams, et al. 1987. "The Commercial Health Insurance Industry in Transition." *Health Affairs* 6, 3: 46–60.

Gabel, Jon, and Dan Ermann. 1985. "Preferred Provider Organizations: Performance, Problems, and Promise." *Health Affairs* 4, 1: 24–40.

Gabel, Jon, Dan Ermann, Thomas Rice, and Greg de Lissovoy. 1986. "The Emergence and Future of PPOs." *Journal of Health Politics, Policy and Law* 11, 2: 305–22.

Ginzberg, Eli. 1985. "The Restructuring of U.S. Health Care." *Inquiry* 22, 3: 272–81.

Ginzberg, Eli. 1986. "The Destabilization of Health Care." *New England Journal of Medicine* 315, 12: 757–61.

Ginzberg, Eli. 1988. "For-Profit Medicine: A Reassessment." *New England Journal of Medicine* 319, 12: 757–61.

Gray, Bradford, and Walter McNerney. 1986. "For-Profit Enterprise in Health Care: The Institute of Medicine Study." *New England Journal of Medicine* 314, 23: 1523–8.

HCFA. 1991. *Health Care Financing. Program Statistics. Medicare and Medicaid Data Book, 1990.* Pub. 03314. Baltimore: HCFA.

HIAA. 1991. *Source Book of Health Insurance Data.* Washington, D.C.: HIAA.

Iglehart, John. 1986. "Early Experience with Prospective Payment of Hospitals." *New England Journal of Medicine* 314, 22: 1460–4.

Kahn, Katherine, Emmett Keeler, Marjorie Sherwood, et al. 1990. "Comparing Outcomes of Care Before and After Implementation of the DRG-Based Prospective Payment System." *Journal of the American Medical Association* 264, 15: 1984–8.

Kane, Nancy, and Paul Manoukian. 1989. "The Effect of the Medicare Prospective Payment System on the Adoption of New Technology: The Case of Cochlear Implants." *New England Journal of Medicine* 321, 20: 1378–83.

Koren, Mary Jane. 1986. "Home Care—Who Cares?" *New England Journal of Medicine* 314, 14: 917–20.

Lawrence, Jean. 1984. "Demand the Right Not to Wait for a Doctor." *Washington Post,* 22 July.

Lefton, Doug. 1985. "Hospitals Score Record Profits Under DRGs." *American Medical News,* 9 August.

Luft, Harold. 1981. *Health Maintenance Organizations: Dimensions of Performance.* New York: Wiley.

Milligan, John. 1985. "Showdown at Medicine Bend." *Institutional Investor,* October: 225–7.

Moxley, John, and Penelope Roeder. 1984. "New Opportunities for Out-of-Hospital Health Services." *New England Journal of Medicine* 310, 3: 193–7.

National Center for Health Statistics. 1991. *Health, United States, 1990.* Hyattsville, Md.: Public Health Service.

"New Sites for Care and Cure." 1985. *New York Times,* Supplement: "Health and Medicine Employment Outlook," 3 November: 15.

Newhouse, Joseph. 1989. "Do Unprofitable Patients Face Access Problems?" *Health Care Financing Review* 11, 2: 33–42.

Relman, Arnold. 1980. "The New Medical-Industrial Complex." *New England Journal of Medicine* 303, 17: 963–70.

Rice, Thomas. 1991. *Containing Health Care Costs in the United States.* Washington, D.C.: Public Policy Institute (AARP).

Richards, Glenn. 1984. "FECs Pose Competition for Hospital EDs: Freestanding Emergency Centers Doubling in Number Yearly." *Hospitals* 58, 6: 77–82.

Roos, Noralou, and Jean Freeman. 1989. "Potential for Inpatient-Outpatient Substitution with Diagnosis-Related Groups." *Health Care Financing Review* 10, 4: 31–8.

Saward, Ernest, and E.K. Gallagher. 1983. "Reflections on Change in Medical Practice: The Current Trend to Large-Scale Medical Organizations." *Journal of the American Medical Association* 250, 20: 2820–5.

Scheier, Ronni. 1986. "HMO Enrollment Drops for First Time." *American Medical News,* 10 January.

Schwartz, William, and Daniel Mendelson. 1991. "Hospital Cost Containment in the 1980s: Hard Lessons Learned and Prospects for the 1990s." *New England Journal of Medicine* 324, 15: 1037–42.

Shaughnessy, Peter, and Andrew Kramer. 1990. "The Increased Needs of Patients in Nursing Homes and Patients Receiving Home Health Care." *New England Journal of Medicine* 322, 1: 21–7.

Shengold, Steven. 1989. "The First Three Years of PPS: Impact on Medicare Costs." *Health Affairs* 8, 3: 191–204.

Smego, Raymond. 1985. "Home Intravenous Antibiotic Therapy." *Archives of Internal Medicine* 145, 6: 1001–2.

Steinwachs, Donald, Jonathan Weiner, Paul Batalden, Kathy Coltin, and Fred Wasserman. 1986. "A Comparison of the Requirements for Primary Care Physicians in HMOs with Projections Made by the GMENAC." *New England Journal of Medicine* 314, 4: 217–22.

Sullivan, Cynthia, and Thomas Rice. 1991. "The Health Insurance Picture in 1990." *Health Affairs* 11, 2: 104–15.

U.S. General Accounting Office. 1985. *Constraining National Health Care Expenditures: Achieving Quality Care at an Affordable Cost.* Pub. GAO/HRD-85-105. Washington, D.C.: Government Accounting Office.

Weiner, Jonathan. 1986. "Assuring Quality of Care in HMOs: Past Lessons, Present Challenges and Future Directions." *Journal of the Group Health Association of America* 7: 10–27.

Wilensky, Gail. 1990. "Medicare at 25: Better Value and Better Care." *Journal of the American Medical Association* 264, 15: 1996–7.

Introduction to Part III

Harris, Louis, and Associates, Inc. 1990. *Trade-offs and Choices: Health Policy Options for the 1990s.* Chicago: Louis Harris and Associates, Inc.

Lister, Eric. 1991. "Can We Find a Reasoned Response to Managed Care?" *Psychiatric Times,* 10 November: 9–10.

Prather, Hugh. 1970. *Notes to Myself.* Moab, Utah: Real People Press.

Chapter 8

Altschule, Mark. 1988. "Wish-Fulfillment as a Determinant in the Interpretation of Technology." *Chest* 93, 5: 1092.

American Child Health Association. 1934. *Physical Defects: The Pathway to Correction.* pp. 80–96.

Bayes, T. 1763. "An Essay Toward Solving a Problem in the Doctrine of Chances." *Philosophical Transactions* 53: 370–418.

Berwick, Donald, and David Wald. 1990. "Hospital Leaders' Opinions of the HCFA Mortality Data." *Journal of the American Medical Association* 263, 2:247–9.

Bleich, Howard. 1991. "Classic Articles in Medical Computing." *M.D. Computing* 8, 3: 132–4.

Charache, Samuel, Lydia Nelson, Edward Keyser, and Paul Metzger. 1985. "A Clinical Trial of Three-Part Electronic Differential White Blood Cell Counts." *Archives of Internal Medicine* 145, 10: 1852–5.

Chassin, Mark. 1988. "Standards of Care in Medicine." *Inquiry* 25, 4: 437–53.

Chassin, Mark, Jacqueline Kosecoff, R.E. Park, et al. 1987. "Does Inappropriate Use Explain Geographic Variations in the Use of Health Care Services?: A Study of Three Procedures." *Journal of the American Medical Association* 258, 18: 2533–7.

Close, Pamela. 1984. "Economic Changes Affecting Medical Practice: What Do Medical Students Need to Know?" *OSR Report* 8, #1.

Conlin, Joseph. 1984. *Morrow Book of Quotations in American History.* New York: William Morrow and Co.

Daniels, Marcia, and Steven Schroeder. 1977. "Variations Among Physicians in Use of Laboratory Tests II: Relation to Clinical Productivity and Outcomes of Care." *Medical Care* 15, 6: 482–7.

Dans, Peter. 1985. "Cost-Effective Management of Pneumonia." *Hospital Therapy* November: 23–44.

Dans, Peter, Jonathan Weiner, Jacques Milan, and Lewis Becker. 1983. "Conditional Probability in the Diagnosis of Coronary Artery Disease: Implications for Eliminating Unnecessary Testing." *Southern Medical Journal* 76: 1118–21.

Dixon, Anthony. 1990. "The Evolution of Clinical Policies." *Medical Care* 28, 3: 201–20.

Donabedian, Avedis. 1980. *Explorations in Quality Assessment and Monitoring,* vol. 1: *The Definition of Quality and Approaches to Its Assessment.* Ann Arbor, Mich.: Health Administration Press.

Donabedian, Avedis. 1988a. "The Assessment of Technology and Quality: A Comparative Study of Certainties and Ambiguities." *International Journal of Technology Assessment in Health Care* 4: 487–96.

Donabedian, Avedis. 1988b. "The Quality of Care: How Can It Be Assessed?" *Journal of the American Medical Association* 260, 12: 1743–8.

Draper, David, Katherine Kahn, Ellen Reimisch, et al. 1990. "Studying the Effects of the DRG-Based Prospective Payment System on Quality of Care: Design, Sampling, and Fieldwork." *Journal of the American Medical Association* 264, 15: 1956–61.

Dubois, Robert, Robert Brook, and William Rogers. 1987. "Adjusted Hospital Death Rates: A Potential Screen for Quality of Medical Care." *American Journal of Public Health* 77, 9: 1162–7.

Egdahl, Richard, and Cynthia Taft. 1986. "Financial Incentives to Physicians." *New England Journal of Medicine* 315, 1: 59–61.

Eisenberg, John. 1986. *Doctors' Decisions and the Cost of Medical Care.* Ann Arbor, Mich.: Health Administration Press.

Eisenberg, John. 1989. "Clinical Economics: A Guide to the Economic Analysis of Clinical Practices." *Journal of the American Medical Association* 262, 20: 2879–86.

Eisenberg, John, and Deborah Kitz. 1986. "Savings From Outpatient Antibiotic Therapy for Osteomyelitis: Economic Analysis of a Therapeutic Strategy." *Journal of the American Medical Association* 255, 12: 1584–8.

Epstein, Arnold. 1990. "The Outcomes Movement—Will It Get Us Where We Want to Go?" *New England Journal of Medicine* 323, 4: 266–70.

Estaugh, Steven. 1981. "Teaching the Principles of Cost-Effective Clinical Decisionmaking to Medical Students." *Inquiry* 18, 1: 28–36.

Fineberg, Harvey. 1985. "Technology Assessment: Motivation, Capability, and Future Directions." *Medical Care* 23, 5: 663–71.

Friedman, Richard, and Jeffrey Katt. 1991. "Cost-Benefit Issues in the Practice of Internal Medicine." *Archives of Internal Medicine* 151, 6: 1165–8.

Fryback, Dennis. 1985. "Decision Maker, Quantify Thyself!" *Medical Decision Making* 5, 1: 51–60.

Fuchs, Victor. 1974. *Who Shall Live? Health, Economics, and Social Choice.* New York: Basic Books.

Geigle, Ron, and Stanley Jones. 1990. "Outcomes Measurement: A Report From the Front." *Inquiry* 27, 1: 7–13.

Geller, Gail, and Neal Holtzman. 1991. "Implications of the Human Genome Initiative for the Primary Care Physician." *Bioethics* 5, 4: 318–25.

Gilson, James, and Kathy Fliehler. 1991. "Evaluating Office-Based Care." *Medical Interface* 4, 4: 59–61.

Ginzberg, Eli. 1986. "The Destabilization of Health Care." *New England Journal of Medicine* 315, 12: 757–61.

Gore, Joel, Robert Goldberg, David Spodick, et al. 1987. "A Community-Wide Assessment of the Use of Pulmonary Artery Catheters in Patients with Acute Myocardial Infarction." *Chest* 92, 4: 721–7.

Greer, Ann. 1988. "The State of the Art versus the State of the Science: The Diffusion of New Medical Technologies into Practice." *International Journal of Technology Assessment in Health Care* 4: 5–26.

Hannan, Edward, Joseph O'Donnell, Harold Kilburn, et al. 1989. "Investigation of the Relationship Between Volume and Mortality for Surgical Procedures Performed in New York State Hospitals." *Journal of the American Medical Association* 262, 4: 503–10.

HCFA. 1986. *Medicare and Medicaid Data Book, 1984.* Pub. 03210. Baltimore: HCFA.

HCFA. 1987. *Medicare Hospital Mortality Information.* Pub. 01-002. Washington, D.C.: HCFA.

HCFA. 1988. *Medicare Hospital Mortality Information.* Pub. 06641. Washington, D.C.: HCFA.

Hubbell, F. Allan, Sheldon Greenfield, Judy Tyler, et al. 1985. "The Impact of Routine Admission Chest X-Ray Films on Patient Care." *New England Journal of Medicine* 312, 4: 209–13.

Huth, Edward. 1985. "Needed: An Economics Approach to Systems for Medical Information." *Annals of Internal Medicine* 103, 4: 617–9.

Iglehart, John. 1986. "Early Experience with Prospective Payment of Hospitals." *New England Journal of Medicine* 314, 22: 1460–4.

Kahn, Katherine, Emmett Keeler, Marjorie Sherwood, et al. 1990. "Comparing Outcomes of Care Before and After Implementation of the DRG-Based Prospective Payment System." *Journal of the American Medical Association* 264, 15: 1984–8.

Kahn, Katherine, Lisa Rubenstein, and David Draper. 1990. "The Effects of the DRG-Based Prospective Payment System on Quality of Care for Hospitalized Medicare Patients." *Journal of the American Medical Association* 264, 15: 1953–5.

Kahn, Katherine, William Rogers, Lisa Rubenstein, et al. 1990. "Measuring Quality of Care with Explicit Process Criteria Before and After Implementation of the DRG-Based Prospective Payment System." *Journal of the American Medical Association* 264, 15: 1969–73.

Kassirer, Jerome. 1989. "Our Stubborn Quest for Diagnostic Certainty: A Cause of Excessive Testing." *New England Journal of Medicine* 320, 22: 1489–91.

Keeler, Emmett, Katherine Kahn, David Draper, et al. 1990. "Changes in Sickness at Admission Following the Introduction of the Prospective Payment System." *Journal of the American Medical Association* 264, 15: 1962–8.

Klinefelter, Harry. 1982. "The Mixed-Blessing of Technology." *The Internist,* March: 9–10.

Komaroff, Anthony. 1985. "Quality Assurance in 1984." *Medical Care* 23, 5: 723–34.

Leape, Lucian, Rolla Park, David Solomon, et al. 1989. "Relation between Surgeons' Practice Volumes and Geographic Variation in the Rate of Carotid Endarterectomy." *New England Journal of Medicine* 321, 10: 653–7.

Lohr, Kathleen, and Steven Schroeder. 1990. "A Strategy for Quality Assurance in Medicare." *New England Journal of Medicine* 322, 10: 707–12.

Lomas, Jonathan, Geoffrey Anderson, Karen Domnick-Pierre, et al. 1989. "Do Practice Guidelines Guide Practice: The Effect of a Consensus Statement on the Practice of Physicians." *New England Journal of Medicine* 321, 19: 1306–11.

Ludmerer, Kenneth. 1985. *Learning to Heal: The Development of American Medical Education.* New York: Basic Books.

MacKenzie, C. Ronald, Mary Charlson, Denise DiGioia, and Kathleen Kelley. 1986. "A Patient-Specific Measure of Change in Maximal Function." *Archives of Internal Medicine* 146, 7: 1325–9.

McCarthy, Eugene, Madelon Finkel, and Hirsch Ruchlin. 1981. "Second Opinions on Elective Surgery." *Lancet,* 20 June: 1352–4.

McNeil, Barbara. 1985. "Hospital Response to DRG-Based Prospective Payment." *Medical Decision Making* 5, 1: 15–21.

McPherson, Klim, John Wennberg, Ole Hovind, and Peter Clifford. 1982. "Small-Area Variations in the Use of Common Surgical Procedures: An International Comparison of New England, England, and Norway." *New England Journal of Medicine* 307, 21: 1310–4.

Morreim, E. Haavi. 1985. "The MD and the DRG." *Hastings Center Report* 15, 3: 30–8.

Nash, David, and Norbert Goldfield. 1989. "Information Needs of Purchasers." In: Goldfield, N., and D. Nash, eds. *Providing Quality Care: The Challenge to Clinicians.* Philadelphia: American College of Physicians, pp. 5–24.

National Academy of Sciences, IOM. 1985. *Assessing Medical Technologies.* Washington, D.C.: National Academy Press.

Neuhauser, Duncan, and Ann Lewicki. 1975. "What Do We Gain from the Sixth Stool Guaiac?" *New England Journal of Medicine* 293, 5: 226–8.

Perry, Seymour. 1986. "Technology Assessment: Continuing Uncertainty." *New England Journal of Medicine* 314, 4: 240–3.

President's Commission for the Study of Ethical Problems in Medicine and Biomedical and Behavioral Research. 1982. USGPO-1982-0383-515/8673. Washington, D.C.: Government Printing Office.

Pryor, David, Robert Califf, Frank Harrell, et al. 1985. "Clinical Data Bases: Accomplishments and Unrealized Potential." *Medical Care* 23, 5: 623–47.

Reinhardt, Uwe. 1985. "Future Trends in the Economics of Medical Practice and Care." *American Journal of Cardiology* 56, 5: 50C–9C.

Relman, Arnold. 1980. "Assessment of Medical Practices: A Simple Proposal." *New England Journal of Medicine* 303, 3: 153–4.

Relman, Arnold. 1985. "Cost Control, Doctors' Ethics and Patient Care." *Issues in Science and Technology,* Winter: 103–11.

Rhyne, Robert, and Stephen Gehlbach. 1979. "Effects of an Educational Feedback Strategy on Physician Utilization of Thyroid Function Panels." *Journal of Family Practice* 8, 5: 1003–7.

Rice, Thomas. 1991. *Containing Health Care Costs in the United States.* Washington, D.C.: Public Policy Institute (AARP).

Robin, Eugene. 1985. "The Cult of the Swan-Ganz Catheter: Overuse and Abuse of Pulmonary Flow Catheters." *Annals of Internal Medicine* 103, 3: 445–9.

Robin, Eugene. 1987. "Death by Pulmonary Artery Flow-Directed Catheter (Editorial): Time for a Moratorium?" *Chest* 92, 4: 727–31.

Robin, Eugene. 1988. "Defenders of the Pulmonary Artery Catheter." *Chest* 93, 5: 1059–66.

Roper, William, William Winkenwerder, Glenn Hackbarth, and Henry Krakauer. 1988. "Effectiveness in Health Care: An Initiative to Evaluate and Improve Medical Practice." *New England Journal of Medicine* 319, 18: 1197–202.

Rubenstein, Lisa, Katherine Kahn, Ellen Reinisch, et al. 1990. "Changes in Quality of Care for Five Diseases Measured by Implicit Review, 1981–1986." *Journal of the American Medical Association* 264, 15: 1974–9.

Sager, Alan. 1988. "Price of Equitable Access: The New Massachusetts Health Insurance Law." *Hastings Center Report* 18, 3: 21–5.

Shortliffe, Edward. 1987. "Computer Programs to Support Clinical Decision Making." *Journal of the American Medical Association* 258, 1: 61–6.

Showstack, Jonathan, Mary Stone, and Steven Schroeder. 1985. "The Role of Changing Clinical Practices in the Rising Costs of Hospital Care." *New England Journal of Medicine* 313, 19: 1201–7.

Sibbald, William, and Charles Sprung. 1988. "The Pulmonary Artery Catheter: The Debate Continues." *Chest* 94, 5: 899–901.

Spodick, David. 1989. "Analysis of Flow-Directed Pulmonary Artery Catheterization." *Journal of the American Medical Association* 261, 13: 1946–7.

Steinwachs, Donald, Jonathan Weiner, and Sam Shapiro. 1989. "Management Information Systems and Quality." In: Goldfield, N., and D. Nash, eds. *Providing Quality Care: The Challenge to Clinicians.* Philadelphia: American College of Physicians, pp. 160–81.

Stern, Robert, and Arnold Epstein. 1985. "Institutional Responses to Prospective Payment Based on Diagnosis-Related Groups: Implications for Cost, Quality, and Access." *New England Journal of Medicine* 312, 10: 621–7.

Tierney, William, Michael Miller, and Clement McDonald. 1990. "The Effect on Test Ordering of Informing Physicians of the Charges for Outpatient Diagnostic Tests." *New England Journal of Medicine* 322, 21: 1499–504.

Tobin, Richard. 1980. "Should Cost Be a Factor in Personal Medical Care?" Letter to the Editor. *New England Journal of Medicine* 303, 5: 288.

U.S. Department of Health and Human Services, National Center for Devices and Radiological Health. 1983. *The Selection of Patients for X-Ray Examinations: Chest X-Ray Screening Examinations.* HHS (FDA) 83-8204. Washington, D.C.: Government Printing Office.

Walsh, Diana, and Richard Egdahl. 1977. *Payer, Provider, Consumer: Industry Confronts Health Care Costs.* New York: Springer-Verlag.

Wasson, John, Harold Sox, Raymond Neff, and Lee Goldman. 1985. "Clinical Prediction Rules: Applications and Methodological Standards." *New England Journal of Medicine* 313, 13: 793–9.

Weiner, Jonathan. 1987. "Balancing Cost and Quality in the New Medical Marketplace." Seminar, 23 November, Baltimore.

Weiner, Jonathan, Neil Powe, Donald Steinwachs, and Greg Dent. 1990. "Applying Insurance Claims Data to Assess Quality of Care: A Compilation of Potential Indicators." *Quality Review Bulletin, Journal of Quality Assurance* 16, 12: 424–38.

Weinstein, Milton, and William Stason. 1977. "Foundations of Cost-Effectiveness Analysis for Health and Medical Practices." *New England Journal of Medicine* 296, 13: 716–21.

Wennberg, John. 1985. "On Patient Need, Equity, Supplier-Induced Demand, and the Need to Assess the Outcome of Common Medical Practices." *Medical Care* 23, 5: 512–20.

Wennberg, John. 1986. "Which Rate Is Right?" *New England Journal of Medicine* 314, 5: 310–1.

Wennberg, John, and Alan Gittelsohn. 1982. "Variations in Medical Care among Small Areas." *Scientific American* 246, 4: 120–32.

Wennberg, John, Jean Freeman, Roxanne Shelton, and Thomas Bubolz. 1989. "Hospital Use and Mortality among Medicare Beneficiaries in Boston and New Haven." *New England Journal of Medicine* 321, 17: 1168–73.

Winslow, Constance, Jacqueline Kosecoff, Mark Chassin, et al. 1988. "The Appropriateness of Performing Coronary Artery Bypass Surgery." *Journal of the American Medical Association* 260, 4: 505–9.

Wyszewianski, Leon. 1988. "The Emphasis on Measurement in Quality Assurance: Reasons and Implications." *Inquiry* 25, 4: p. 424–33.

Young, David. 1985. "Physician Accountability for Health Care Costs." *Business and Health,* November: 16–8.

Chapter 9

AMA. 1986a. *Physician Characteristics and Distribution in the U.S.* Chicago: AMA.

AMA. 1986b. *Socioeconomic Characteristics of Medical Practice, 1986.* Chicago: AMA.

AMA, Council on Ethical and Judicial Affairs. 1992. "Conflicts of Interest: Physician Ownership of Medical Facilities" *Journal of the American Medical Association* 267, 17: 2366–9.

Angell, Marcia. 1985. "Cost Containment and the Physician." *Journal of the American Medical Association* 254, 9: 1203–7.

Bakken, Eljon. 1991. "Cigna Subsidiary Denied Payments for Needed Care, Panel Finds." *Psychiatric Times,* September: 86.

Bell, Nancy. 1991. "The AAPI Accreditation Program." *Medical Interface* 4, 4: 22–7, 39.

Berger, Stanley, and Amy Roth. 1984. "Prospective Payment and the University Hospital." *New England Journal of Medicine* 310, 5: 316–8.

Breo, Dennis. 1985. "Band Together or Lose Professional Freedom, Physicians Warned." *American Medical News,* 19 July: 2, 19–21.

Brook, Robert, and Kathleen Lohr. 1985. "Efficiency, Effectiveness, Variations, and Quality: Boundary-Crossing Research." *Medical Care* 23, 5: 710–22.

Cameron, James. 1985. "The Indirect Costs of Graduate Medical Education." *New England Journal of Medicine* 312, 19: 1233–8.

Daniels, Norman. 1986. "Why Saying No to Patients in the United States Is So Hard: Cost Containment, Justice, and Provider Autonomy." *New England Journal of Medicine* 314, 21: 1380–3.

Des Harnais, Susan, Edward Kobrinski, James Chesney, et al. 1987. "The Early Effects of the Prospective Payment System on Inpatient Utilization and the Quality of Care." *Inquiry* 24, 1: 7–16.

"Doctor-Owned Labs in Florida Perform More Tests at Greater Cost, Study Finds." 1991. *Baltimore Sun,* 9 August: A19.

Dolenc, Danielle, and Charles Dougherty. 1985. "DRGs: The Counterrevolution in Financing Health Care." *Hastings Center Report* 15, 3: 19–29.

Durenburger, David. 1985. "Who, How, and When to Pay for Physicians' Training." *Business and Health,* April: 7–11.

Dyer, Allen. 1986. "Patients, Not Costs, Come First." *Hastings Center Report* 16, 1: 5–7.

Eisenberg, John. 1989. "Clinical Economics: A Guide to the Economic Analysis of Clinical Practices." *Journal of the American Medical Association* 262, 20: 2879–86.

Elstein, Arthur. 1985. "Consultation and Referral in New Medical-Practice Environments: A Gloomy Outlook?" *Annals of Internal Medicine* 85, 4: 616–7.

Enthoven, Alain. 1989. "A 'Cost-Unconscious' Medical System." *New York Times,* 13 July: A23.

Fineberg, Harvey. 1985. "Future Directions for Research." *Medical Decision Making* 5, 1: 35–8.

Ginzberg, Eli. 1983. "Cost Containment—Imaginary and Real." *New England Journal of Medicine* 308, 20: 1220–4.

Gray, Bradford, ed. 1986. *For-Profit Enterprise in Health Care.* Washington, D.C.: National Academy Press.

Health Care Cost Containment Board. 1992. *Joint Ventures among Health Care Providers in Florida.* Draft report. Tallahassee: State of Florida.

Herzlinger, Regina, and William Krasker. 1987. "Who Profits from Non-Profits?" *Harvard Business Review,* January-February: 93–106.

Hillman, Alan. 1987. "Financial Incentives for Physicians in HMOs: Is There a Conflict of Interest?" *New England Journal of Medicine* 317, 27: 1743–8.

Horn, Susan, Pheobe Sharkey, Angela Chambers, and Roger Horn. 1985. "Severity of Illness Within DRGs: Impact on Prospective Payment." *American Journal of Public Health* 75, 10: 1195–9.

Hyman, David, and Joel Williamson. 1989. "Fraud and Abuse: Setting the Limits on Physicians' Entrepreneurship." *New England Journal of Medicine* 320, 19: 1275–8.

Iglehart, John. 1986. "Early Experience with Prospective Payment of Hospitals." *New England Journal of Medicine* 314, 22: 1460–4.

Jones, Laurie. 1991. "Surveys Show that Costs Keep Cancer Patients from Getting Optimal Care." *American Medical News,* 1 April: 3, 29.

Juba, David. 1985. "Medicare Part B: A Time for Reform." *Business and Health,* November: 5–8.

Kahn, Henry, and Peter Orris. 1982. "The Emerging Role of Salaried Physicians: An Organizational Proposal." *Journal of Public Health Policy* 3, 3: 284–92.

Kahn, Katherine, Emmett Keeler, Marjorie Sherwood, et al. 1990. "Comparing Outcomes of Care Before and After Implementation of the DRG-Based Prospective Payment System." *Journal of the American Medical Association* 264, 15: 1984–8.

Kahn, Katherine, William Rogers, Lisa Rubenstein, et al. 1990. "Measuring Quality of Care with Explicit Process Criteria Before and After Implementation of the DRG-Based Prospective Payment System." *Journal of the American Medical Association* 264, 15: 1969–73.

King, Lester. 1985. "Medicine—Trade or Profession?" *Journal of the American Medical Association* 253, 18: 2709–10.

Korcok, Milan. 1986. "From Patient Advocate to 'Gatekeeper.'" *American Medical News,* 4 April: 21–3.

"Lawyer Can Help MD Navigate to 'Safe Harbors' for Investments." 1991. *Clinical Psychiatry News,* September: 2.

Levinsky, Norman. 1984. "The Doctor's Master." *New England Journal of Medicine* 311, 24: 1573–5.

Lister, Eric. 1991. "Can We Find a Reasoned Response to Managed Care?" *Psychiatric Times,* November: 9–10.

Loewy, Erich. 1980. "Should Cost Be a Factor in Personal Medical Care?" Letter to the Editor. *New England Journal of Medicine* 303, 5: 288.

LoGerfo, James. 1990. "The Prospective Payment System and Quality: No Skeletons in the Closet." *Journal of the American Medical Association* 264, 15: 1995–6.

Lowenstein, Steven, Lisa Iezzoni, and Mark Moskowitz. 1985. "Prospective Payment for Physician Services: Impact on Medical Consultation Practices." *Journal of the American Medical Association* 254, 18: 2632–7.

Ludmerer, Kenneth. 1985. *Learning to Heal: The Development of American Medical Education.* New York: Basic Books.

Luft, Harold. 1982. "Health Maintenance Organizations and the Rationing of Medical Care." *Milbank Quarterly* 60, 2: 268–306.

Morreim, E. Haavi. 1985. "The MD and the DRG." *Hastings Center Report* 15, 3: 30–8.

National Academy of Sciences, IOM. 1985. *Assessing Medical Technologies.* Washington, D.C.: National Academy Press.

Newhouse, Joseph. 1989. "Do Unprofitable Patients Face Access Problems?" *Health Care Financing Review* 11, 2: 33–42.

Nutter, Donald. 1984. "Access to Care and the Evolution of Corporate, For-Profit Medicine." *New England Journal of Medicine* 311, 14: 917–9.

Omenn, Gilbert, and Douglas Conrad. 1984. "Implications of DRGs for Clinicians." *New England Journal of Medicine* 311, 20: 1314–7.

Petersdorf, Robert. 1985. "Current and Future Directions for Hospital and Physician Reimbursement: Effect on the Academic Medical Center." *Journal of the American Medical Association* 253, 17: 2543–8.

Rabkin, Mitchell. 1982. "The SAG Index." *New England Journal of Medicine* 307, 21: 1350–1.

Reinhardt, Uwe. 1982. "Table Manners at the Health Care Feast." In: Yaggy, D., and W. Anylan, eds. *Financing Health Care: Competition vs. Regulation.* Cambridge Mass.: Ballinger Publishing.

Reinhardt, Uwe. 1985. "Future Trends in the Economics of Medical Practice and Care." *American Journal of Cardiology* 56, 5: 50C–9C.

Relman, Arnold. 1980. "The New Medical-Industrial Complex." *New England Journal of Medicine* 303, 17: 963–70.

Rice, Thomas. 1991. *Containing Health Care Costs in the United States.* Washington, D.C.: Public Policy Institute (AARP).

Rock, Robert. 1985. "Assuring Quality of Care under DRG-Based Prospective Payment." *Medical Decision Making* 5, 1: 31–4.

Rogers, William, David Draper, Katherine Kahn, et al. 1990. "Quality of Care Before and After Implementation of the DRG-Based Prospective Payment System." *Journal of the American Medical Association* 264, 15: 1989–94.

Saward, Ernest, and E.K. Gallagher. 1983. "Reflections on Change in Medical Practice: The Current Trend to Large-Scale Medical Organizations." *Journal of the American Medical Association* 350, 20: 2820–5.

Schroeder, James, John Clarke, and James Webster. 1985. "Prepaid Entitlements: A New Challenge for Physician-Patient Relationships." *Journal of the American Medical Association* 254, 21: 3080–2.

Shortell, Stephen, Michael Morrisey, and Douglas Conrad. 1985. "Economic Regulation and Hospital Behavior: The Effects on Medical Staff Organization and Hospital-Physician Relationships." *Health Services Research* 20, 5: 597–628.

Simborg, Donald. 1981. "DRG Creep: A New Hospital-Acquired Disease." *New England Journal of Medicine* 304, 26: 1602–4.

Smits, Helen, and Rita Watson. 1984. "DRGs and the Future of Surgical Practice." *New England Journal of Medicine* 311, 25: 1612–5.

Steinwald, Bruce. 1986. "The Impact of New Reimbursement Schemes on Clinical Research in Hospitals: The Case of the Prospective Payment System." *Journal of General Internal Medicine* 1, Supplement: S56-9.

Swick, Thomas. 1986. "The Emergence of Physician Unions . . . Can They Balance Economic and Public Interests?" *American College of Physicians Observer*, March: 4–5.

Thomasma, David, Kenneth Micetich, and Patricia Steinecker. 1985. "Social Censorship of Medical and Ethical Decisions." *The Pharos* 48, 3: 22–6.

Thurow, Lester. 1984. "Learning to Say No." *New England Journal of Medicine* 311, 24: 1569–72.

Veatch, Robert. 1986. "DRGs and the Ethical Allocation of Resources." *Hastings Center Report* 16, 3: 32–40.

Weiner, Jonathan. 1987. "Balancing Cost and Quality in the New Medical Marketplace." Seminar, 23 November, Baltimore.

Wennberg, John, Klim McPherson, and Philip Capter. 1984. "Will Payment Based on Diagnosis-Related Groups Control Hospital Costs?" *New England Journal of Medicine* 311, 5: 295–300.

Westermeyer, Joseph. 1991. "Problems With Managed Psychiatric Care Without a Psychiatrist-Manager." *Hospital and Community Psychiatry* 42, 12: 1221–4.

Wilensky, Gail. 1990. "Medicare at 25: Better Value and Better Care." *Journal of the American Medical Association* 264, 15: 1996–7.

Williams, Sankey. 1985. "The Impact of DRG-Based Prospective Payment on Clinical Decision Making." *Medical Decision Making* 5, 2: 23–9.

Yarbro, John, and Lee Mortenson. 1985. "The Need for Diagnosis-Related Group 471: Protection for Clinical Research." *Journal of the American Medical Association* 253, 2: 684–5.

Young, David, and Richard Saltman. 1985. *The Hospital Power Equilibrium: Physician Behavior and Cost Control.* Baltimore: Johns Hopkins University Press.

Chapter 10

AMA. 1987. *The Health Policy Agenda for the American People; Final Report.* Chicago: AMA.

Beauchamp, Tom, and James Childress. 1989. *Principles of Biomedical Ethics,* 3rd ed. New York: Oxford University Press.

Bovbjerg, Randall, Philip Held, and Louis Diamond. 1987. "Provider-Patient Relations and Treatment Choice in the Era of Fiscal Incentives: The Case of the End-Stage Renal Disease Program." *Milbank Quarterly* 65, 2: 177–202.

Colombotos, John, and Corinne Kirchner. 1986. *Physicians and Social Change.* New York: Oxford University Press.

Eddy, David. 1990. "Connecting Value and Costs: Whom Do We Ask, and What Do We Ask Them?" *Journal of the American Medical Association* 264, 13: 1737–9.

Eisenberg, John. 1989. "Clinical Economics: A Guide to the Economic Analysis of Clinical Practices." *Journal of the American Medical Association* 262, 20: 2879–86.

Eisenberg, John, and Sankey Williams. 1981. "Cost Containment and Changing Physicians' Practice Behavior: Can the Fox Learn to Guard the Chicken Coop?" *Journal of the American Medical Association* 246, 19: 2195–201.

Engelhardt, H. Tristram, and Michael Rie. 1988. "Morality for the Medical-Industrial Complex: A Code of Ethics for the Mass Marketing of Health Care." *New England Journal of Medicine* 319, 16: 1086–9.

Faden, Ruth, Gail Geller, Madison Powers, eds. 1991. *AIDS, Women and the Next Generation.* New York: Oxford University Press.

Geller, Gail, and Nancy Kass. 1991. "Informed Consent in the Context of Prenatal HIV Screening." In: Faden, Ruth, Gail Geller, and Madison Powers, eds. *AIDS, Women and the Next Generation*. New York: Oxford University Press, pp. 288–307.

Iglehart, John. 1984. "Opinion Polls on Health Care." *New England Journal of Medicine* 310, 24: 1616–20.

Katz, Jay. 1984. *The Silent World of Doctor and Patient*. New York: Free Press.

King, Lester. 1985. "Medicine—Trade or Profession." *Journal of the American Medical Association* 253, 18: 2709–10.

Kramon, Glenn. 1988. "Insurance Rates for Health Care Increase Sharply." *New York Times*, 12 January: 1.

Louis Harris and Associates. 1983. *The Equitable Healthcare Survey: Options for Controlling Costs*. New York: Louis Harris and Associates.

Louis Harris and Associates. 1984. *The Equitable Healthcare Survey II: Physicians' Attitudes Toward Cost Containment*. New York: Louis Harris and Associates.

McCullough, Laurence. 1988. "An Ethical Model for Improving the Patient-Physician Relationship." *Inquiry* 25, 4: 454–68.

Pellegrino, Edmund. 1987. "Toward a Reconstruction of Medical Morality." *Journal of Medical Humanities and Bioethics* 8, 1: 7–20.

Radovsky, Saul. 1990. "U.S. Medical Practice Before Medicare and Now—Differences and Consequences." *New England Journal of Medicine* 322, 4: 263–7.

Redelmeier, Donald, and Amos Tversky. 1990. "Discrepancy Between Medical Decisions for Individual Patients and for Groups." *New England Journal of Medicine* 322, 16: 1162–4

Relman, Arnold. 1983. "The Future of Medical Practice." *Health Affairs* 2, 2: 5–19.

Relman, Arnold. 1985. "Cost Control, Doctors' Ethics, and Patient Care." *Issues in Science and Technology*, Winter: 103–11.

Relman, Arnold. 1987. "Practicing Medicine in the New Business Climate." *New England Journal of Medicine* 316, 18: 1150–1.

Thomasma, David, Kenneth Micetich, and Patricia Steinecker. 1985. "Social Censorship of Medical and Ethical Decisions." *The Pharos* 48, 3: 22–6.

Veatch, Robert. 1991. "Allocating Health Resources Ethically: New Roles for Administrators and Clinicians." *Frontiers of Health Services Management* 8, 1: 3–44.

Young, David. 1985. "Physician Accountability for Health Care Costs." *Business and Health*, November: 16–8.

Introduction to Part IV

Dass, Ram, and Paul Gorman. 1990. *How Can I Help?*, 7th ed. New York: Alfred A. Knopf.

Chapter 11

AMA. 1986. *Socioeconomic Characteristics of Medical Practice 1986*. Chicago: AMA.

AMA, Office of Socioeconomic Research Information. 1991. *Trends in U.S. Health Care 1990*. Chicago: AMA Center for Health Policy Research.

AMA, Special Task Force on Professional Liability and Insurance. 1984. *Professional Liability in the '80s*, reports 1–3. Chicago: AMA.

"AMA Statement Rebuts Claims by Trial Lawyers' Association." 1985. *American Medical News*, 4 October: 36–9.

Anderson, Eugene. 1986. "Compensation, Without Lawyers." *New York Times*, 1 May: Y29.

Anderson, Robert, Rolla Hill, and Charles Key. 1991. "The Sensitivity and Specificity of Clinical Diagnostics During Five Decades: Toward an Understanding of Necessary Fallibility." *Journal of the American Medical Association* 261, 11: 1610–7.

Angell, Marcia. 1985. "Cost Containment and the Physician." *Journal of the American Medical Association* 254, 9: 1203–12.

Baily, Mary Ann, and Warren Cikins, eds. 1985. *The Effects of Litigation on Health Care Costs*. Washington, D.C.: Brookings Institution.

Berwick, Donald. 1991. "The Double Edge of Knowledge." *New England Journal of Medicine* 266, 6: 841–2.

Bosk, Charles. 1986. "Professional Responsibility and Medical Error." In: Aiken, Linda, and David Mechanic, eds. *Applications of Social Science to Clinical Medicine and Health Policy*. New Brunswick, N.J.: Rutgers University Press, pp. 460–77.

Bovbjerg, Randall. 1991. "Lessons for Tort Reform from Indiana." *Journal of Health Policy, Politics and Law* 16, 3: 466.

Bovbjerg, Randall, and Clark Havighurst. 1985. "Medical Malpractice: An Update for Noncombatants." *Business and Health*, September: 38–42.

Brennan, Troyen. 1991. In: Robert Wood Johnson Foundation Communications Office. 1991. "A Special Edition on Medical Malpractice." *ABridge*, Spring.

Brennan, Troyen, Lucian Leape, Nan Laird, et al. 1991. "Incidence of Adverse Events and Negligence in Hospitalized Patients: Results of the

Harvard Medical Practice Study I." *New England Journal of Medicine* 324, 6: 370–6.

Brightbill, Tim. 1991. "Jury Still Out on Tort Reform as Malpractice Fix." *Health Week* 5, 3: 1, 31–2.

Cheney, Frederick, Karen Posner, Robert Caplan, and Richard Ward. 1989. "Standard of Care and Anesthesia Liability." *Journal of the American Medical Association* 361, 11: 1599–603.

Crane, Mark. 1986. "Malpractice: The Most Dangerous Places to Practice." *Medical Economics,* 3 February: 65–71.

Creasey, Daniel. 1991. In: Robert Wood Johnson Foundation Communications Office. 1991. "A Special Edition on Medical Malpractice." *ABridge,* Spring, p. 1.

"Disciplinary Actions by State Boards Up 9%." 1991. *Clinical Psychiatry News* 19, 11: 3.

"Doctors and Lawyers Square Off on Lawsuits." 1985. *New York Times,* 26 December.

Dolin, Leigh. 1985. "Antitrust Law Versus Peer Review." *New England Journal of Medicine* 313, 18: 1156–7.

Gonzalez, Martin, ed. 1991. *Socioeconomic Characteristics of Medical Practice 1990/1991.* Chicago. AMA Center for Health Policy Research.

Gorovitz, Samuel, and Alisdair MacIntyre. 1986. "Toward a Theory of Medical Fallibility." In: Engelhard, H.T., and D. Callahan, eds. *The Foundations of Ethics and Its Relationship to Science.* Hastings-on-Hudson, N.Y.: Hastings Center, pp. 248–74.

Gronfein, William, and Eleanor Kinnoy. 1991. "Controlling Large Malpractice Claims: the Unexpected Impact of Damage Caps." *Journal of Health Policy, Politics and Law* 16, 3: 441–64.

Gutheil, Thomas, Harold Bursztajn, and Archie Brodsky. 1984. "Malpractice Prevention Through the Sharing of Uncertainty." *New England Journal of Medicine* 311, 1: 49–51.

Henderson, Charles. 1986. "A Medical Malpractice Primer." *Maryland Medical Journal* 35, 1: 38–42.

Hunter, Robert. 1986. "Taming the Latest Insurance 'Crisis.'" *New York Times,* 13 April: F3.

"Insurance Monitor." 1986. *Maryland Medical Journal* 35, 1: 10.

Jury Verdict Research. 1985. *Current Award Trends,* January. Solon, Ohio.

Leape, Lucian, Troyen Brennan, Nan Laird, et al. 1991. "The Nature of Adverse Events in Hospitalized Patients." *New England Journal of Medicine* 324, 6: 377–84.

Lee, Richard. 1986. "The Jaundiced View: Malpractice Malaise." *American Journal of Medicine* 30, 2: 159–60.

McHugh, Paul. 1991. Personal Communication, 30 October.

Mussman, Mary, Lu Zawistowich, Carol Weisman, et al. 1991. "Medical Malpractice Claims Filed by Medicaid and Non-Medicaid Recipients in Maryland." *Journal of the American Medical Association* 265, 22: 2992–4.

O'Connell, Jeffrey. 1985. "The Case Against the Current Malpractice System." Presentation at The Urban Institute's National Medical Malpractice Conference, "Can the Private Sector Find Relief?" 21–22 February.

Pauker, Stephen, and Jerome Kassirer. 1987. "Decision Analysis." *New England Journal of Medicine* 316, 5: 250–8.

Rawls, John. 1971. *A Theory of Justice.* Cambridge, Mass.: Harvard University Press.

Robert Wood Johnson Foundation Communications Office. 1991. "A Special Edition on Medical Malpractice." *ABridge,* Spring.

Rostow, Victoria, Marian Osterweis, and Roger Bulger. 1989. "Medical Professional Liability and the Delivery of Obstetrical Care." *New England Journal of Medicine* 321, 15: 1057–60.

Rust, Mark. 1985. "MDs Cease High-Risk Care in N.Y." *American Medical News,* 21 June: 1, 26.

Rust, Mark. 1986a. "MDs No Longer Alone in Tort Reform Fight." *American Medical News,* 14 February: 1, 23, 25–6.

Rust, Mark. 1986b. "Tort Reform Legislation Gains Momentum." *American Medical News,* 25 April: 1, 28–9.

Rust, Mark. 1987. "Malpractice: New Alliances Aid in Passage of Tort Reforms." *American Medical News,* 2 January: 3, 35.

Schwartz, William, and Henry Aaron. 1984. "Rationing Hospital Care: Lessons from Britain." *New England Journal of Medicine* 310, 1: 52–6.

Siden, Harold, Benjamin Ticho, and Mitchell Kopnick. 1986. "Malpractice Concerns Enter the Medical School Classroom." Letter to the Editor. *New England Journal of Medicine* 314, 8: 522–3.

Stempfer, Meir, Walter Willet, Graham Colditz, et al. 1985. "A Prospective Study of Postmenopausal Estrogen Therapy and Coronary Heart Disease." *New England Journal of Medicine* 313, 17: 1044–9.

Weiler, Paul, Joseph Newhouse, and Howard Hiatt. 1992. "Proposal for Medical Liability Reform." *Journal of the American Medical Association* 267, 17: 2355–8.

Williams, Sarah, ed. 1985. "Medical Malpractice Resurfacing as Issue for States." *Alpha Centerpiece,* October. Washington, D.C.: The Alpha Center.

Wilson, Peter, Robert Garrison, and William Castelli. 1985. "Post-menopausal Estrogen Use, Cigarette Smoking, and Cardiovascular Morbidity in Women Over 50: The Framingham Study." *New England Journal of Medicine* 313, 17: 1038–43.

Chapter 12

Aday, Lu Ann, and Ronald Anderson. 1975. *Access to Medical Care.* Ann Arbor, Mich.: Health Administration Press.

AMA Office of Socioeconomic Research Information. 1991. *Trends in U.S. Health Care 1990.* Chicago: AMA Center for Health Policy Research.

American Association of Medical Colleges. 1992. *AAMC Data Book: Statistical Information Related to Medical Education.* Washington, D.C.: AAMC.

"American Health Care: Paying More and Getting Less." *The Economist,* 25 November: 17–9.

American Public Health Association. 1985. *Washington News Letter,* #9. Washington, D.C.: APHA.

Annas, George. 1986. "Your Money or Your Life: 'Dumping' Uninsured Patients from Hospital Emergency Wards." *American Journal of Public Health* 76, 1: 74–7.

Beauchamp, Dan, and Ronald Rouse. 1990. "Universal New York Health Care: A Single-Payer Strategy Linking Cost Control and Universal Access." *New England Journal of Medicine* 323, 10: 640–4.

Berman, Neal, and Phyllis Lauro. 1985. "Determining the True Cost of Graduate Medical Education." *Business and Health,* April: 12–3.

Blendon, Robert, and Jennifer Edwards. 1991. "Caring for the Uninsured: Choices for Reform." *Journal of the American Medical Association* 265, 19: 2563–5.

Blendon, Robert, Linda Aiken, Howard Freeman, et al. 1986. "Uncompensated Care by Hospitals or Public Insurance for the Poor: Does it Make a Difference?" *New England Journal of Medicine* 314, 18: 1160–3.

Blumenthal, David, Mark Schlesinger, Pamela Drumheller, and the Harvard Medicare Project. 1986. "The Future of Medicare." *New England Journal of Medicine* 314, 11: 722–8.

Brandon, William. 1982. "Health-Related Tax Subsidies: Government Handouts for the Affluent." *New England Journal of Medicine* 307, 15: 947–50.

Brook, Robert, John Ware, William Rogers, et al. 1983. "Does Free Care Improve Adults' Health?: Results from a Randomized Controlled Trial." *New England Journal of Medicine* 309, 23: 1426–34.

Bronow Ronald, Robert Beltran, Stephen Cohen, et al. 1991. "The Physicians Who Care Plan: Preserving Quality and Equitability in American Medicine." *Journal of the American Medical Association* 265, 19: 2511–5.

Brown, E. Richard. 1988. "Principles for a National Health Program: A Framework for Analysis and Development." *Milbank Quarterly* 66, 4: 573–617.

Butler, Stuart. 1991. "A Tax Reform Strategy to Deal with the Uninsured." *Journal of the American Medical Association* 265, 19: 2541–4.

Calkins, David, Linda Burns, and Thomas Delbanco. 1986. "Ambulatory Care and the Poor: Tracking the Impact of Changes in Federal Policy." *Journal of General Internal Medicine* 1, 2: 109–15.

Census Bureau, Washington, D.C.

Citrin, Toby. 1985. "Trustees at the Focal Point." *New England Journal of Medicine* 313, 19: 1223–6.

Colburn, Don, and Richard Morin. 1991. "Americans Grade Their Health Care." *Washington Post,* Health Section, 31 December: 6–9.

Daniels, Norman. 1986. "Why Saying No to Patients in the United States is So Hard: Cost Containment, Justice, and Provider Autonomy." *New England Journal of Medicine* 314, 21: 1380–3.

Davidson, Stephen, Jerry Cromwell, and Rachel Shurman. 1986. "Medicaid Myths: Trends in Medicaid Expenditures and the Prospects for Reform." *Journal of Health Politics, Policy and Law* 10, 4: 699–728.

Davis, Karen. 1985. "Access to Health Care: A Matter of Fairness." In: *Health Care: How to Improve It and Pay for It.* Washington, D.C.: Center for National Policy, pp. 45–57.

Davis, Karen. 1991. "Expanding Medicare and Employer Plans to Achieve Universal Health Insurance." *Journal of the American Medical Association* 265, 19: 2525–8.

Davis, Karen, and Cathy Schoen. 1978. *Health and the War on Poverty: A Ten-Year Appraisal.* Washington, D.C.: Brookings Institution.

Davis, Karen, and Diane Rowland. 1983. "Uninsured and Underserved: Inequality in Health Care in the United States." *Milbank Quarterly* 61, 2: 149–76.

Employee Benefits Research Institute. 1992. *Sources of Health Insurance and Characteristics of the Uninsured: Analysis of March, 1991 Current Population Survey.* Washington, D.C.

Enthoven, Alain, and Richard Kronick. 1989. "A Consumer-Choice Health Plan For the 1990s: Universal Health Insurance in a System Designed to Promote Quality and Economy (First of Two Parts)." *New England Journal of Medicine* 320, 1: 29–37; 2: 94–101.

Enthoven, Alain, and Richard Kronick. 1991. "Universal Health Insurance through Incentives Reform." *Journal of the American Medical Association* 265, 19: 2532–6.

Epstein, Arnold, Robert Stern, and Joel Weissman. 1990. "Do the Poor Cost More? A Multihospital Study of Patients' Socioeconomic Status and Use of Hospital Resources." *New England Journal of Medicine* 322, 16: 1122–8.

Fein, Rashi. 1991. "The Health Security Partnership." *Journal of the American Medical Association* 265, 19: 2555–8.

Freeman, Howard, Robert Blendon, Linda Aiken, et al. 1987. "Americans Report on Their Access to Health Care." *Health Affairs* 6, 1: 6–18.

Friedman, Emily. 1991. "The Uninsured: From Dilemma to Crisis." *Journal of the American Medical Association* 265, 19: 2491–5.

Ginsburg, Paul, and Frank Sloan. 1984. "Hospital Cost Shifting." *New England Journal of Medicine* 310, 14: 893–8.

Ginzberg, Eli, and Miriam Ostow. 1991. "Beyond Universal Health Insurance to Effective Health Care." *Journal of the American Medical Association* 265, 19: 2559–62.

Greenblatt, Milton. 1983. "Point of View." In: Upton, David, ed. *Mental Health Care and National Health Insurance.* New York: Plenum Press, pp. 227–39.

Grumbach, Kevin, Thomas Bodenheimer, David Himmelstein, and Steffie Woolhandler. 1991. "Liberal Benefits, Conservative Spending: the Physicians for a National Health Program Proposal." *Journal of the American Medical Association* 265, 19: 2549–54.

Hadley, Jack, Earl Steinberg, and Judith Feder. 1991. "Comparison of Uninsured and Privately Insured Hospital Patients: Condition on Admission, Resource Use and Outcome." *Journal of the American Medical Association* 265, 3: 374–9.

Health Policy Alternatives. 1985. "Paying for Physicians' Services Under Medicare: Issues and Reform Options for the American Association of Retired Persons." A Report to the AARP on Medicare Physician Payment Reform.

Himmelstein, David, Steffie Woolhandler, and the Writing Committee of the Working Group on Program Design. 1989. "A National Health Program for the United States." *New England Journal of Medicine* 320, 2: 102–3.

Holahan, John, and Sheila Zedlewski. 1991. "Expanding Medicaid to Cover Uninsured Americans." *Health Affairs* 10, 1: 45–61.

Iglehart, John. 1985. "U.S. Health Care System: A Look to the 1990s." *Health Affairs* 4, 3: 120–7.

Iglehart, John. 1986. "Canada's Health Care System." *New England Journal of Medicine* 315, 3: 202–8; 12: 778–84; 25: 1623–8.

Iglehart, John. 1989. "The United States Looks at Canadian Health Care." *New England Journal of Medicine* 321, 25: 1767–72.

Johns, Lucy. 1985. "Selective Contracting in California." *Health Affairs* 4, 3: 32–48.

Jolly, Paul, Leon Taskel, and David Baime. 1986. "U.S. Medical School Finances." *Journal of the American Medical Association* 256, 12: 1570–80.

Kellermann, Arthur, and Terrence Ackerman. 1988. "Interhospital Patient Transfer: The Case for Informed Consent." *New England Journal of Medicine* 319, 10: 643–6.

Kimball, Merit. 1991. "Governors Say Medicare Shifts Strain Medicaid." *HealthWeek* 5, 3: 1, 34.

King, Wayne. 1985. "Texas Adopts Stringent Rules on Rights of Poor at Hospitals." *New York Times,* 15 December: 30.

Kronick, Richard. 1991. "Can Massachusetts Pay for Health Care for All?" *Health Affairs* 10, 1: 26–44.

Lee, Philip, and Carroll Estes, eds. 1990. *The Nation's Health.* Boston: Jones and Bartlett Publishers.

Levey, Samuel, and James Hill. 1989. "National Health Insurance—The Triumph of Equivocation." *New England Journal of Medicine* 321, 25: 1750–4.

Lewin, Lawrence, and Marion Lewin. 1987. "Financing Charity Care in an Era of Competition." *Health Affairs* 6, 1: 47–60.

Linton, Adam. 1990. "The Canadian Health Care System: A Physician's Perspective." *New England Journal of Medicine* 322, 3: 197–9.

Louis Harris and Associates. 1984. *The Equitable Healthcare Survey II: Physicians' Attitudes Toward Cost Containment.* New York: Louis Harris and Associates.

Lundberg, George. 1991. "National Health Care Reform: An Aura of Inevitability is Upon Us." *Journal of the American Medical Association* 265, 19: 2566–7.

Lurie, Nicole, Nancy Ward, Martin Shapiro, and Robert Brook. 1984. "Termination From Medi-Cal—Does It Affect Health?" *New England Journal of Medicine* 311, 7: 480–4.

Means, James. 1953. *Doctors, People, and Government.* Boston: Little, Brown and Co.

Miller, Seymour. 1987. "Race in the Health of America." *Milbank Quarterly* 65, Supplement 2: 500–31.

National Center for Health Services Research. 1980. "Who Are the Uninsured?" Data Preview 1 from the National Health Care Expenditures Study, PHS, DHHS. Washington, D.C.: Government Printing Office.

National Center for Health Statistics. 1991. *Health, United States, 1990.* Hyattsville, Md.: Public Health Service.

National Mental Health Association. 1991. *Legislative Alert.* #102-4. Alexandria, Va.

Navarro, Vicente. 1987. "Federal Health Policies in the United States: An Alternative Explanation." *Milbank Quarterly* 65, 1: 81–111.

Neuschler, Edward. 1990. "Canadian Health Care: The Implications of Public Health Insurance." *Research Bulletin* (HIAA), June.

Newhouse, Joseph. 1989. "Do Unprofitable Patients Face Access Problems?" *Health Care Financing Review* 11, 2: 33–42.

Nutter, Donald. 1984. "Access to Care and the Evolution of Corporate, For-Profit Medicine." *New England Journal of Medicine* 311, 14: 917–9.

Nutter, Donald. 1987. "Medical Indigency and the Public Health Care Crisis: The Need for a Definitive Solution." *New England Journal of Medicine* 316, 18: 1156–8.

Pauly, Mark, Patricia Danzon, Paul Feldstein, and John Hoff. 1991. "A Plan for 'Responsible National Health Insurance.'" *Health Affairs* 10, 1: 5–25.

Penchansky, Roy, and J. William Thomas. 1981. "The Concept of Access: Definition and Relationship to Consumer Satisfaction." *Medical Care* 19, 2: 127–40.

PPRC. 1991. *Annual Report to Congress 1991.* Washington, D.C.: Government Printing Office.

Pollack, Andrew. 1991. "Medical Technology 'Arms Race' Adds Billions to the Nation's Bills." *New York Times,* 29 April: A1, B8.

Reinhardt, Uwe. 1986a. "Rationing the Health-Care Surplus: An American Tragedy." *Nursing Economics* 4, 3: 101–8.

Reinhardt, Uwe. 1986b. "Rationing the Nation's Health-Care Surplus: A Paradox? Or as American as Apple Pie?" Statement before the House Select Committee on Aging, U.S. Congress. Washington, D.C.

Relman, Arnold, and Uwe Reinhardt. 1986. "Debating For-Profit Health Care." *Health Affairs* 5, 2: 5–31.

Rice, Dorothy. 1990. "The Medical Care System: Past Trends and Future Projections." In: Lee, Philip, and Carroll Estes, eds. *The Nation's Health.* Boston: Jones and Bartlett Publishers, pp. 72–93.

Rice, Thomas. 1991. *Containing Health Care Costs in the United States.* Washington, D.C.: Public Policy Institute (AARP).

Richards, Glenn. 1984. "FECs Pose Competition for Hospital EDs." *Hospitals* 58, 6: 77–82.

Ries, Peter. 1991. *Characteristics of Persons With and Without Health Care Coverage: United States, 1989.* Advance Data from Vital and Health Statistics, #201. Hyattsville, Md.: National Center for Health Statistics.

Robert Wood Johnson Foundation. 1987. *Access to Health Care in the U.S.* Special Report #2. Princeton, N.J.: RWJ.

Rockefeller, John. 1991. "A Call for Action: The Pepper Commission's Blueprint for Health Care Reform." *Journal of the American Medical Association* 265, 19: 2507–10.

Roybal, Edward. 1991. "The 'US Health Act': Comprehensive Reform for a Caring America." *Journal of the American Medical Association* 265, 19: 2545–8.

Scheier, Ronni. 1986a. "Hospital's Burden: The Rising Uninsured." *American Medical News,* 4 April: 3, 39–40.

Scheier, Ronni. 1986b. "States Continue Expansion of Medicaid Programs" *American Medical News,* 9 May: 9.

Schieber, George, 1990. "Health Expenditures in Major Industrialized Countries, 1960–1987." *Health Care Financing Review* 11, 4: 159–67.

Schieff, Robert, David Ansell, James Schlosser, et al. 1986. "Transfers to a Public Hospital: A Prospective Study of 467 Patients." *New England Journal of Medicine* 314, 9: 552–7.

Schramm, Carl. 1983. "The Teaching Hospital and the Future Role of State Government." *New England Journal of Medicine* 308, 1: 41–5.

Sharfstein, Steven, Anne Stoline, and Howard Goldman. 1993. "Psychiatric Care and Health Insurance Reform." *American Journal of Psychiatry,* 150, 1:7–18.

Sloan, Frank, James Blumstein, and James Perrin, eds. 1986. *Uncompensated Hospital Care: Rights and Responsibilities.* Baltimore: Johns Hopkins University Press.

Stevens, Robert, and Rosemary Stevens. 1974. *Welfare Medicine in America: A Case Study of Medicaid.* New York: Free Press.

Sulvetta, Margaret, and Katherine Swartz. 1986. *The Uninsured and Uncompensated Care.* Washington, D.C.: National Health Policy Forum.

Todd, James, Steven Seekins, John Krichbaum, and Lynn Harvey. 1991. "Health Access America—Strengthening the US Health Care System." *Journal of the American Medical Association* 265, 19: 2503–6.

Treviño, Fernando, M. Eugene Moyer, R. Burciaga Valdez, and Christine Stroup-Benham. 1991. "Health Insurance Coverage and Utilization of Health Services by Mexican Americans, Mainland Puerto Ricans, and Cuban Americans." *Journal of the American Medical Association* 265, 2: 233–7.

Upton, David. 1983. *Mental Health Care and National Health Insurance.* New York: Plenum Press.

U.S. Department of Health and Human Services. 1986. *Health of the Disadvantaged.* Pub. HRS-P-DV86-2. Washington, D.C.: Government Printing Office.

Weiner, Jonathan. 1987. "Primary Care Delivery in the United States and Four Northwest European Countries: Comparing the 'Corporatized' with the 'Socialized.'" *Milbank Quarterly* 65, 3: 426–61.

Weissman, Joel, and Arnold Epstein. 1989. "Case Mix and Resource Utilization by Uninsured Hospital Patients in the Boston Metropolitan Area." *Journal of the American Medical Association* 261, 24: 3572–6.

Welch, H. Gilbert. 1989. "Health Care Tickets for the Uninsured: First Class, Coach, or Standby?" *New England Journal of Medicine* 321, 18: 1261–4.

Chapter 13

Aaron, Henry, and William Schwartz. 1984. *The Painful Prescription.* Washington, D.C.: Brookings Institution.

AMA Office of Socioeconomic Research Information. 1991. *Trends in U.S. Health Care 1990.* Chicago: AMA Center for Health Policy Research.

Angell, Marcia. 1985. "Cost Containment and the Physician." *Journal of the American Medical Association* 254, 9: 1203–7.

Annas, George. 1986. "Your Money or Your Life: 'Dumping' Uninsured Patients from Hospital Emergency Wards." *American Journal of Public Health* 76, 1: 74–7.

Anonymous in Ram Dass and Paul Gorman. 1990. *How Can I Help?,* 7th ed. New York: Alfred A. Knopf.

Bayer, Ronald, Daniel Callahan, John Fletcher, et al. 1983. "The Care of the Terminally Ill: Morality and Economics." *New England Journal of Medicine* 309, 24: 1490–4.

Bennett, Ivan. 1977. "Technology as Shaping Force." In: Knowles, John, ed. *Doing Better and Feeling Worse: Health in the United States.* New York: W.W. Norton, pp. 125–33.

Bentley, James, Richard Knapp, and Robert Petersdorf. 1989. "Education in Ambulatory Care—Financing is One Piece of the Puzzle." *New England Journal of Medicine* 320, 23: 1531–4.

Blainpain, Jan. 1985. "The Changing Environment of Health Care." *International Journal of Technology Assessment in Health Care* 1, 2: 271–7.

Blendon, Robert, and David Rogers. 1983. "Cutting Medical Care Costs: *Primum Non Nocere.*" *Journal of the American Medical Association* 250, 14: 1880–5.

Blendon, Robert, and Drew Altman. 1984. "Public Attitudes About Health Care Costs: A Lesson in National Schizophrenia." *New England Journal of Medicine* 311, 9: 613–6.

Brook, Robert, and Kathleen Lohr. 1986. "Will We Need to Ration Effective Health Care?" *Issues in Science and Technology*, Fall: 68–77.

Callahan, Daniel. 1987. *Setting Limits: Medical Goals in an Aging Society.* New York: Simon and Schuster.

Callahan, Daniel. 1990. "Rationing Medical Progress: The Way to Affordable Medical Care." *New England Journal of Medicine* 322, 25: 1810–3.

Calmes, Selma. 1984. "Memories of Polio." *Archives of Internal Medicine* 144, 6: 1273.

Comptroller General of the U.S. Charles Bowsher addressing the House Committee on Ways and Means, April 17, 1991. *U.S. Health Care Spending.* GAO/HRD-91-104. Washington, D.C.: General Accounting Office.

Daniels, Norman. 1985. *Just Health Care.* New York: Cambridge University Press.

Daniels, Norman. 1986. "Why Saying No to Patients in the United States Is So Hard: Cost Containment, Justice, and Provider Autonomy." *New England Journal of Medicine* 314, 21: 1380–3.

Davis, William. 1986. "'THEY' Threaten Medical System." *American Medical News*, 5 September: 29.

Dolenc, Danielle, and Charles Dougherty. 1985. "DRGs: The Counterrevolution in Financing Health Care." *Hastings Center Report* 15, 3: 19–29.

Donabedian, Avedis. 1980. *Explorations in Quality Assessment and Monitoring,* vol. 1: *The Definition of Quality and Approaches to Its Assessment.* Ann Arbor, Mich.: Health Administration Press.

Eddy, David. 1990. "Connecting Value and Costs: Whom Do We Ask, and What Do We Ask Them?" *Journal of the American Medical Association* 264, 13: 1737–9.

Eisenberg, Carola. 1986. "It is Still a Privilege to Be a Doctor." *New England Journal of Medicine* 314, 17: 1113–4.

Eisenberg, John. 1989a. "Clinical Economics: A Guide to the Economic Analysis of Clinical Practices." *Journal of the American Medical Association* 262, 20: 2879–86.

Eisenberg, John. 1989b. "How Can We Pay for Graduate Medical Education in Ambulatory Care." *New England Journal of Medicine* 320, 23: 1525–31.

Fishman, Linda, ed. 1991. *COTH Report* 25, #1. Council of Teaching Hospitals.

Foege, William, Robert Amler, and Craig White. 1985. "Closing the Gap: Report of the Carter Center Health Policy Consultation." *Journal of the American Medical Association* 254, 10: 1355–8.

Freymann, John. 1989. "The Public's Health Care Paradigm is Shifting: Medicine Must Swing With It." *Journal of General Internal Medicine* 4, 4: 313–9.

Fuchs, Victor. 1984. "The Rationing of Medical Care." *New England Journal of Medicine* 311, 24: 1572–3.

Fuchs, Victor. 1986. "Has Cost Containment Gone Too Far?" *Milbank Quarterly* 64, 3: 479–88.

Fuchs, Victor. 1987. "A Hard Look at Cost Containment." *New England Journal of Medicine* 316, 18: 1151–6.

Ginzberg, Eli. 1990. "Health Care Reform—Why So Slow?" *New England Journal of Medicine* 322, 20: 1464–6.

Goldfield, Norbert, and David Nash, eds. 1989. *Providing Quality Care: The Challenge to Clinicians.* Philadelphia: American College of Physicians.

Green, Josephine. 1990. "Calming or Harming? A Critical Review of Psychological Effects of Prenatal Diagnosis on Pregnant Women." Galton Institute Occasional Papers, Second Series, #2, Paris.

Hellinger, Fred. 1988. "National Forecasts of the Medical Care Costs of AIDS: 1988–1992." *Inquiry* 25, 4: 469–84.

Hughes, Robert, Dianne Barker, and Richard Reynolds. 1991. "Are We Mortgaging the Medical Profession?" *New England Journal of Medicine* 325, 6: 404–7.

Iglehart, John. 1984. "Opinion Polls on Health Care." *New England Journal of Medicine* 310, 24: 1616–20.

Iglehart, John. 1986. "Early Experience with Prospective Payment of Hospitals." *New England Journal of Medicine* 314, 22: 1460–4.

Iglehart, John. 1991. "The Struggle over Physician-Payment Reform." *New England Journal of Medicine* 325, 11: 823–8.

Jolly, Paul. 1988. "Medical Education in the United States, 1960–1987." *Health Affairs,* Supplement: 144–57.

King, Lester. 1985. "Medicine—Trade or Profession?" *Journal of the American Medical Association* 253, 18: 2709–10.

Lee, Philip, and Carroll Estes, eds. 1990. *The Nation's Health,* 3rd ed. Boston: Jones and Bartlett Publishers.

Lee, Philip, Kevin Grumbach, and Wendy Jameson. 1990. "Physician Payment in the 1990s: Factors that Will Shape the Future." *Annual Review of Public Health* 11: 297–318.

Levinsky, Norman. 1984. "The Doctor's Master." *New England Journal of Medicine* 311, 24: 1573–5.

Levinsky, Norman. 1990. "Age as a Criterion for Rationing Health Care." *New England Journal of Medicine* 322, 25: 1813–5.

Lewis, Irving, and Cecil Sheps. 1983. *The Sick Citadel.* Cambridge, Mass.: Oelgeschlager, Gunn and Hain.

Lind, Stuart. 1986. "Fee-for-Service Research." *New England Journal of Medicine* 314, 5: 312–5.

Lister, Eric. 1991. "Can We Find a Reasoned Response to Managed Care?" *Psychiatric Times,* November: 9–10.

Loewy, Erich. 1980. "Cost Should Not Be a Factor in Medical Care." Letter to the Editor. *New England Journal of Medicine* 302, 12: 697.

Louis Harris and Associates. 1983. *The Equitable Healthcare Survey: Options for Controlling Costs.* New York: Louis Harris and Associates.

Louis Harris and Associates. 1984. *The Equitable Healthcare Survey II: Physicians' Attitudes Toward Cost Containment.* New York: Louis Harris and Associates.

Louis Harris and Associates. 1990. "Trade-Offs and Choices: Health Policy Options for the 1990s." Survey for Metropolitan Life. New York. New York: Louis Harris and Associates.

Ludmerer, Kenneth. 1985. *Learning to Heal: The Development of American Medical Education.* New York: Basic Books.

McCormick, Brian. 1991. "Medicare Rules Would Fold Capital Costs into PPS." *American Medical News,* 8 April: 5.

Mechanic, David. 1991. "Changing Our Health Care System." *Medical Care Review* 48, 3: 247–60.

Miller, Frances, and Graham Miller. 1986. "The Painful Prescription: A Procrustean Perspective?" *New England Journal of Medicine* 303, 5: 288.

Navarro, Vicente. 1990. "Federal Health Policies in the United States: An Alternative Explanation." In: Lee, Philip, and Carroll Estes, eds. *The Nation's Health*. Boston: Jones and Bartlett Publishers, pp. 154–63.

O'Day, Steven. 1984. "The Hospice Movement: An Alternative to Euthanasia." Unpublished.

Radovsky, Saul. 1990. "U.S. Medical Practice before Medicare and Now—Differences and Consequences." *New England Journal of Medicine* 22, 4: 263–7.

Redelmeier, Donald, and Amos Tversky. 1990. "Discrepancy between Medical Decisions for Individual Patients and for Groups." *New England Journal of Medicine* 322, 16: 1162–4.

Reed, David. 1980. "Should Cost Be a Factor in Personal Medical Care?" Letter to the Editor. *New England Journal of Medicine* 303, 5: 288.

Reinhardt, Uwe. 1987. "Resource Allocation in Health Care: The Allocation of Lifestyles to Providers." *Milbank Quarterly* 65, 2: 153–76.

Schwartz, William, and Henry Aaron. 1984. "Rationing Hospital Care: Lessons from Britain." *New England Journal of Medicine* 310, 1: 52–6.

Shenkin, Henry. 1986. *Clinical Practice and Cost Containment: A Physician's Perspective*. New York: Praeger Publishers.

Somers, Anne. 1986. "The Changing Demand for Health Services: A Historical Perspective and Some Thoughts for the Future." *Inquiry* 23, 4: 395–402.

Steinberg, Earl, Jane Sisk, and Katherine Locke. 1985. "X-Ray CT and Magnetic Resonance Imagers: Diffusion Patterns and Policy Issues." *New England Journal of Medicine* 313, 14: 859–64.

Thurow, Lester. 1984. "Learning to Say No." *New England Journal of Medicine* 311, 24: 1569–72.

Veatch, Robert. 1986. "DRGs and the Ethical Allocation of Resources." *Hastings Center Report* 16, 3: 32–40.

Watts, Malcolm. 1985. "Dealing With a Stereotype." *American Medical News,* 27 September: 4.

Weiner, Jonathan. 1987. "Primary Care Delivery in the U.S. and Four Northwest European Countries: Comparing the 'Corporatized' With the 'Socialized.'" *Milbank Quarterly* 65, 3: 426–61.

Wilensky, Gail. 1985. "Making Decisions on Rationing." *Business and Health*, November: 36–8.

Glossary

Weiner, Jonathan and Grey deLissovoy. In press. "Raising a Tower of Babel: A Taxonomy for Managed Care and Health Insurance Plans." *Journal of Health Politics, Policy, and Law*.

INDEX

Access to medical care: 228–246;
1900–1945, 17–20; 1946–1978,
27–28; 1990s, 133; health and,
238–239; malpractice and,
217–219
Advertising, 54–55, 127, 133
Agency for Health Care Policy and
Research (AHCPR), 160–161
All-payer reimbursement systems,
113–114
Ambulatory Patient Groups (APGs),
106
American Association of Retired Per-
sons (AARP), 38, 250
American Medical Association
(AMA), 7, 21, 29, 34, 81, 108,
190, 191
American Tort Reform Association
(ATRA), 221
Antitrust law, 55
Assignment, 85–86
Autonomy: clinician, 176–177,
193–194; patient, 22, 187,
193–195, 252–253

Balance billing, 86
Behavioral offset, 111
Beneficence, 186
Blue Cross and Blue Shield Insurance
Company: cost-based reimburse-
ment, 82; cost-sharing in, 63; ori-
gins, 18

Canadian health care system, 242
Capitation: cost advantages, 89–91;
definition, 64
Case management, 73–74
Case-mix reimbursement system,
103

Certificate of Need (CON) Program,
95–96
Charity care: 1900–1945, 16–18;
pre-1900, 10; PPS and, 234;
providers and, 244–246
Clinical decision-making (*see also*
Quality of care, Outcomes of care,
Protocols): 143–167; uncertainty
in, 146–151; variations in,
143–144
Co-insurance, 62
Committee on Costs of Medical
Care, 19
Competition: Enthoven Plan, 55–56;
factors affecting, 54
Competitive Medical Plans (CMPs),
76
Computers, use of, 162–163
Convenience-care centers, 123
Co-payment, 63
Cost-benefit analysis (CBA), 156
Cost-effectiveness analysis (CEA),
156
Cost-plus reimbursement: 31; infla-
tionary effect of, 90
Cost-sharing: definition, 62; effect
on demand, 67–68; for cost con-
trol, 70–71
Cost-shifting, 113–14, 233
Costs of health care: 1930–1990, 34,
36; 1990s, 135; causes of increas-
ing, 31–35; effects of cost control,
133–135; future forecast, 2; mal-
practice and, 219
Cross-subsidization, 113–114, 233
Customary-Prevailing-Reasonable
(CPR) payment, 82–84

Decision-making, *see* Clinical decision-making